Writings for a Liberation Psychoanalysis

In *Writings for a Liberation Psychoanalysis*, Robert K. Beshara establishes a groundbreaking framework that links the Freudo–Lacanian tradition directly to transmodernity and decoloniality. Traditional psychoanalytic institutions have long been tethered to colonial logic, often pathologizing the marginalized rather than challenging the structures that oppress them, but Beshara shows how psychoanalysis can be a tool for liberation.

By re-thinking psychoanalysis from the Exterior perspective of the oppressed, Beshara argues that the radical seeds of liberation are extimate or already present within the praxis—waiting to be activated through ethical listening and free association. This work synthesizes the transformative insights of scholars such as Edward Said, Paulo Freire, and Enrique Dussel to develop a "Psychoanalysis of the Oppressed" or "Liberation Psychoanalysis." More than just a theoretical intervention, this book offers a roadmap for liberation as an analectical materialist praxis—a way to theorize oppression and prefigure a concrete utopian horizon by politicizing the unconscious from within the core of a crumbling empire.

This book is designed for undergraduate and postgraduate students, scholars, and professionals interested in psychoanalysis, liberation, and decoloniality. It would be particularly suitable for courses on Liberation Philosophy, Liberation Psychology, Decoloniality, Postcolonialism, and Radical Psychoanalysis.

Robert K. Beshara is the founder of the Critical Psychology website, www.criticalpsychology.org. In addition to being an Associate Professor of Psychology and Humanities at Northern New Mexico College, he is a psychoanalyst-in-formation with the Lacanian School of Psychoanalysis. He is also the author or editor of numerous books, *Decolonial Psychoanalysis: Towards Critical Islamophobia Studies* (Routledge, 2019), *Critical Psychology Praxis: Psychosocial Non-Alignment to Modernity/Coloniality* (Routledge, 2021), and *Radical Humanism: Decolonizing Perspectives in Critical Psychology* (Routledge, 2026).

The Lines of the Symbolic in Psychoanalysis Series

Series Editor:
Ian Parker, *Manchester Psychoanalytic Matrix*

Psychoanalytic clinical and theoretical work is always embedded in specific linguistic and cultural contexts and carries their traces, traces which this series attends to in its focus on multiple contradictory and antagonistic 'lines of the Symbolic'. This series takes its cue from Lacan's psychoanalytic work on three registers of human experience, the Symbolic, the Imaginary and the Real, and employs this distinctive understanding of cultural, communication and embodiment to link with other traditions of cultural, clinical and theoretical practice beyond the Lacanian symbolic universe. The Lines of the Symbolic in Psychoanalysis Series provides a reflexive reworking of theoretical and practical issues, translating psychoanalytic writing from different contexts, grounding that work in the specific histories and politics that provide the conditions of possibility for its descriptions and interventions to function. The series makes connections between different cultural and disciplinary sites in which psychoanalysis operates, questioning the idea that there could be one single correct reading and application of Lacan. Its authors trace their own path, their own line through the Symbolic, situating psychoanalysis in relation to debates which intersect with Lacanian work, explicating it, extending it and challenging it.

On the Theory and Clinic of Lacanian Psychoanalysis: Speaking of Lacan
Chris Vanderwees

Queer Psychoanalysis: Minor Clinic and Deconstruction of Gender
Fabrice Bourlez

A Contemporary Return to the Lacanian Mirror: You Are That
Sergio J. Aguilar Alcalá

Writings for a Liberation Psychoanalysis: Politicizing the Unconscious from the Core of a Crumbling Empire
Robert K. Beshara

For more information about the series, please visit: https://www.routledge.com/The-Lines-of-the-Symbolic-in-Psychoanalysis-Series/book-series/KARNLOS

Writings for a Liberation Psychoanalysis

Politicizing the Unconscious from the Core of a Crumbling Empire

Robert K. Beshara

Routledge
Taylor & Francis Group
LONDON AND NEW YORK

Designed cover image: Getty Images

First published 2027
by Routledge
4 Park Square, Milton Park, Abingdon, Oxon OX14 4RN

and by Routledge
605 Third Avenue, New York, NY 10158

Routledge is an imprint of the Taylor & Francis Group, an informa business

British Library Cataloguing-in-Publication Data
A catalogue record for this book is available from the British Library

ISBN: 9781041291169 (hbk)
ISBN: 9781041291138 (pbk)
ISBN: 9781003768104 (ebk)

DOI: 10.4324/9781003768104

Typeset in Times New Roman
by KnowledgeWorks Global Ltd.

This book is dedicated to oppressed peoples of the world, particularly in Palestine, Sudan, Congo, Syria, Afghanistan, Yemen, and Haiti. Liberation is possible.

It is also dedicated to the memory of my father-in-law, Antonio Luis Garrido Acuña.

Contents

Series Preface

Psychoanalysis has been intimately connected with colonialism, but has also always been at the edge of empire, and it has attracted anti-colonial and decolonial activists to the idea that oppression runs deeper than the professed conscious wishes of masters and slaves. That contradiction at the heart of psychoanalytic theory and practice, a contradiction consonant with Sigmund Freud's attention to unconscious ambivalence, is now at the heart of this book, an impressive reclamation work, taking us from an alliance with power to a resource for resistance.

Decolonization is not a metaphor, though it is often reduced to being a mere linguistic trope, just as material processes of colonial subjugation are too-often reduced inside the psychoanalytic clinic to expressions of suffering on the part of the individual analysand. In Robert Beshara's hands, in detailed readings of texts that range from classical psychoanalytic pronouncements to Arabic theological treatise to African-American music, this materiality of colonization and decolonization is put at the forefront; we meet the Real of oppression and resistance that undergirds its Symbolic contours and its Imaginary replication in the consciousness and unconsciousness of rulers and ruled.

To accomplish this task means mining the manifold significations of Freud's text, returning to Freud in such a way as to open up the contradictions, and doing so with the help of Jacques Lacan. For instance, a popular, and colonial reading of Freud's famous phrase to describe the task of psychoanalysis, 'Where id is, there ego shall be', is to treat nature, the 'id', as the untamed wasteland that must be driven back, occupied, by the rational civilized self, the 'ego'. That, indeed, has, in Freud's metaphor, borrowed from the draining of the Zuider Zee, been one kind of 'reclamation work'. The now naturalized term 'id' to signify what Freud, in the original German actually specified as 'it', and the 'ego' to translate the German 'I', drums home this image of the treatment.

This project, metaphorized in many ways over the course of colonial history, is a very real one, of dispossession and control. This book's sensitivity to ecology, to the ongoing destruction of the planet, makes that characterization of psychoanalysis all the more pertinent. Lacan re-reads the Freudian phrase, even though, plot spoiler, Lacan himself was not the most ardent of anti-colonialists. A Lacanian re-reading of the phrase now has it that 'where it was, there I should become'. And so, in place of the triumphant driving back of barbarian nature, and, by implication, the barbarian others, we have a call that we ally with decolonial struggle to find ourselves there.

This is a Lacanian re-reading of Freud that now, in this book, harnesses a range of theoreticians and activists, enabling us to show solidarity with, even at times identify with, peoples who have been at the sharp end of the so-called 'war on terror' and of the ongoing genocide in Gaza. Beyond Lacan, we arrive at what Beshara calls 'pluriversal solidarity', liberation psychoanalysis rooted in a collective approach to liberation, redeeming the promise of many psychoanalysts working in the orbit of Freud, that we might arrive at the impossibility psychoanalysis speaks of, but now in an 'impossible republic' rebuilt from the ruins of crumbling empire, where we speak and act across difference to remake the world.

Psychoanalytic clinical and theoretical work circulates through multiple intersecting antagonistic symbolic universes. This series opens connections between different cultural sites in which Lacanian work has developed in distinctive ways, in forms of work that question the idea that there could be single correct reading and application. The Lines of the Symbolic in Psychoanalysis series provides a reflexive reworking of psychoanalysis that transmits Lacanian writing from around the world, steering a course between the temptations of a metalanguage and Imaginary reduction, between the claim to provide a god's eye view of psychoanalysis and the idea that psychoanalysis must everywhere be the same. And the elaboration of psychoanalysis in the Symbolic here grounds its theory and practice in the history and politics of the work in a variety of interventions that touch the Real.

Ian Parker
Manchester Psychoanalytic Matrix

Acknowledgments

I deeply appreciate the editors of *Stillpoint Magazine, Awry*: *Journal of Critical Psychology, European Journal of Psychoanalysis*, and *(Des)troços: Revista de Pensamento Radical*, who permitted me to re-publish four of my articles as Chapters 5, 6, 8, and 10. A special mention to the Lacan School of Psychoanalysis, Gohar Homayounpour of the Freudian Group of Tehran, Ivan Ward and Anshu Srivistava of the Guild of Psychotherapists, Minorities and Philosophy at the University of New Mexico, Dwayne Monroe, Calum Neill of Lacan in Scotland, and Nadia Bou Ali of BICAR. Special thanks to my editors: Eleanor Taylor and Ian Parker, Saloni Singhania and Yvonne Doney. Finally, I am grateful to my wife (Cony), my daughter (Sofia Nur), and my two cats (Marx and Freud) for always being there and supporting me in various ways.

Chapter 1

Introducing *Writings for a Liberation Psychoanalysis*

Since this book is the third and final installment in a trilogy that began with *Decolonial Psychoanalysis* and was followed by *Freud and Said*, I want to sketch the contours of my project in the first two books before explicating how this third book advances the main arguments I have made so far. My current research is situated within the Freudo–Lacanian leftist tradition of psychoanalytic political theory (Apollon & Feldstein, 1996; Stavrakakis, 2002; Žižek, 1989, 2002), particularly since the decolonial turn (Boutebal, 2020; Gaztambide, 2024; Gaztambide et al., 2024; Iwuanyanwu, 2015; Maldonado-Torres et al., 2021; Rahmat, 2021, 2025; Rolnik, 2023; Sheehi & Sheehi, 2021; Swartz, 2022; Togashi, 2020; Tummala-Narra, 2022). Before I begin my theoretical analysis, I wish to frame the current political moment, since my attempt in this work is to politicize the unconscious from the core of a crumbling empire.

Nathan Akehurst (2026) argues that the United States has shifted from being a confident "hyperpower" to a "weakened and dangerous empire," marked by a "chaotic and violent decline." Using the kidnapping of Venezuelan President Nicolás Maduro as a key example, Akehurst posits that contemporary U.S. foreign policy has forsaken the "liberal world order" in favor of "parochial and defensive" strategies shaped by "strategic ambiguity." Interventions, often justified by the "War on Drugs" or immigration control, illustrate this shift. He notes that this change signifies a "striking reduction in material capacities" and depicts a "flailing empire" that compensates for its diminishing resources by reacting unpredictably and immorally—an "imperial theater," aimed at managing the optics of decline by projecting hyperpower as a spectacle through the politics of fear. Akehurst concludes that while the U.S. continues to focus on "resource control" and extrajudicial actions, the lack of a cognitive map for strategy fosters a volatile global environment where "constant imitative displays of aggression" are normalized for maintaining global hegemony. This is the precarious moment contextualizing my theorization of liberation psychoanalysis.

The decolonial turn, in my view, affirms postcolonialism or postcolonial studies, but negates *postcoloniality*, which often takes the form of the postcolonial nation-state, particularly in the aftermath of decolonization in Africa and Asia (1945–1960). Postcoloniality signifies political decolonization, which was not

DOI: 10.4324/9781003768104-1

accompanied by economic decolonization. This led Kwame Nkrumah (1965) to characterize postcoloniality as a form of neo-colonialism. Therefore, this text is concerned with the question of *what happens after political decolonization*? Revolutionary zeal produces an idealization or romanticization of violence, but, as Hannah Arendt (1969) shows, violence is just a *means* to an end, and not an end in itself. The end must be *power*, which necessitates *legitimacy*. Violence, on the other hand, requires *justification*. While revolutionary violence may be, in some instances, justified as a humanizing counter-force to dehumanization, I believe it is not the only, or most effective, path of liberation. Let us recall how Maximilien Robespierre was hoisted by his own petard during the French Revolution when he was executed by the guillotine, the primary tool of the Terror he oversaw.

Consequently, my position leans toward *strategic nonviolence* as opposed to absolute pacifism; the latter is not a pragmatic stance given that the history of emancipatory struggles includes numerous successful examples of the oppressed liberating themselves through the instrumental use of revolutionary violence, such as the Haitian Revolution (1791–1804), the Algerian War of Independence (1954–1962), the Cuban Revolution (1952–1959), the Vietnamese Revolution (1945–1975), and the Angolan War of Independence (1961–1974). Having acknowledged the force of revolutionary violence, I shall now explore some of the tenets of strategic nonviolence, particularly from a psychoanalytic perspective.

Mohandas Gandhi's (2001) word for nonviolent resistance is *Satyagraha*, which he translates as "Truth-force" (p. 3), "Love-force or Soul-force" (p. 6). Since the Other is "the place of truth" (Safouan, 2004, p. 11), psychoanalytically speaking, one can then argue that *Satyagraha* is also *Unconscious-force* as in *Other-force*. Furthermore, nonviolent resistance, in this context, "is a function of the progress of the analysand's discourse, that is, a function of its proximity to truth" (Safouan, 2004, p. 10). But which truth is the subject nonviolently resisting? The truth of unconscious desire (p. 14).

The problem here is that desire can only be half-said, which points to the difference between unconscious truth and paranoid knowledge, for "desire is an interpretation of the Other's desire" (p. 24), but "*as* an interpretation it gives [us] a false certitude of what the Other desires of [us]. It gives [us] a kind of knowledge ... that deserves to be described as paranoid" (p. 25, emphasis in original). But there is another conundrum: liberation is an *objet a*; therefore, as the cause of revolutionary desire, liberation "is neither a sign of love nor an object of need" (p. 62). We can schematize this second predicament as follows: Demand (for love) – Need (for survival) = Desire (for liberation). My reading of this Lacanian formulation from *Écrits* maps neatly onto Abraham Maslow's (1943) hierarchy of needs, which, I would argue, is *a hierarchy of needs, demands, and desire* since the first two levels (physiological and safety needs) concern basic needs, while the third and fourth levels (love and esteem needs) involve psychological demands. Finally, self-actualization is the place of desire. In liberation praxis, it entails community-actualization, too.

While Gandhi's praxis of *Satyagraha* was informed by his experiences with apartheid in South Africa and British colonialism in India, Zen Buddhist master Thích Nhất Hạnh's praxis of nonviolent social action was shaped by the context of the Vietnam War, which was known as the American War in Vietnam. When Hạnh (1993) writes, "The essence of nonviolence is love" (p. 39), he is arguing that the essence of nonviolence is a demand from the subject and the Other to be loved for their lack. However, this demand, he clarifies, "is not a dogma," but "a process" (p. 39). For Hạnh, nonviolence is also an action that "requires a thorough understanding of the situation and of the psychology of the people" (p. 40). In other words, nonviolence is a praxis, too: a theorization of oppression that is meant to drive our actions toward liberation. From a Buddhist perspective, liberation demands "true love" (Hạnh, 1998), which is comprised of four elements: *maitri* (loving-kindness), *karuna* (compassion), *mudita* (joy), and *upeksha* (equanimity). In humanistic psychology, true or unconditional love has been popularized by Carl Rogers as unconditional positive regard; however, we should not shy away from using the signifier 'love,' which Jacques Lacan (2015) defines as "giving what you don't have" (p. 129). One question remains: what makes unconditional love possible in light of the fact that *conditional love is the gifting of lack*? Whereas conditional love is transactional, unconditional love is ontological. In other words, unconditional love is not about giving or having, but about being. What kind of being? A forgiving, or a light-hearted, being.

Edith Stauffer (1987), drawing equally from psychosynthesis and the mystical teachings of the Essenes, as expressed in the Khaboris Codex, writes about the interdependence between unconditional love and forgiveness, which "fit like hand and glove" (p. 133). The Aramaic word for forgiveness is *shavaq*, which means untying the knot or letting go. In a Lacanian sense, this untying functions as a structural intervention in the Borromean knot of the subject, wherein releasing the Symbolic debt of suffering through speech prevents the Imaginary ego—the body—from remaining perpetually captive to the traumatic Real in the form of the symptom.

Stauffer defines forgiveness, accordingly, as "canceling expectations" (p. 128). As such, forgiveness, for her, is not a question of moral obligation, but a psychospiritual technique for energetic release. If libido is not expressed or released, then it is repressed and repeated symptomatically. Forgiveness, in Essene mysticism, is the process of clearing the *naphsha* (soul or *nafs* in Arabic) from the entanglements of trauma and resentment in order to restore the *rukha* (spirit or *ruh* in Arabic) to its natural state of unconditional love. The Order of the Essenes was a Jewish ascetic sect that existed between the 2nd century BCE and the 1st century CE. Its teachings were likely a source of inspiration for Jesus through John the Baptist. Interestingly, the Essenes may have been influenced by Buddhism—which reached the Levant via Ashoka's missionaries in the 3rd century BCE—and by Ancient Egyptian ascetic traditions, as practiced by the kindred Therapeutae sect.

From an Ancient Egyptian perspective, the *Ka* (the life force or double), which is symbolized by two upraised arms, represents the part of the *naphsha* that remains tied to the physical realm and requires sustenance, while the *Ba* (personality) represents the wandering soul—in the form of a bird—that must be freed from earthly weight. The *Akh*—denoted by a crested ibis—corresponds directly to *rukha*. In Ancient Egypt, the *House of Ka* (the tomb) served as the sacred space for this psychospiritual process; here, the *Ka* resided and received the ritual offerings that sustained the deceased, allowing it to reunite nightly with the *Ba*. It was only through this successful reunion—and the clearing of the heart's debts in divine judgment—that the deceased was transfigured into an *Akh*: an effective spirit capable of dwelling among the gods. Thus, whether viewed as the untying of a knot, or the transfiguration of the *Ka* and the *Ba* into an *Akh*, forgiveness acts as the essential clearing that allows the divided subject to return to their singularity of being, in order for them to assume their rightful place among the ancestors.

Stauffer's (1987) definition of forgiveness as canceling expectations stems from the linguistic fact that the Aramaic word for love (*khuba*) and debt (*khaba*) are spelled identically: ܚܘܒܐ. By releasing our expectations and the debts (*khaba*) we feel others have incurred against us, we return to a state of *khuba*. This Symbolic debt (*khaba*) is what Stauffer means by "expectation." When we forgive, or cancel expectations, we are essentially deleting a Symbolic ledger that was keeping the (k)not—the subject—in a perpetual state of anxiety. Once we have cleared the *naphsha* of trauma and resentment, we become capable of not only *khuba*, "pure love" as an intention, but also *rakhma*, "transpersonal love" as a method (p. 117)—the Arabic equivalents are *hob* (love, desire) and *rahma* (compassion, mercy), respectively.

Rahma shares its root with the Arabic word for womb (*rahim*), suggesting that transpersonal love is a generative space of rebirth. This shift from the personal to the transpersonal, or from unconscious desire (*khuba*) to unconditional love (*rakhma*) mirrors the psychospiritual journey of the dead toward the Hall of Two Truths. There, *psychostasia*, the literal weight of the *Ib* (heart or *qalb* in Arabic), acts as the ultimate psychological ledger; the *Ba* is the part of the soul that carries the weight of the *Ib* to the scales. Only a heart unburdened by the density of *khaba* (debt) could balance perfectly against the feather of Maat (truth and justice), allowing the *Ba* to return to the tomb—not as a place of death, but as a *rahim* (womb), a place of rebirth—and successfully reunite with its *Ka*. This is how the *Ka* and the *Ba* are transfigured into an *Akh*, which also means brother in Arabic—a comrade to the gods, an ancestor.

Essentially, this untying of the Symbolic debt does more than just release the ego, it is a traversal of fantasy that collapses the distance between the fragmented parts of the subject, such as the *Khet* (physical body), the *Sah* (spiritual body), the *Ren* (name), and the *Shuyet* (shadow). By clearing the ledger of the heart from debt, the subject of the unconscious is no longer held captive by the demands or desires of the Other, allowing their symptomatic knot to be reconfigured into the singularity of the *Akh*—the subject-as-drive, who is finally reborn as a compassionate being by subjectifying the cause of *rakhma*. In 1967, Hạnh recognized Martin Luther King Jr. as a *bodhisattva*, "an enlightened being trying to awaken other living beings and help them move toward more compassion and understanding" (as cited in Hạnh, 2016, p. 73).

In turn, King Jr. was inspired by both Gandhi and Hạnh to embrace nonviolence, from a Christian perspective, as a form of resistance against racism and segregation in the U.S. King Jr. (1991) identified five points to the method of nonviolent resistance: (1) "this is not a method for cowards; it *does* resist" (p. 7, emphasis in original); (2) "nonviolent resistance does not seek to defeat or humiliate the opponent, but to win his [or her] friendship and understanding" (p. 7); (3) "the attack is directed against forces of evil rather than against persons who are caught in those forces" (p. 8); (4) "it avoids not only external physical violence but also internal violence of the spirit" (p. 8); and (5) "the method of nonviolence is based on the conviction that the universe is on the side of truth" (p. 9).

In summary, there is an isomorphism between nonviolent resistance and the Ancient Egyptian principle of *mꜣꜥt* (truth and justice). The oppressed resist because justice is on their side and they employ the method of nonviolence to articulate the truth of their unconscious desire. However, justice is not an abstract ideal; it is the concrete, collective construction of a just society, which is achieved through the abolition of systemic oppression. Justice is a liberatory network, wherein economic relations, social status, and political power are fundamentally structured around principles of equity in material well-being—ensuring all basic needs are met for everyone—and genuine equality of opportunity and voice for all; in other words, liberation is a demand for unconditional love and a desire for self-/community-actualization.

While the dimension of justice has to do with economic, social, and political decolonizations, the dimension of truth concerns psychic decolonization, which follows a psychoanalytic sequential logic (alienation → separation → the traversal of fantasy) *vis-à-vis* three forms of lack: Imaginary frustration, Symbolic castration, and Real privation. In alienation, the modern subject is frustrated with the Other's demand and often projects this frustration narcissistically through aggressive relations with other egos (an either/or logic that pervades the conservative politics of us vs. them); in separation, the postmodern subject is castrated by the Other's desire and has taken responsibility for neither their desire nor their *jouissance* (a neither/nor logic that permeates the liberal politics of recognition); and, finally, in the traversal of fantasy, the transmodern subject comes to terms with the Other's lack and views the *objet a* as a placeholder for their Real lack-of-being or *manque-à-être* (a both/and logic that animates the radical politics of reconciliation). In radical politics, truth and justice necessitate unconditional love and forgiveness.

Both the Other and the Other of the Other do not exist, except as necessary fictions. As such, the traversal of fantasy entails subjectifying the cause of liberation, which results in a state of desirousness that then drives the speaking being's (*parlêtre*) ethico-political acts toward the self-/community-actualization of transmodernity, as the analectical sublation of Totality and Exteriority. To put it differently, the transmodern subject asks: what desires are covered over by colonial and (anti) modern fantasies?

Acting out colonial and (anti)modern fantasies is the death of decolonial desire. The situation is similar with the *passage à l'acte.* According to Safouan (2004), "acting out is going into the [Imaginary] scene to signify something. *Passage à l'acte* is throwing oneself outside the scene" (p. 28, emphasis in original). While acting out is a non-discursive message, in *passage à l'acte* the subject ejects themself from the Symbolic circuit altogether and is left with nothing but the Real weight of existential dread. Both acts are forms of autoimmunity, but the latter is a much more violent act since it often involves self-harm and/or harming the community. Traversing the fantasy, on the other hand, entails delinking desire from fantasy, that is, not conflating or integrating the two.

The Imaginary is the level of ideological fantasy, which covers over sexual impotence, non-rapport, or frustration with the oppressive logics of coloniality and/or (anti)modernity—both being two sides of a parallax view. This dual problem can be stated as *the challenge of transmodernity*, and it must be inspected from two different perspectives: Totality and Exteriority. These Imaginary scenes or stages of colonial and/or (anti)modern ideological fantasies sustain the Symbolic order of racial capitalism, an impossible or inconsistent order, which is why it is replete with the passions of love, hate, and ignorance (cf. Soler, 2015), particularly as discursive-practices or cultural demands.

The Symbolic is the dimension where an abstract (civilizational) line is drawn between friend (civilized) and enemy (savage) following the binary rhetoric of Totality vs. Exteriority, or the west vs. the rest. This Symbolic cut produces the analectics of colonial desire vs. decolonial desire. My term for the abstract (civilizational) line is *colonial difference*; as history shows, civilization is often invoked to morally justify *(post)modern forms of violence* (e.g., state terrorism and religious terrorism by non-state actors)—Sayyid Qutb's category of *jāhiliyyah* (pre-Islamic ignorance), for example, is the antimodern equivalent of savagery. Consequently, the Crusades, for instance, may be framed as *a clash of fantasies*, a war between the Other and the Other of the Other, but as I argue throughout the book, both Symbolic representatives ($\not{A}$ and $\not{A}^2$) are barred, and this is what I mean by *cultural difference* as a sociopolitical ontology of Symbolic castration. Since postcoloniality is at the threshold between Totality and Exteriority, I put the prefix (post) in parentheses to signify both the coloniality of Euromodernity and the antimodernity of the (non)European, whom I say more about later. Similarly, by occasionally writing (anti)modern, I am underscoring the non-rational and irrational tendencies within modernity.

The traumatic Real is the hole structuring both subjectivity and ideology, an abyss of anxiety *qua* being; it is in this realm of lack, void, or privation, where we encounter biological needs and the drives, especially in relation to both empirical objects and the *objet a*. If the Imaginary is the fantasmatic world of alienation and the Symbolic is the discursive world of separation, then the Real is the otherworld of *jouissance*, wherein lies the possibility of traversing both colonial and (anti) modern fantasies.

Because the Real can neither be Imaginarized nor fully Symbolized, the Praxis of Learned Ignorance—understood as a psychosocial ontology of Real privation and structurally akin to Lacan's *la passe*—serves as the transversal line enabling the Transmodern Subject to confront the impasses of coloniality and (anti)modernity: $P_{LI}(T\$: I \rightarrow S) = R$. This praxis positions the transmodern Other as the subject-supposed-to-know, embodying a precise non-knowledge, which structures the transmodern subject's division and the impossibility of decolonial desire; in this way, transmodernity emerges as the collective equivalent of the end of analysis—a traversal that can sinthomize the wounds of coloniality and (anti)modernity, as irreducible kernels of the Real, which Totality perpetually occludes. In other words, the transmodern subject starts in the Imaginary, but through analysis (embodied in the praxis of learned ignorance as sustained non-knowledge), the subject traverses the symbolic circuit (demand → desire → drive) and converts the demand for recognition into the drive for reconciliation—a passage that prevents re-totalization by keeping the space open for decolonial desirousness. Transmodernity rejects the dialectical recuperation of the Real (Exteriority) into a totalizing order, opting instead for an analectical materialism wherein a Symbolic pluriverse is knotted—at the site of the traumatic Real—via the transmodern subject's singularity of being.

Learned ignorance resonates with Karl Popper's (2013) notion of "critical rationalism," which, for him, is not only just, or morally superior to both irrationalism and uncritical/comprehensive rationalism, but also true. For Popper, critical rationalism is the closest position to the "scientific attitude," wherein "I may be wrong and you may be right, and by an effort we may get nearer to the truth" (p. 442). This is so because critical rationalism "recognizes the fact that the fundamental rationalist attitude results from an (at least tentative) act of faith—from faith in reason" (p. 437). However, unlike comprehensive rationalism, critical rationalism "frankly admits its origin in an irrational decision (and which, to that extent, admits a certain priority of irrationalism)" (p. 437). This acknowledgement of a non-rational foundation for logic aligns with the paradoxical nature of historical reason: it is (trans)rational, integrating magical and mythic forms of thinking within a scientific framework.

Popper accuses Hegel, Marx, and Freud of being unscientific. For him, their works are unfalsifiable because they commit the sin of comprehensive rationalism:

> By making argument and criticism impossible, he [Hegel] intends to make his own philosophy proof against all criticism, so that it may establish itself as a *reinforced dogmatism*, secure from every attack, and the unsurmountable summit of all philosophical development.
>
> (pp. 253–54)

For Popper, reinforced dogmatism "opens wide the door to the enemy, deeply significant metaphysical nonsense, and throws out, by the same door, the best friend, that is to say, scientific hypothesis" (p. 659). Unlike Popper, I contend that socialism and psychoanalysis are indeed falsifiable. Socialism and psychoanalysis are not dogmatic systems; rather, they are (trans)rational inquiries into truth and justice. Because they dialectically integrate three layers of historical reason—the magical, the mythic, and the rational—they serve as the foundation for liberation praxis. This praxis is defined by its capacity for empirical correction and its orientation toward transmodernity.

As I will show, liberation is a praxis, which drives the oppressed in a variety of ways. As an *objet a*, liberation is a source of *divine jouissance*. However, liberation is not an empirical object to be realized for the sake of satisfaction; it is a cause that can never be fulfilled. The end goal of liberation is power, which is a shifting target because the way to get there is through "a zigzag movement" like "the movements of the horse in a game of chess" (Safouan, 2004, p. 5); therefore, the desire for liberation is a circuitous or nonlinear journey. This is what I mean by "decolonization is a metonym."

There are four dimensions to liberation psychoanalysis, and some are more emphasized than others throughout the text: (1) psychic liberation, (2) social liberation, (3) political liberation, and (4) economic liberation. *Psychic liberation* entails a release from distress through the assumption of the *manque-à-être* (want-to-be) at the core of our existence—a lack sustained by an ethics of unconscious desire. Psychic liberation restores the *psykhe* to its traditional sense as a spiritual awareness of our fundamental emptiness. Because form is emptiness (*śūnyatā*) and emptiness is form, this process simultaneously liberates the *soma*, effectively sublimating *eros*. *Social liberation* is ending oppression and violence through an anti-oppressive and nonviolent praxis, which includes dialogue, civil disobedience, and boycott among other tactics. *Political liberation* is the dissolution of authoritarianism—be that right-wing fascism or left-wing totalitarianism—through ideology critique and anarchist power. *Economic liberation* requires transcending the lure of surplus-*jouissance* promised by capital, effectively breaking the superegoic injunction to 'Enjoy!' at all costs. Rather than being amused to death through the illusory possession of the phallus, we achieve a radical cessation of consumption by defetishizing the commodity form. This pivots the transmodern subject toward a divine *jouissance* of the socialist variety—*a collective enjoyment of the commons* that exists beyond the reach of exploitation. The four dimensions of liberation are interdependent and necessary for organizing the international as not all, the community-actualization of lack.

Our current moment, as the oppressed, may be characterized by the failures of postcoloniality, a function of its compromised position at the edge of Totality. This book enacts a decolonial doubling from a (non)European perspective: *a critique of Totality* and *a self-criticism of Exteriority*. The aim of this double work is to affirm both Euromodernity and the alter-modernity of the (non)European. This is the pluriversal spirit of transmodernity: a liberatory and (non)violent sublation of the analectical kind, wherein *the method of analectics is isomorphic to the cause of liberation* (cf. Marcuse, 2015, p. 163).

Furthermore, this parallel processing negates coloniality and (anti)modernity, thereby undermining the *mythic jouissance* derived from (post)colonial violence and (post)modern oppression. The dual task of decoloniality then falls primarily on (non)European analysands, who have the potential to become *transmodern subjects of liberation* and secondarily on (non)European analysts, who possess the capacity to become *decolonial objects* that can cause the desire of (non)Europeans for liberation.

Before I move to the next section, I wish to briefly explore the question of modernity—for a more in-depth treatment, see Beshara (2024). If coloniality is the worst of modernity, then what is the best? Euromodernity is a structure of being, which totalizes the subject. It marks the eclipse of the Ancient *Logos*—which sought to reveal *Alētheia* as an eternal and undivided cosmic order—by a relentless instrumental reason. This eclipse fractured a kinship-based communalist world through the prisms of class struggle, racism, and sexist oppression, leaving the divided subject to bear the scars of this historical trauma. Furthermore, the eclipse of historical reason produced the fractal subject of modernity: a fractured individual, who fancies themself the architect of their reality, unaware that their subjective experience is merely a self-similar iteration of an objective topology. Rather than disclosing the world as a pluriversal cosmos, the modern subject constitutes it as an ideological hall of mirrors. Within this infinite reflection, the fractal subject bifurcates: reiterating the colonial desire of the modern Other for everything while deploying ideological fantasy to mask their fundamental nothingness. This dual operation clarifies the mechanics of Orientalism (Said, 1978): it functions as an ideological fantasy structure, allowing the modern subject to project their own lack onto the Oriental Other of the Other. Through this projection, the Other of the Other is cast into a contradictory, exotic status—simultaneously a desirable object of fantasy and a repulsive subject of alterity.

Yet, to understand the fractal entrapment of the modern subject, one must first recognize the emancipatory fire from which it was forged: the wisdom of the Ancients. If coloniality is the shadow of Euromodernity, its light is found in the rebirth of the classical spirit—specifically its humanistic commitment to the authority of reason over tradition. In this light, the modern project is the inherent negation of authoritarianism. Historically, this Promethean spirit re-emerged in opposition to the institutional dogmatism of the Medieval Church, yet the conflict was nuanced: the Church had effectively canonized Aristotelian philosophy and Ptolemaic cosmology as dogma. Consequently, the fiery spirit of modernity re-emerged as a double affirmation: the democratic secularization of *Nomos* (human order) and the empirical interrogation of *Physis* (natural order).

Galileo and Descartes are often considered the 'fathers' of Euromodernity. Galileo changed the object of *Physis* through his desacralization of nature. Descartes changed the subject of *Nomos* through the method of radical doubt. If Galileo's support of the heliocentric model physically displaced the Earth from the center of the cosmos, the later Copernican Revolution of psychoanalysis completed the decentering of consciousness. While the Cartesian *cogito* attempted to ground certainty by applying radical doubt to conscious thought, Freud's invention of the unconscious revealed that the "I," which is actually doing the thinking, is not the ego in a position of mastery. As such, these hysterical 'fathers' had (non)European 'grandfathers,' who pioneered the paradigm shifts of modernity. In Baghdad, Ibn al-Haytham, the first true scientist, established the method of empiricism in his *Book of Optics*, effectively overturning Aristotelian authority by prioritizing evidence over syllogism.

In Córdoba, Ibn Rushd's insistence on the harmony between *revelation* and *reason* prefigured the *double-truth theory* of later Latin Averroists. This separation of *theological truth*—revealed directly to the faithful—from *demonstrative truth*—arrived at through reason—provided the early blueprint for secularization: the separation of Church and State. The double-truth theory was foundational for the development of the Cartesian *cogito*, as the theoretical beginning of the modern subject of science. This is the ancestor of the psychoanalytic subject of the signifier, who is divided between *false being* and *unconscious thinking*. By establishing substance dualism—the split between *res extensa* and *res cogitans*—Descartes enacted the division of labor between *theology* and *philosophy*. The Copernican Revolution of psychoanalysis suggests that modernity is defined by a *double-decentering*: just as the Earth was moved from the center of the heavens, the conscious ego was moved from the center of subjectivity.

This double-decentering speaks to the atheological and antiphilosophical core of psychoanalysis as a secular and materialist praxis driven by *historical reason*, or "rationality as a project for the liberation of society" (Quijano, 1993, p. 147). To that end, historical reason entails *the systematic analysis of how the human subject negotiates (non)meaning within the constraints of space–time*. By *systematic analysis*, I mean psychoanalysis in tandem with social, political, and economic analyses. By *(non)meaning*, I am acknowledging *the vel of alienation*, wherein the modern subject must choose between *being* and *meaning*. If the subject chooses being, they succumb to non-meaning. And if they choose the Other's meaning, they lose their trans-linguistic experience with being. Consequently, the modern subject of the unconscious is defined by the nonsensical signifiers that history imposes upon them via the Symbolic order. While these cultural signifiers initially appear as symptoms of alienation, they ultimately function as *sinthomes*—singular knots that prevent the total collapse of the subject into non-meaning.

Historical reason—unlike the detached abstractions of pure reason—is a concrete form of reason: embodied, situated, and engaged with the task of liberation. It stands in sharp relief to instrumental reason, which functions as the logic of coloniality, reducing the modern subject to a calculable unit within the apparatus of racial capitalism. In *Dialectic of Enlightenment*, Horkheimer and Adorno (2002) refer to the instrumentalization of reason as "technical rationality," or "the rationality of domination" (p. 95). Furthermore, Horkeimer and Adorno argue that instrumental reason is inherently irrationalist:

> This irrationality of reason has been precipitated in cunning, as the adaptation of bourgeois reason to any unreason which confronts it as a stronger power. The lone voyager armed with cunning is already *homo oeconomicus*, whom all reasonable people will one day resemble: for this reason the Odyssey is already a Robinsonade. Both these prototypical shipwrecked sailors make their

> weakness—that of the individual who breaks away from the collective—their social strength. Abandoned to the vagaries of the waves, helplessly cut off, they are forced by their isolation into a ruthless pursuit of their atomistic interest. They embody the principle of the capitalist economy even before they make use of any worker; but the salvaged goods they bring with them to the new venture idealize the truth that the entrepreneur has always entered the competition armed with more than the industry of his hands. Their powerlessness in face of nature already functions as an ideology for their social predominance. Odysseus's defenselessness against the foaming sea sounds like a legitimation of the enrichment of the voyager at the expense of indigenous inhabitants. Bourgeois economics later enshrined this principle in the concept of risk: the possibility of foundering is seen as a moral justification for profit. From the standpoint of the developed exchange society and its individuals, the adventures of Odysseus are no more than a depiction of the risks which line the path to success. Odysseus lives according to the ancient principle which originally constituted bourgeois society. One had to choose between cheating and going under. Fraud was the stigma of reason, which betrayed its particular interest. The universal socialization for which the globetrotter Odysseus and the solo manufacturer Robinson Crusoe provide a preliminary sketch was attended from the first by the absolute loneliness which at the end of the bourgeois era is becoming overt. Radical socialization means radical alienation. Both Odysseus and Crusoe deal in totality: the former measures it out; the latter fabricates it. They can do so only in total isolation from all other human beings, who appear to both men only in estranged forms, as enemies or allies, but always as instruments, things.
>
> (pp. 48–49, emphasis in original)

The promise of reason was liberation from magical thinking, but when reason is instrumentalized, it becomes a mythic tool for domination. Instrumental reason is not a pursuit of wisdom or morality, but the exercise of cunning or shrewdness in the service of "atomistic interest." Odysseus survives not through strength alone, but through the deception of mythic unreason itself. Yet, while Odysseus return a winner, or at least alive, from a series of zero-sum games that characterize his tumultuous voyage, he loses his soul (*psykhe*) in the process. He was forced to negate his humanity in order to calculate his survival. Thus, instrumental reason reveals its irrational core: it reduces life to a relentless game of calculation, displacing the holistic *vita activa* (Arendt, 2019)—a mode of being that integrates the ethical necessity of *labor* (basic needs), the political necessity of *action* (the need for unconditional love), and the aesthetic necessity of *work* (the desire for self-/community-actualization).

"Radical socialization means radical alienation" because *there is no such thing as society*: "There are individual men and women and there are families" (Thatcher, as cited in Keay, 1987). The logic of Thatcherism echoes the Lacanian axiom *il n'y a pas de rapport sexuel*, revealing a profound overlap between neoliberal ideology and psychoanalytic theory. Both suggest that the ontological One we fantasize about—be it a cohesive Society or the perfect Couple—is a structural impossibility. For Thatcher, Society is a myth used to abdicate individual responsibility; for Lacan, sexual rapport is a myth masking the lack of any organic unity between sexed subjects. This is the paradox of the Symbolic order: to become a social being, the subject must enter into language and Law. Yet, because language is Other—a "virus from outer space"—the act of speaking through the Other's signifiers renders the subject fundamentally alienated. Thatcherism suggests that the more we lean on Society, the more we alienate ourselves from the drive for self-reliance. This is the death drive *par excellence*. The Robinsonade story of Chuck Noland and Wilson (the volleyball) from the film *Cast Away* (2000) deconstructs this ego-driven notion of a self without an Other. Contrary to the main character's last name, there was land, but no one else was there, except Wilson, of course. Even though the Other does not exist, we cannot but be in an interdependent relationship with this non-existent Other, and Wilson, as an *objet a*, is proof of that.

In essence, Thatcher argues, like Lacan, that the Other does not exist. However, by ignoring the unconscious, she posits the individual as a substantial, self-identical ego, a move akin to Jungian individuation—hence, the contemporary appeal of analytical psychology to conservatives like Jordan Peterson and his followers. Conversely, for Lacan, Horkheimer, and Adorno, this individual is not a refuge from Society, but a symptom of radical socialization/alienation: an egoic mask (*persona*) fashioned through the instrumental destruction of reason.

Horkheimer and Adorno argue that Odysseus is the proto-bourgeois individual celebrated by Thatcher. While Thatcher champions the individual *qua* consumer, for Horkheimer and Adorno, the bourgeois individual only emerges through the cunning of self-preservation, an ideological process that requires dehumanizing oneself and others into mere tool-beings: Odysseus *as* the bow, for instance. Therefore, whereas the individual is the symptom of alienation, the subject is the *sinthome* of disalienation—a singular way of sublimating the drives, which refuses the instrumental reason of the free market. Contra Althusser, we are not interpellated, by ideology, as subjects, but as individuals; therefore, subjectification is a process of de-ideologization. Only by traversing the fantasy of the self-made individual can we move from *the alienating socialization of market freedom* toward *the disalienating socialism of collective liberation*.

Within the apparatus of racial capitalism, socialization requires that the subject be made fungible—exchangeable units of labor. Everything, from our relationships to our lack of being, is commodified. We view our lives refracted through a spectacle calibrated by market value, our singularity flattened until we fit the self-similar iteration of Totality's ideological topology. To break this fractal loop requires more than mere resistance; it demands an *un-thinking* of the Odyssean cunning that defines the survival of the fittest. This un-thinking is an unconscious act of relinquishing the individual's death drive for mastery.

Odysseus survives under the guise of Nobody, but a Nobody who owns many things, hence, we must distinguish between *nihilistic nothingness* (the void of the market) and *existential emptiness* (the abyss of freedom)—the latter is the basis for *commoning*. The analectical turn requires us to be Nobody in a different sense: not as a cunning mask, but as a lack of being, which I interpret as *interbeing* (Hạnh, 1998). This is how we move beyond the zero-sum games of colonial difference and toward a re-sacralized engagement with the world (*Physis* → *Gaia*)—one that recognizes our lack of being not as a void to be filled with commodities, but as the very groundless ground, where the pluriversal cosmos of transmodernity is disclosed (*Nomos* → Commons). Only through the integral analectical materialist framework of historical reason can we reclaim the *vita activa* and restore the *Alētheia* eclipsed by instrumental reason and irrationalism. Why? Because if we do not enact systemic decolonization, "risk colonization" (Rothstein et al., 2006) will always be "at the expense of indigenous inhabitants" and other oppressed groups.

The modern political landscape is not a spectrum of opinions, but a collision of three distinct forms of reason that drive the three ideologies of the modern world-system. Liberalism is driven by instrumental reason, employing bureaucratic management as its means to achieve a global technocracy. Within this framework, the reification of the subject is operationalized through racial capitalism, wherein the logic of the market and the State-machine intersect to produce a hierarchy of human value, justifying extraction, over-exploitation, and extermination along racist and sexist lines to sustain the engine of capital. Under this regime, democracy is reduced to an Imaginary spectacle—a periodic ritual that masks the reification of the subject as a quantifiable resource. For example, while the world is burning, Congressional Democrats in the U.S. held a vapid candlelight vigil on January 6, 2026. Because the masses eventually revolt against being treated as soulless components of a megamachine, this technocratic nonsense inherently generates its own antithesis: conservatism. Driven by irrationalism, conservatism uses romanticism as its means to reach fascism, offering a violent restoration of instinct, myth, and vitality against the megamachine.

While liberals and conservatives appear as adversaries, they represent the cold and hot phases of the same apparatus; both are anchored in racial capitalism and rely on the instrumental reason of the State-machine to mediate the fractal subject's desire through oppression and violence. Liberalism and conservatism are essentially two different ways of regulating mythic *jouissance*—the extraction of surplus-*jouissance* from racism and sexist oppression during the extraction of surplus-value. The Totality of the modern world-system converts this excess of human suffering into the libidinal energy required to stabilize a reified Symbolic order, a crumbling empire. This conversion functions as a suture, using the surplus-*jouissance* of the oppressed to patch the paradoxical logic of the colonial unconscious, thereby tricking the modern subject into believing that the State-machine is a consistent and necessary Totality rather than a hollow artifice.

Furthermore, this ideological process reveals that the State-machine is powered by *the obscene underside of the Law* (Žižek, 1989), wherein the liberal facade of technocratic neutrality (democracy, freedom, rights) is secretly animated by a fascist, mythic violence that the apparatus disavows in principle but requires in practice to anchor the modern subject's libidinal investment in mythic *jouissance*. This investment is necessary because it transforms the fractal subject's crisis of meaning into an ideology of non-meaning in the form of *the colonial desire for everything*. Fascism serves as the aesthetic mask for the void at the core of a crumbling empire. It validates the old adage: *scratch a liberal and a fascist bleeds*. While liberalism functions as a metaphysics of presence—the Emperor's new clothes—fascism operates as the phallus, the fundamental signifier of lack. It is a violent overcompensation that emerges to suture the gap between the empire's nihilism and the sovereign's castration.

Radicalism offers a third path through historical reason, which seeks to make humanity the unconscious author of its destiny, aiming for *communism as the self-actualized society*. However, when historical reason is sucked into the vortex of instrumental reason to survive the threat of irrationalism, the logic short-circuits. The result is totalitarianism (e.g., Stalinism)—a catastrophic distortion, where the State adopts the cold efficiency of the megamachine to enforce a paranoid, pseudo-radical myth. Finally, libertarianism acts as the deconvolution of historical reason. It is the anti-authoritarian effort to delink the liberatory logic of history from the instrumental reason of the State. By stripping away the mediating structures of both the technocrat and the vanguard, libertarianism attempts to achieve the radical goal of autonomy without falling into the trap of totalitarianism.

This is the crisis of Totality, which is manifesting in the form of a crumbling empire. Now, let us turn to four critiques of modernity/coloniality: (1) *critical modernity* aligns with the path of historical reason, though it remains tethered to a Eurocentric horizon that often mistakes the ideology of western secularism for the process of decolonial secularization. In contrast, (2) *postmodernity* acts as a solvent for instrumental reason, though it often risks feeding the irrationalism of the conservative pole by dissolving all objective ground. Meanwhile, (3) *antimodernity* provides the philosophical backbone for the conservatives' irrationalist revolt by rejecting the trajectory of reason entirely. (4) *Transmodernity* is the bridge for libertarian deconvolution, seeking a way out of the State-machine by integrating non-European ways of knowing and being, thereby, moving beyond Totality without abandoning the liberatory logic of history.

History is liberatory because it is the unfolding of the transmodern subject-as-drive. If history had no logic, we would be eternally suspended in the technocratic coldness of a perfect Symbolic order. The persistent revolt of the masses against their own reification—their refusal to function as soulless components of a megamachine—is the insistence of the Letter within the historical process. This radical humanistic logic proves that there is a structural lack within Totality that no instrumental reason can close; this lack gets irrationally projected onto Exteriority. Therefore, the liberatory logic of history points in the direction of a collective traversal of ideological fantasies, which is the realization that the imperial Other does not exist, leading us toward a *communism of autonomy*, wherein social organization no longer attempts to fill the void of the subject—its lack of being—with technocratic management or fascist myth. Instead, lack becomes the very ground of our collective liberation.

For Horkheimer and Adorno, Odysseus, being an economic man who calculates his actions to maximize his own profit or utility, is the first modern man. He treats the world and himself as resources to be exploited. Even in ancient Greek myth, we see the blueprint for the bourgeois individual: A Robinson Crusoe type of subject, who survives by using the cunning of instrumental reason. Odysseus is not a hero; he is a manager. He manages his crew, his risks, and his own identity, such as when he tells the Cyclops his name is "Nobody." Odysseus's technical rationality can be formalized as such: Nobody (deception) ∴ no ego (self-abnegation) ∴ false being (alienation) ∴ unconscious thinking (instrumental reason). The irrationality of instrumental reason is summarized perfectly by this cunning of (un)reason: *To save his life, Odysseus has to pretend he does not exist.* By the time he gets home to Ithaca, he has spent so much time being "Nobody" that he is effectively a stranger to himself. Adorno and Horkheimer believe this is the paradoxical tragedy of the modern subject: we are so crafty at surviving the world that we eventually have no *body* left to enjoy the life we saved. This is the pathological logic of retirement—the perpetual postponement of joy in service of a future that has already been hollowed out. The lone voyager is the predecessor to the modern worker, who views the entire world as something to be conquered through cunning, yet is alienated by this technical rationality of domination.

The Odyssey is not a myth of homecoming, but a founding document of proprietary sovereignty. It serves as a bridge between historical stages, illustrating how an ancient slave mode of production can prefigure the predatory logic of modern capitalism. While Odysseus is technically a slave-owner in a proto-feudal setting, his actions align with that of a monopolist protecting their capital. Odysseus's return—after ten years of fighting in the Trojan War and ten years of trials and tribulations on his journey back home—functions as a violent re-establishment of his power over Ithaca's means of production.

Odysseus's outward journey represents the primitive accumulation of a colonizer. Here are Odysseus's words about his raid of the city of Ismarus, for example: "I destroyed the city there, killed the men, seized their wives, and captured lots of treasure, which we divided up" (Homer, 2002, p. 147). Consequently, his return signifies a violent consolidation of capital through the brutal killing of a rising class of parasitic suitors. Ithaca was in a state of anarchy. Odysseus's mythic violence, therefore, is the Law-making and Law-preserving violence of an authoritarian legal order: hierarchy. After all, Odysseus is an archer. He bows to no one; he is a King without a crown, a Nobody wielding the bow. In this economy of power, the bow—not the crown—functions as the phallus, the instrument of sovereignty that facilitates his psychopathic killing spree.

Although Ithacan society is fundamentally a slave economy—relying on the total ownership and extraction of surplus from an enslaved class—it exhibits the shrewd instrumental reason found in later capitalist societies. While Ithaca predates modern jurisprudence, Odysseus's trajectory from a raider of cities to a warrior-King illustrates the metamorphosis of the *oikos* (household) into a proto-corporate entity. In this transition, Odysseus mutates from a metonymic *aristocrat*—relying on the mythic natural right of blood evidenced by his ancestral scar—to a metaphorical *oligarch*, who ignores the sentiment of homecoming to conduct a cold capital audit of his Phaeacian gold, treating the household as a private firm and its resources as capital to be secured. The suitors represented a distorted version of communal kinship. They occupied the *oikos*, ate from a shared table, and treated the household resources as free commodities to be consumed, but they did so parasitically, rendering them a perverse commune.

Odysseus completes his mutation by becoming a literal *autocrat*: the sovereign higher-archer, who uses the mechanical technology of the bow to codify his dominance. This final mutation—achieved through the systematic liquidation of the parasitic suitors and disloyal slaves—marks the foreclosure of communal kinship, replacing it with a tyrannical hierarchy, where the bow serves as the absolute arbiter of the Law. The possibility of communal kinship is what makes the ending so tragic.

Therefore, Odysseus's killing of the suitors is not a moral triumph but a brutal enforcement of private property rights, demonstrating that the domestic order is maintained through a State-like monopoly on mythic violence. Here is Odysseus addressing the suitors before killing most of them single-handedly: "You dogs, because you thought I'd not come back from Troy to my own home, you've been ravaging my house, raping women, and, in devious ways, wooing my wife, while I was still alive" (Homer, 2002, p. 389).

In Horkheimer and Adorno's reading, the institution of marriage is stripped of its romantic veneer and revealed as a socio-economic contract designed to ensure the orderly inheritance of wealth. Penelope serves as the title deed to Ithaca; her fidelity is not a matter of sentiment, but the essential mechanism for preserving the patriarchal bloodline and the continuity of the Ithaca estate. The predatory logic of this proto-capitalist order reaches its zenith through the execution of twelve female slaves for enjoying sex with the parasitic suitors during Odysseus's twenty-year absence. Odysseus decrees:

> You three men [Telemachus, Eumaeus, and Philoetius], start carrying these corpses [of the suitors] outside now, then punish those shameless servant women. Have them clean these splendid chairs and tables, and wipe them with sponges soaked in water. Once you've put the entire house in order, then take those servants from the well-built hall to a spot outside between the roundhouse and the sturdy courtyard wall and kill them. Slash them with long swords, until life is gone from all of them, and they cannot recall Aphrodite and how they loved the suitors when they enjoyed sex with them in secret.
>
> (Homer, 2002, p. 403)

Just as the mythic hero's bow functions as a phallic instrument for reclaiming a fractured hierarchy, the modern conservative's curation of arms serves as a fractal enactment of the State's monopoly on mythic violence. This spectacle of weaponry transcends mere utility; it is a Symbolic performance intended to purge the *oikos* of those deemed illegal. This impulse finds its systemic realization in the current actions of federal law enforcement; for instance, the aggressive operations of ICE against immigrants from the Global South mirror this colonial desire to 'civilize' the *oikos* by terrorizing the 'savage' Other.

This problem of purification invites a critical departure from Fanon's (1961/2004) argument for violence as "a cleansing force" (p. 94). While Odysseus represents a colonizer *par excellence* and Fanon a colonized revolutionary, the metaphorical glorification of violence, as a sanitizing act, remains fundamentally mythic, whether Law-making or Law-preserving. Odysseus does not achieve justice with his mythic violence; he merely re-establishes a hegemonic order that relies on the negation of the Other of the Other. As such, one must question whether revolutionary violence can ever truly be emancipatory, or if it merely serves to re-install a new—but equally brutal—logic of power.

By contrast, divine violence does not seek to dismantle the master's house, but to undo the borders that define the *oikos* as private property. This requires the transformation of Ithaca into an *agora*: a commons, where Penelope is no longer property and the labor of the slaves ceases to be over-exploited. Justice, in this light, is found not in the clean halls of power, but in the messy abyss of freedom. This political transition from private property to the commons is the concrete utopian alternative to the mythic violence required for Odysseus to assert his sovereignty over the Kingdom of Ithaca. To be clear, Odysseus and Penelope can have personal property; the seizing of the Kingdom's means of production actualizes *the Commons of Ithaca.*

In the Lacanian reading of the homecoming, Ithaca functions not as a literal destination, but as the phallus, signifying a lost greatness that Odysseus believes will finally fill his lack of being, a self-inflicted alienation resulting from war trauma—today's equivalent would be the post traumatic-stress disorder experienced by veterans of imperial conquests. The Other's demand, in the Symbolic form of a debt of honor—an oath sworn to Helen's father, Tyndareus, to defend Helen's marriage to Menelaus—forced Odysseus to leave Ithaca. After his return, to constitute himself as the restored King and rightful owner of the Ithaca estate, Odysseus had to endure a radical separation from the Other as Law (the Name-of-the-Father), arriving on his shores stripped of his ships, men, and name; he returns as a remainder, a destitute subject defined by his status as less than nothing: a beggar.

It is in this fragile state that Odysseus encounters the *objet a*, embodied in Penelope's incomplete shroud for lord Laertes and the bed he carved out of a living olive tree. Both the shroud and the bed function as extimate objects that stabilize Odysseus's subjectivity against the Real void of his twenty-year absence. Penelope's weaving and unweaving is a metaphor for *différance*—the constant deferral of meaning. By unweaving the shroud every night for two decades, Penelope ensured that the master-signifier (the choice of a new King) is strategically deferred, keeping Ithaca in a state of undecidability, where Odysseus is neither dead nor alive, and the throne is neither occupied nor empty. While the incompleteness of the shroud functions as a hole in the Symbolic order of Ithaca that cannot be filled, the tree-bed is a metonym of hospitality, being the material proof of the host's mastery over his *oikos*. This mastery is further affirmed through the absurd act of killing all of the parasitic suitors. While the shroud represents a deferral of the Law, the bed signifies laying down the Law. The former is divine, and the latter is mythic.

As such, the topology of the Ithaca estate (*oikos*) is that of a tube torus: a closed circuit of the drive, endlessly circling a central absence. Odysseus is this absence at the heart of the torus, the void that frames the suitors' excessive *jouissance.* Penelope constitutes the toroidal body, her weaving and unweaving functioning as the repetitive circuit of the drive preserving the hole that marks Odysseus's absence. Against this structural void, the suitors appear as the toroidal flow—the kinetic, noisy, and parasitic energy that occupies the surface of the donut.

Yet, the tragedy of the shrewd subject is that the homecoming can resolve neither his lack of being nor the impossibility of his sovereignty. Even when he reclaims his throne, Odysseus finds that the Ithaca of his memory—the place of plenitude—is a fantasy. Hence, the necessity of the traversal of fantasy: the prophecy that he must depart once more. This is the metonymy of his colonial desire: he chases an *objet a* (*oikos*) to fill a lack of being that is, by definition, structurally unfillable. The *oikos* was never a home but a decoy. Odysseus's colonial desire was a failed attempt to escape the toroidal loop of his mythic existence. This is why the phallic search for a lost greatness produces nothing but a fascist politics of sameness, wherein difference must be forcefully exterminated.

The crisis of modernity is a dialectical trap: instrumental reason, exhausted by its own drive for mastery, regresses into a reactionary irrationalism. This is no exit from coloniality, but rather its postcolonial mutation into a mystical, primordial hierarchy—the precise tyranny Plato foretold as the successor to a hollowed-out democracy. Liberation requires a transition to transmodernity, which is driven by the feminine (*not all*) logic of historical reason. This nonlinear path constitutes the decolonial unconscious as a double-negation of both the suffocating Totality of the colonizer and the essentialist Exteriority of the reactionary. In doing so, it clears the ground for the pluriverse of radical humanism: a radical politics of reconciliation understood as a politics of difference.

Lest I be misunderstood, I wish to emphasize that there are non-European critical modernities beyond the Frankfurt School—such as Latin American decoloniality and the Black Radical Tradition. Furthermore, there is no shortage of irrationalist tendencies within Euromodernity itself (e.g., Völkisch nationalism and market fundamentalism), where reason is often emptied of ethical substance and refilled with myth. This internal decay within Totality highlights that even postmodernity—the very discourse dedicated to deconstructing Euromodernity—is not a purely European phenomenon.

It is historically significant that one of the progenitors of the concept, in a literary and philosophical sense, was Ihab Hassan, an Egyptian scholar. Hassan's intervention, particularly his essay from 1971 titled "POSTmodernISM", suggests that the exhaustion of the Enlightenment project was perhaps most visible to those standing at its borders. His subjectivity (border thinking) and scholarship (border methodology) serve as a reminder that the critique of Totality has always been co-authored by Exteriority, proving that the 'post' in postmodernity is an extimate product of a transmodern encounter rather than a closed European monologue.

In addition to Cairo, Perry Anderson (1998) shows, in *The Origins of Postmodernity*, that other non-European cities also contributed to the birth of postmodernity at the threshold between Totality and Exteriority: Lima, Shaanxi, Angkor, and Yucatan. In Anderson's words:

> 'Postmodernism' as term and idea supposes the currency of 'modernism'. Contrary to conventional expectation, both were born in a distant *periphery* rather than at the centre of the cultural system of the time: they come not from Europe or the United States.
>
> (p. 3, emphasis added)

However, the peripheral origins of postmodernity do not resolve the core problem of postmodernity: "The movement of religious reform began with the breaking of images; the arrival of the postmodern has installed *the rule of images* as never before" (p. 114, emphasis added). As such, one ought not to be lured by the multicultural origins of postmodernity, for they are essentially "oligopolies of the spectacle" (p. 105). Consequently, for Anderson, as for Frederic Jameson, postmodernity is "the cultural signal [and logic] of a new stage in the history of the regnant mode of production [i.e., late capitalism]" (p. 55). Therefore, postmodernity, as a critique of modernity, signifies the historical defeat of the Left:

> The universal triumph of capital signifies more than just a defeat for all those forces once arrayed against it, although it is also that. Its deeper sense lies in the cancellation of political alternatives. Modernity comes to an end, as Jameson observes, when it loses any antonym. The possibility of other social orders was an essential horizon of modernism. Once that vanishes, something like postmodernism is in place. This is the unspoken moment of truth in Lyotard's original construction. How, then, should the conjuncture of the postmodern be summed up? A capsule comparison with modernism might run: postmodernism emerged from the constellation of a *déclassé* ruling order, a mediatized technology and a monochrome politics.
>
> (pp. 91–92, emphasis in original)

The multicultural logic of postmodernity results from the failure of the old Left—the radical tradition originating in the French Revolution—to achieve rapid social transformation on an international scale. This defeat of the old Left—not only by external liberal and conservative forces, but also by internal schisms—instigated a mutation of radical socialist politics into a new Left since the 1960s, a global movement characterized by its commitment to anti-imperialism and student activism, yet one that Anderson suggests often acts as the "immediate vector'" (p. 62) for a newly affluent stratum: the Professional-Managerial Class (PMC).

In this context, a critical distinction must be made between multiculturalism and cultural pluralism: while multiculturalism—particularly the metaphor of the melting pot—often functions as a monochrome symptom of a market-saturated society, where genuine political alternatives have vanished, cultural pluralism—when guided by historical reason—recognizes these "segmented identities and localized groups, typically based on ethnic or sexual differences" (p. 62) as objective results of racial capitalism's totalization. Cultural pluralism is not a mere celebration of diversity among the high bourgeoisie, or even a democratization, but a "plebeianization," a dialectical concept from Bertolt Brecht, which Anderson interprets, with ambivalence, to mean: "*a vast broadening of the social basis of modern culture*; but by the same token also *a great thinning of its critical substance*, to yield the flat postmodern potion" (p. 113, emphasis added). Because postmodern multiculture is now so integrated into the market, it lacks the adversarial edge that modernism once possessed, resulting in a flat ideological world. However, this flatland is not universal, for the pluriverse is multidimensional.

The Zapatista movement in Chiapas, Mexico, is perhaps the clearest example of historical reason in action. On January 1, 1994—the day NAFTA went into effect—they declared "Enough!" (*¡Ya Basta!*). They rejected the instrumental reason of neoliberalism, which viewed their ancestral lands as mere commodities. They did not retreat into a romantic past by demanding a return to pre-colonial monarchies. Instead, they used the Women's Revolutionary Laws to challenge traditional hierarchies within their own communities (e.g., patriarchy). Subsequently, they developed a form of horizontal governance that is deeply rooted in Maya communal traditions, but also used modern tools (the internet, international law, and human rights discourse) to protect their autonomy.

Historical reason is (trans)rational as opposed to irrational (Gebser, 1986): it transcends and includes—or integrates—esotericism, such as magical and mythical forms of thinking. The (trans)rationality of historical reason ought not be confused with the obscene underside of instrumental reason: authoritarian mysticism, which is the reactionary marriage between high-tech efficiency and predatory occultism. Instrumental reason justifies systemic (extractive, settler-colonial, and genocidal) violence and intersectional (racist, sexist, and exploitative) oppressions. Authoritarian mysticism—an irrationalism in service of a fragile yet narcissistic ego that survives only by inflating itself through over-identification with the Leader or the Nation—does the dirty work for instrumental reason.

For example, the Nazis instrumentalized the predatory occult ideas of the Thule Society regarding Ariosophy to justify their racial supremacist ideology of Aryanism. Similarly, Silicon Valley today seems enamored with right-wing accelerationism, particularly the transhumanist philosophy of Nick Land. However, esotericism without historical reason, becomes a techno-myth, a colonial ideology, which has *the power of a daimōn but the amorality of an algorithm*.

All of these examples demonstrate that modernity and westernization—or, even, colonization—are not identical (cf. Eisenstadt, 2000). Islamic medievalism was, in many respects, more modern than its Christian counterpart between the 9th and

12th centuries. While medieval Europe was a world of agrarian villages, the Abbasid and Umayyad Caliphates were metropolitan hubs of institutionalized knowledge. This is exemplified by Fatima al-Fihriya, a 'grandmother' of modernity, who founded the University of al-Qarawiyyin, establishing the academic infrastructure—the degree and the chair—that allowed the authority of reason to outlive its authors (Abdouni, 2021).

Modernity, then, deconstructs our notions of linear time and Eurocentric geography; there are "multiple modernities" (Eisenstadt, 2000) before the Renaissance and beyond Europe—for example, Adonis (2003) traces Arab modernity to the eighth century. As such, Hypatia and Hildegard of Bingen served as 'mothers' to the modern spirit, preserving a commitment to observation and reason that would later become the bedrock of the Enlightenment (Dzielska, 1995; Newman, 1998); Princess Elisabeth of the Palatinate dismantled Cartesian dualism by demanding a more integrated view of the mind–body connection, thereby, predicting the crisis of the subject that Freud eventually solved (Shapiro, 2007); and Margaret Cavendish and Émilie du Châtelet challenged the mechanistic worldview by reintroducing the concepts of vitality and kinetic energy into the physical laws of nature (Merchant, 1980; O'Neill, 1997). Modernity, in this light, is a pluriversal project defined by its commitment to scientific rigor, humanistic inquiry, and the secularization of truth. Taken together, this incomplete lineage suggests that the true spirit of modernity is found in the courage to de-center the world and our place in it—to trade the comfort of dogma for the analectical, or polycentric, authority of historical reason. It is here that the contradictions of racial capitalism are resolved into a new ethical horizon: transmodernity, where truth meets justice, love meets forgiveness, radicalism meets humanism, and past meets future; where pluriversality meets singularity, poetics meets praxis, ecology meets the body, and order meets complexity; and where the collective care of socialism finally meets the radical freedom of libertarianism.

Decolonial Psychoanalysis

Decolonial Psychoanalysis (Beshara, 2019) is an ideology critique of the "war on terror" (WOT) discourse and the Islamophobia/Islamophilia fantasy. In the book, I theorize the relationship between (counter)terrorism and Islamophobia through a radical qualitative methodology: Lacanian discourse analysis. To psychoanalyze the fantasmatic dimension of the WOT discourse, I drew on Žižekian ideology critique. However, since my topic was cathected with Orientalist signifiers, I chose to ground my analysis on *an empirical basis* and *a decolonial footing*.

I accomplished the empirical portion by interviewing 19 U.S. Muslims regarding both their accounts of Islamophobia and how they resisted it. These were discursive accounts as opposed to phenomenological experiences. My words, as the interviewer, were part of the analysis, which entailed critical reflexivity. One of my findings was crystallized in the psychoanalytic concept of *internalized Islamophobia*. I used *decoloniality* as an Exterior framework with which I could keep psychoanalysis in check to make sure that I was not excessively or uncritically burdening my analysis with psychoanalytic jargon. *Decolonial Psychoanalysis* was about decolonizing psychoanalysis, and this book, in a sense, is about psychoanalyzing decoloniality. Both projects share an engagement in immanent critique, which I also phrase as *a critique from a place of love*. Immanent critiques of psychoanalysis and decoloniality are critiques from within that necessitate working through the internal logics of these fields as opposed to merely rejecting or refusing them from an external perspective of crass ignorance—and this is one of the main reasons I am against the liberal approach of cancelation.

The question of resistance was crucial for me back then because the psychological literature during the time of my research was foregrounding 'coping' as the most appropriate response to Islamophobia, which I read as *complicity with oppression*. The majority of the psychological studies on Islamophobia were quantitative and quasi-experimental in their aspiration to 'measure' Islamophobia through scales administered to potential Islamophobes. I, on the other hand, chose to tread a qualitative, or human scientific, path with a firm sense that Muslim voices must be centered in my analysis, if I am to adequately describe and explain the complex psychosocial phenomenon of Islamophobia. In sum, *Decolonial Psychoanalysis* explains the alienation of *the (post)colonial subject as demand*, particularly when they are interpellated by a master's discourse like the WOT: "Either you are with us, or you are with the terrorists" (Bush, 2001).

Decolonial Psychoanalysis rejects the false dichotomy implied by the contrary relationship between these two subject-positions in Bush's speech and locates itself in the negative (but ethical) space of anti-terrorism, an Exteriority that implicates two decolonial subject-positions, that of *not-terrorist* and *not-counterterrorist*. These implicated decolonial subject-positions, while in a contrary relationship to one another, converge in their contradictory relationship to violence and oppression, so they are subject-positions, which are inherently for (non)violence and liberation, as new master-signifiers.

The project of decolonizing psychoanalysis fundamentally begins with a critique of the inherent European bias and supposed universal applicability of psychoanalytic theory. This process demands a radical decentering of the field from Exteriority, moving away from a theory heavily shaped by "the cultural, social, and economic capital of Western paternalism" (Togashi, 2020, p. xiii). Decolonization insists that psychoanalysis must "replace the coercions of apparent 'universals' with the infinite choice of the particular, the variable, the multiple routes to spontaneity and freedom" (Swartz, 2018, p. 143). This skepticism extends to the field's most foundational concepts, such as the Oedipus Complex, which Wapeemukwa (2022) critiques as being so "inextricable from civilization" in Freud's view that its challenge appears to require "civilizational annihilation" (p. 95). This false assumption on the part of the "Oedipal Empire" is rejected by (non)Europeans who assert that "[d]ecolonization is not the death of civilization but its rebirth," which is achievable through alternative relational models like "Indigenous kinship relations" (Wapeemukwa, 2022, p. 95). The overall objective of decolonizing psychoanalysis is to dismantle the theoretical structures that have historically excluded and "devalue[d] the experiences of racial minorities, and more broadly people who are socially and economically marginalized" (Tummala-Narra, 2022, p. 232).

Decolonizing psychoanalysis mandates a re-theorization of the modern subject, who is invested in a colonial unconscious. This re-theorization is necessary to adequately work through the traumatic Real of coloniality. Andréa Guerra (2024), for instance, theorizes the traumatic Real of coloniality through two key terms: "linguicide" or "the suppression of language, culture, family, economy, physical, and symbolic territory of belonging" (p. 7) and "the crypt," as "a phantasmagorical inheritance of the colonised unconscious" (p. 15). Fanon (1952) initiated this decolonial shift toward analyzing the colonial unconscious of modernity by insisting that understanding the colonized subject requires moving beyond "phylogeny and ontogeny" to embrace "sociogeny" (p. 4), thus recognizing that alienation is a collective rather than a purely individual condition, which echoes the Marxist thesis in many ways. Fanon's sociogenic principle is the foundation of decolonial psychoanalysis; it asserts that the psyche is not a closed circuit but is constitutively perforated and shaped by different forms of oppression, rendering alienation a social problem requiring a political solution, not just a clinical one: *disalienation* qua *liberation.*

Decolonial psychoanalysis, according to Stephen Sheehi (2018), aims to reach "beyond a Manichean condition of two-ness, beyond a two-state condition to a one-state condition," tackling how "binary identity structures" are normalized to produce "subjects of coloniality" (p. 319). Crucially, decolonial psychoanalysis requires an integrative approach that posits the unconscious as an embodied, socially embedded phenomenon. This integrative approach challenges the Cartesian dualism that reinforces colonial divisions of mind over body (Gaztambide et al., 2024, p. 332), a dualism that justifies the civilizational logic of 'man' over 'nature,' wherein the former is presumed to be the modern subject of psychoanalysis (i.e., male, European, secular Christian, bourgeois intellectual, liberal humanist, etc.) and the latter signifies the savage, the primitive, or the barbarian as a violent site of extraction, over-exploitation, and extermination—Fanon's zone of nonbeing. Man thinks; nature is unthought. Man is; nature is nought. This is why decolonial psychoanalysis—unlike orthodox Marxism—is concerned not only with class struggle, but also with other forms of oppression like racism and sexism.

Accordingly, Evzonas (2020) contends that to "queer and decolonize psychoanalysis" promotes an "overinclusive, non-hegemonic, and non-axiological way of thinking about sexualities, gender, class, and, race" (pp. 576–577), allowing for "a different understanding of integration" (Dadlani, 2020, p. 125). Theoretically, this integration extends even to Lacan's L-schema, of which Burnham (2022) proposes a decolonial reading that recasts *the Other as decoloniality*, representing "the insistence on a politics of revolt and resurgence" (p. 60); a decolonial Other grounded in *the materiality of language* as the basis for a revolutionary standpoint (Rahmat, 2025, pp. 1–2).

The decolonization effort, however, must move beyond theory into the realm of practice and institutional structures, for the "psychoanalysis of colonization and decolonizing psychoanalysis are one and the same process" (Chen, 2010, p. 73). This requires "facing past and ongoing oppressive ideologies and practices" with an attitude of humility to "challenge systemic racism" (Tummala-Narra, 2022, p. 232). This is described as a two-part process by Swartz (2018): one part involves the historical analysis of theory's colonial influences, while the second concerns the "practices of transmitting psychoanalytic DNA from centre to periphery," which involves "quarrelling with authorities guarding the gates of psychoanalytic theory," including "licensing bodies, editorial boards and conference committees, everywhere" (p. 143). Essentially, the call of decoloniality is for *an insurgent (re) reading and practice* (Maldonado-Torres et al., 2021, p. 248) that focuses on "decolonizing the subjectivity of both patient and therapist" (Gaztambide et al., 2024, p. 332), ensuring that the clinical space itself becomes a political site of challenging, rather than reproducing, colonial power dynamics.

If coloniality is the psychic remainder of colonialism, then decoloniality—as the negation of coloniality—is essentially *an analectical praxis*, not an (anti)modern Luddite attitude. Rather, decoloniality is the project of *delinking modernity from coloniality* in both Totality and Exteriority, materially and ideologically. Decoloniality is a complex, long-term process of political, economic, psychic, and social liberation, particularly *the decoloniality of power, knowledge, and being*. The decolonial affirmation of modernity, while negating coloniality, is a crucial theoretical move to prevent decolonization from regressing to a form of (anti)modernity as a nostalgic/romantic retreat to a pre-modern past, which never existed, except as an ahistorical object of fantasy. Furthermore, now that the signifier 'decolonization' is a buzzword coopted by liberal capitalists and applied to everything from marketing to diet, I share Gheorghe's (2022) concern:

> there is no decolonization if that process results into a new class of colonizers imposing their paradigm. Decolonial thinking doesn't mean exchanging one dogma with another; but rather striving to escape the rigidity and simplism of binary thinking and learning to see the world as macro and micro networks of systems, deeply interconnected at multiple levels.
>
> (p. 133)

Therefore, I do not simply regard modernity as a tragic historical event, which began with the colonization of the Americas in the 15th century; however, I do concur with Enrique Dussel (1985) that 1492 specifically marks the birth of *modernity/coloniality* as a world system that inaugurated *the Totality of the racial capitalist apparatus*. As such, I recognize the theoretical modernity or contemporaneity of ancient philosophy as an early documented example of radical humanism: a non-dogmatic or critical—i.e., scientific—attitude *vis-à-vis* Truth. This is why, for example, we continue to read and think with Plato and Aristotle thousands of years later. Their thinking still speaks to us today. The decolonial move, of course, is to read Plato and Aristotle alongside Lǎozǐ and Ptahhotep, for instance. In other words, decoloniality is not about throwing out the baby (modernity) with the bathwater (coloniality), but about *delinking the modern subject from the colonial unconscious* to construct *the transmodern subject*. My notion of double-unconsciousness stems from the ambivalence of the (de)colonial unconscious—being de- and colonial, an (un)doing. This is why I consider antimodernity to be a decolonial fantasy: a reactionary stance that purports to be anti-, but is nothing but the return of the repressed: modernity. In other words, there is no *pure* decoloniality, for the very notion of *purity* is irrational and, as I showed before, the act of *purification* is mythic violence *par excellence*. This is why transmodernity cannot repeat the error of Euromodernity, for the ideological purity of modernization justified the cruelty of colonization.

Modernity is a global project, as opposed to a European one. The signifier 'transmodernity,' which was popularized by Dussel (1985), makes the pluriversality of decoloniality explicit. Like modernity, psychoanalysis is a transmodern project; as such, decolonial psychoanalysis is an analectical materialist praxis that has a twofold aim, according to Ranjan Khanna (2003): "It documents the world events through which psychoanalysis was produced, and it also offers a critical reading practice which itself is a product of that initial violent projective saying. Worlding [psychoanalysis] is the understanding of global strife in the production of textuality" (p. 5). I read *worlding* beyond Khanna's invocation of Heidegger and in light of Said's (1983) arguments around secular criticism in *The World, the Text, and the Critic*.

Contrapuntal Psychoanalysis

Building on this foundation of decolonizing psychoanalysis, my next work, *Freud and Said* (Beshara, 2021a) expands the scope of my research in various ways. First, I invoke the notion of *apparatus* to account for not only capitalist ideology but also the materiality of exploitation and other forms of oppression. I home in on the apparatus of *racial capitalism*, in particular, as the material context that must be historicized so that a discourse like the WOT can be situated and explained in terms of the politico-libidinal economy (cf. Lyotard, 1993). Then I juxtapose the thinking of Edward Said with that of Sigmund Freud to show how the latter influenced the former and why reading the latter through the former is fecund, which challenges the widespread assumption that postcolonialism and psychoanalysis are somehow incompatible fields, wherein Said is reduced to strictly being a Foucaultian when he was influenced by a variety of thinkers and practitioners, such as Giambattista Vico, Antonio Gramsci, Eqbal Ahmad, Theodor Adorno, Jean-Paul Sartre, Simone de Beauvoir, Taheyya Kariokka, Virginia Woolf, Jacques Derrida, James Baldwin, Noam Chomsky, C. L. R James, Frantz Fanon, Malcolm X, and, of course, Sigmund Freud and Jacques Lacan.

As such, my effort was to bridge the theoretical gap between postcolonialism and psychoanalysis by highlighting that this gap may be nonexistent or illusory since psychoanalysis was fundamental, for example, in Said's theorization of Orientalism. The dialectics of contrapuntal psychoanalysis move us toward *the decolonial subject as desire*. The contrapuntal subject is a decolonial subject that follows the psychoanalytic or negative logic of separation: neither terrorist nor counterterrorist. This contrapuntal subject desires anti-terrorism (and, by extension, anticapitalism, antiracism, and antisexism), that is, *a non-hierarchical world characterized by (non)violence and liberation*.

If decolonial psychoanalysis critiques (post)colonial psychoanalysis from an Exterior vantage point, then contrapuntal psychoanalysis—defined as liberation praxis—is a further sublation, which entails *the immanent critique of psychoanalysis from within Totality* and *the self-criticism of decoloniality from within Exteriority*. In sum, *Decolonial Psychoanalysis* dealt with the ethics of liberation (i.e., resistance), and *Freud and Said* was about the aesthetics of liberation (i.e., counterpoint). In this book, I am concerned with *the politics of liberation* (i.e., the politico-libidinal economy).

Liberation Psychoanalysis

With the ethics and aesthetics of liberation established in the first two books, this third book is concerned with *the politics of liberation*, or liberation psychoanalysis; after all, *the unconscious is politics*, as Lacan suggests in Seminar XIII. For Mladen Dolar (2008), psychoanalysis prepares us for political action but leaves us at a threshold "without prescription and without guarantee" and "this circumscribing a place is itself a political gesture, a political opening, the opening of a door through which we must make a step" (p. 29).

Liberation Psychoanalysis stages a further separation and prefigures *the transmodern subject as drive*. This transmodern subject is driven by collective liberation (i.e., the cause of historical reason). The transmodern subject can be characterized by their traversal of the racial capitalist fantasies of both coloniality and (anti) modernity. The colonial fantasy is at work in racial capitalist modernization in the form of instrumental reason. The (anti)modern fantasy tends to be irrationalist, a nostalgia for a 'greatness' that never was.

Modernity, however, follows historical reason, which is *the use of reason for liberation*. In contrast, instrumental reason is *the use of reason for domination* (Quijano, 1989). C. L. R. James et al. (2006) make a similar distinction between two philosophies of rationalism: "mastery over men [and women]" and "mastery over things" (p. 69). They qualify the former as a "bourgeois morality" and the latter as a "collective morality" (p. 70). To echo their socialist argument regarding *rationalism as a philosophy of life*, liberation psychoanalysis "must become proletarian" (p. 66).

Transmodernity recognizes modernity within Totality *and* Exteriority. Liberation is the antithesis of oppression, so if we are the define oppression as *dehumanization through exploitation, racism, sexism* (cf. Young, 1990), and other means, then liberation would concretely signify *socialism + humanism*. Socialism refers to an economic system that does not exist yet and which will surpass capitalism by resolving its central contradiction: labor exploitation. Similarly, humanism is the resolution of racism and sexism, which are forms of dehumanization weaponized by the ruling class. My invocation of the signifier 'socialism' is an anti-campist attempt to unite the three schools of socialist thought (i.e., revolutionary socialism, democratic socialism, and libertarian socialism) against capitalist realism through the concept of *dual power*, which emphasizes prefigurative politics, as the unifying basis for all socialist action; sublating, for example, the strategies of reform and revolution. By 'humanism,' I mean a commitment to radical, transformative becoming—a political imperative to liberate human potential, which is fundamentally distinct from the colonial archive of liberal humanism and its passive moralism. Not to mention that radical humanism is also opposed to the nihilism of both anti-humanism and trans-humanism.

Figure 1.1 summarizes my theory of liberation psychoanalysis in a diagrammatic form. To begin, the semiotic square (cf. Greimas & Rastier, 1968) is structured by the apparatus of racial capitalism–the invisible hand of the market, which informs the politico-libidinal economy of the global market. As such, the x-axis signifies class struggle and divided subjectivity, wherein coloniality ($\sim S_2$), for example, functions as the unconscious of modernity (S_1) and as the zone of nonbeing occupied by the oppressed, who are either over-exploited or exterminated.

The left half of the square represents the Totality of modernity/coloniality, wherein coloniality implicates modernity and is in a contradictory relationship with transmodernity. The right half indexes the Exteriority of transmodernity/decoloniality, wherein decoloniality ($\sim S_1$) implicates transmodernity (S_2) and is in a contrary relationship with coloniality. It is important to note that coloniality ≠ modernity, and decoloniality ≠ (anti)modernity. As such, I distinguish between modernity and the colonial fantasy, on the one hand, and between decoloniality and the (anti)modern fantasy, on the other hand.

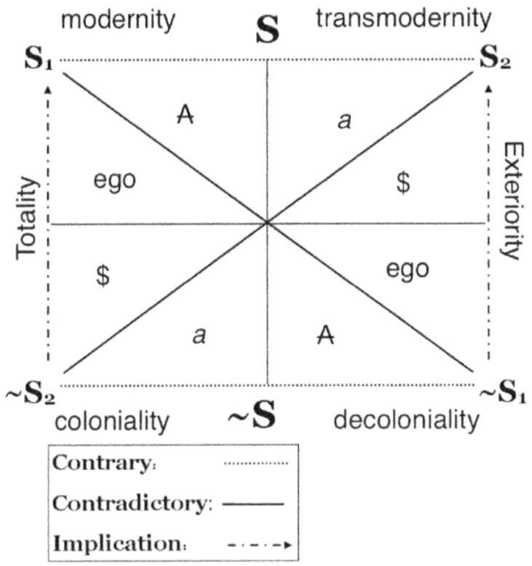

Figure 1.1 Mapping coloniality/modernity and transmodernity/decoloniality

S refers to (trans)modernity, the sublation of modernity and its alterity. For me, modernity is a function of historical reason—for a sustained overview of modernity and historical reason, see Beshara (2024b). As such, (trans)modernity is the scientific but pluriversal quest for Truth, which began with the ancient philosophers, who were driven by their love of wisdom (cf. Adonis, 2003). ~S indicates (de)coloniality as the (ideo)logical fantasy sustaining the discourse of (trans)modernity.

The question of sexual difference concerns the upper left quadrant (the zone of being) and also informs the upper right quadrant (the zone of becoming); however, sexual difference is structured by colonial difference, which is the difference between the zones of being and nonbeing in Totality; a colonial difference that then gets projected as a cultural difference between 'civilized' Totality and 'savage' Exteriority, which are separated by the y-axis. It is worth noting that the relations within the semiotic square are extimate because the center and the periphery are not pure, for "the center itself has its organized enclaves of underdevelopment, its reservations and its ghettos as interior peripheries" (Deleuze & Guattari, 1983, p. 231), and the periphery has its Exterior version of the center.

Finally, modernity/coloniality follows the oppressive and violent logic of the master's discourse, wherein the modern ego functions as a master-signifier propelling modern knowledge (A̶), which paranoically excludes Exterior ways of knowing and being. The colonial fantasy ($ ◊ *a*) materializes this negation, which is then projected onto Exteriority as the space–time of savagery, barbarism, and/or primitivity. Attempts at critiquing modernity/coloniality from within Totality result in either postmodernity or critical modernity. While Totality disavows its foundations, and postmodernity represses its symptoms, critical modernity forecloses the very possibility of coloniality; thus, each position is coextensive with a specific mode of colonial negation.

While schizoanalysis offers a postmodernist dismantling of (post)colonial psychoanalysis, Erich Fromm's (1955) "humanistic psychoanalysis" represents the critical modernism of the Frankfurt School—a tradition rooted in a Freudian humanism that Lacan famously rejected. Indeed, Lacan's anti-humanism, underscored by his rigorous deployments of structural linguistics, topology, and symbolic logic, appears at first glance to be an inhospitable site for decoloniality. One might reasonably ask: Why stretch the Freudo–Lacanian tradition at all? Why not begin with Fanon, who already actualized psychoanalysis as a transmodern praxis from the Exteriority of Martinique and Algeria? While Fanon successfully reconciled decolonial structuralism with radical humanism, my project seeks a different fecundity. I argue that the radical potential of Freudo–Lacanian psychoanalysis lies in its formalist tools, which—when delinked from the logic of coloniality—provide the necessary meta-theoretical conditions for a liberation psychoanalysis capable of navigating the complexities of a transmodern world.

Throughout this book, I argue for the radical potential of psychoanalysis via Freud's Exteriority—a concept Frosh (2020) frames as "decolonial Judaism." This positioning echoes the Exteriority of Moses, yet Freud's specific location inverts the analectical relationship. Where Moses, as an Egyptian outsider, stood in an analectical relationship to the nascent Totality of Judaism, Freud's Exteriority as a Jew stands in an analectical relationship to the expansive Totality of modernity/ coloniality. This parallax explains Freud's paradoxical double-bind: his conscious commitment to methodological atheism functioned as a protective veneer for his deeper investment in a Kabbalistic unconscious (Bakan, 1958). As an Egyptian scholar seeking to pluriversalize the field, I extend this analysis to propose that liberation psychoanalysis be understood as a *decolonial secularization*—a process that strips the colonial mask from universal science to reveal a radical and esoteric Exteriority.

If Freud's project was rooted in a hidden Exteriority, what then of Lacan? Unlike Freud, Lacan did not doubly negate the Exteriority of the Other of the Other; instead, he viewed non-European Exteriority through a parallectic lens from within Totality. For Lacan, the Other was often reduced to a structural necessity of the Symbolic order, viewed from a distance rather than engaged as a living Exteriority. It is precisely here—at the junction where Lacan observes but does not inhabit the Exteriority—that I find the space to stretch his formal logic into a transmodern praxis.

In *Decolonial Psychoanalysis* (2019a), I have pointed to a minor but significant reference in Lacan's (2007) Seminar XVII to "the real of decolonization" (p. 34) *vis-à-vis* French colonialism in Algeria, for example, but that is merely a taste; I have three arguments in favor of Lacan. (1) In Seminar XVIII, Lacan (2025) explores the question of the Chinese unconscious, in a non-Orientalist fashion, through both a close reading of Chinese characters—with which he has familiarity—and a deep engagement with Chinese philosophy, particularly the work of Mèngzǐ.

In addition to this radical affirmation of a major Asian language and the Ru school of thought, there are also (2) Lacan's connections with Africa, namely through the liberatory reflections of Beninese psychoanalyst Solange Faladé and the sub-oppressive actions of Congolese psychoanalyst Yerodia. As Sinan Richards (2023) shows, despite Lacan's final instructions that Solange Faladé, Charles Melman, and Jacques-Alain Miller should collectively lead *La Fondation de la Cause Freudienne*, Miller disregarded Faladé and established *L'École de la Cause Freudienne* (ECF) instead. In response to this exclusion, Faladé founded her own separate institution and psychoanalytic school, known as *L'École Freudienne*, in Dakar, Senegal. According to Richards (2023),

> Faladé chose to exemplify the psychoanalytical and racial implications of her orthodox Lacanian teachings by discussing the end of negotiations between Nelson Mandela and Frederik De Klerk that inaugurated the beginning of the end of apartheid in South Africa, creating with it a multiracial state and democracy. (pg. 436)

Now, we turn to the Yerodia controversy. According to Dany Nobus (2016), before becoming an analyst, Yerodia was Lacan's "butler and right-hand man, driving him back and forth between his house and the lecture theatre, and looking after the day-to-day running of his private affairs and public engagements" (p. 4). Subsequently, after completing his analytic formation, Yerodia became, first, the Minister of Foreign Affairs, then, the Vice-President of the Democratic Republic of Congo.

In 2000, the International Court of Justice issued an arrest warrant against Yerodia in Belgium—which, of course, colonized the Congo for 52 years—for his crimes against humanity since he encouraged the Congolese people to commit genocide against the Tutsis. What is of concern to us here is Yerodia's psychoanalytic justification for his war crimes, which raises a question about how the discourse of the analyst can metamorphose into "a discourse of terror" (Nobus, 2016, p. 6). Nobus (2016) writes:

> In Yerodia's outlook, however, Lacanian psychoanalysis epitomizes exactly the kind of discourse from which his ideological stance can derive theoretical legitimacy and moral strength … "a psychoanalyst must refuse rabble … When there are rabble, one has to condemn them to be rabble, and the psychoanalyst can do nothing…I'm a psychoanalyst. I know what exclusion is" … he subsequently divulged in February 2001 that he had only met two people in his entire life who had made a lasting impression on him, his (recently assassinated) comrade Laurent-Désiré Kabila and his French master Jacques Lacan.
>
> (Nobus, 2016, p. 5)

In addition to Faladé and Yerodia, there is also a third Lacanian progeny, an Other African: Moustafa Safouan. Safouan, whose ideas are weaved through this text, was labeled "the Egyptian Oedipus" (Tresilian, 2020) in his obituary by Al-Ahram Weekly. Furthermore, Iwuanyanwu (2015) argues that Lacan's theoretical development was deeply intertwined with his African travels, where he sought "a physical pilgrimage" (p. 77) to the lands that informed the ethnographic works of Freud.

In Egypt, he focused on the structural depth of hieroglyphs eventually positing that the "dream is constructed like hieroglyphics" (p. 91) and comparing the deciphering of the unconscious to the work of Jean-François Champollion on the Rosetta Stone. His time in Morocco led to an interest in the Saadian Tombs and complex genealogies, providing a historical and physical backdrop for his theories on the "dead father" (p. 85) and the Name-of-the-Father as a symbolic myth essential to the human experience. Furthermore, Lacan used observations from the African landscape, such as comparing the "elephant track of an equatorial forest" (p. 86) to the Parisian highway, to illustrate how the "undeniable signifier" (p. 87) of a pathway gives meaning to procreation, paternity, and death. These experiences also shaped his views on the "master-slave Hegelian myth" (p. 93), where he echoed André Gide's observations on the frustration of labor and the alienation of desire within the colonial context to refine his clinical concept of *jouissance*.

Finally, (3) Lacan is more influential in Latin America, particularly in Argentina and Brazil, than he is in France (cf. Bosteels, 2012). Buenos Aires is known, for example, as the capital of psychoanalysis. However, as is the case in Africa, in Latin America, there is the radical work of Lacan's translator and interpreter Oscar Masotta (an Argentine psychoanalyst), but then there is a reactionary figure like Amilcar Lobo Moreira, a Brazilian psychoanalyst who actively participated in torture sessions, in the early 1970s, during the dictatorship of the military junta. Arguments 2 and 3 demonstrate that Exteriority is not inherently more ethical or moral than Totality, for the oppressed internalize oppression and can subsequently engage in sub-oppressive or horizontal violence. However, the internalization of oppression implies a preceding colonial violence that then gets internalized.

For this reason, I maintain that liberation psychoanalysis must resist being used to justify violence, revolutionary or otherwise. Here, I diverge from many contemporary interpreters of Fanon: while I share their admiration for his decolonial insights, I argue that *Fanon-the-analyst* and *Fanon-the-revolutionary* represent distinct theoretical modalities that have been too easily conflated. *Peau Noire, Masques Blancs* and *Les Damnés de la Terre* deploy disparate methodologies regarding the nature of liberation. Fundamentally, I contend that the ethical position of the decolonial psychoanalyst is distinct from that of the political revolutionary; to merge them risks collapsing the delicate clinical work of psychic liberation into the totalizing mechanics of political force. This does not mean that psychoanalysis and revolution are disconnected, but, rather, that they are not the same.

Transmodernity/decoloniality follows the logic of the analyst's discourse, wherein *a* represents the liberation psychoanalyst's position, the cause of the transmodern subject's ($) desire. As such, $a \lozenge \$$ indicates a traversal of the colonial fantasy. However, *the problem of the (anti)modern fantasy* remains as a result of the transmodern subject's excessive over-hystericization of the master-signifiers of modernity to the extent that decoloniality becomes a solidified (anti)modern ego formation through identification with new master-signifiers that blind the transmodern subject from the incompleteness of decolonial forms of knowing (Ⱥ). This is the dimension of the traumatic Real, or the death drive, which affects subjects in both Totality and Exteriority, but in different ways. The death drive must be worked through and integrated analytically as a structural cut: the limit of knowledge and the lack of being.

In *Beyond the Pleasure Principle*, Freud (1920/1961) distinguishes between the ego/death drive (Thanatos) and the life/sex drive (Eros). For him, they are two sides of the same coin (repetition-compulsion), but they express themselves differently in relation to the *objet a*. The repetitions of the drives speak to their "conservative" or "regressive" nature, and they are often visualized by Lacanians as orbiting the *objet a* the way the planets orbit the sun. In desire, the relationship with the *objet a* is also nonlinear, but not necessarily following an elliptical or spiral topology, which opens up nondual forms of enjoyment beyond sexual and colonial difference, such as cultural difference as *the decolonial sublimation of ethics, aesthetics, and politics*.

Whereas the ego/death drive is a destructive downward spiral, the life/sex drive is a creative upward spiral. The relationship between conservatism and the drives is interesting to ponder, even if Freud's use of the term was technical and not political.

Freud (1923/1961) returns to the conservative dialectics of the drives in *The Ego and the Id* when he writes that the drives are

> conservative in the strictest sense of the word, since both (the ego/death and the life/sex drives) would be endeavouring to re-establish a state of things that was disturbed by the emergence of life. The emergence of life would thus be the cause of the continuance of life and also at the same time of the striving towards death; and life itself would be a conflict and compromise between these two trends. The problem of the origin of life would remain a cosmological one; and the problem of the goal and purpose of life would be answered dualistically.
>
> (pp. 40–41)

Speaking of the drives, the dominant form of enjoyment within Totality (modernity/coloniality) is *mythic jouissance*—the enjoyment of oppression and violence. Conversely, transmodernity/decoloniality is characterized by *divine jouissance*, the enjoyment of liberation and (non)violence (Sharp, 2005). My theoretical distinction between these two modes of *jouissance* stems from my juxtaposition of the thinking of Benjamin and Lacan, an effort to historicize and politicize the question of sexual difference through my conception of colonial difference, which opens up the vertical or hierarchical dimension of subjugation underlying subjectification. For Lacan, whereas phallic or masculine *jouissance* follows the structure of Aristotle's logic of the all (i.e., universal Law), Other or feminine *jouissance* represents the particular negative, the logic of exception; in other words, singularity, or the *sinthome*, is the not all. As such, we can explain the continuity of patriarchy, or the sexist oppression of women, as an asymmetrical system of power, which is a function of the dominance of Aristotle's totalizing logic. The logic of the all has been internalized and sedimented over millennia that it constitutes the political unconscious of Totality, which often manifests as a colonial unconscious.

Accordingly, ~~Woman~~ does not exist because universality is phallogocentric and excludes singularity; "man is the measure of all things," as Protagoras claimed. This also explains the negation of the ~~Man~~ (or ~~Black~~) within Totality—I extend Curry's category of the Man-Not by invoking the racialized and the politicized, to consider the exclusion of ~~Brown~~, ~~LGBTQ~~, etc. In other words, sexist oppression and racism are symptoms of syllogism (e.g., "All Lives Matter"). Conversely, pluriversality follows the liberatory logic of the not all, which affirms the transmodern subject's singularity of being, or their *sinthome* (e.g., "Black Lives Matter").

Is there mythic *jouissance* in Exteriority? Absolutely. The problems of authoritarianism and fundamentalism in the Global South (Wahba, 2022), for example, stem from sub-oppression, which is an effect of (neo)colonialism (Nkrumah, 1965). These problems undoubtedly require *self-criticism* in order for them to be resolved or, at least, reckoned with (Al-Azm, 2012). Is there divine *jouissance* in Totality (cf. Musser, 2018)? Of course. The best example of divine *jouissance* in the Global North is African American music, a form of ethico-political resistance that sublimates the traumatic Real of slavery and racism through liberation aesthetics—this is what Benjamin (1935) meant by *the politicization of aesthetics*. But even liberation aesthetics can get coopted, hence the necessity of ideology critique and liberation praxis, particularly in the face of fascist reversals, which aestheticize (and anesthetize) politics. This leads Barnaby Barratt (2011), for example, to argue that Martín-Baró's liberation psychology facilitates "the potential of psychoanalysis as ideology critique" (p. 129).

The title of my book is, of course, a variation on Ignacio Martín-Baró's (1996) *Writings for a Liberation Psychology*—a foundational text in the Latin American critical psychology canon. The book could have also been titled *Fragments of a Libertarian Psychoanalysis* (cf. Graeber, 2004). As such, my book is also a collection of selected works under the theme of liberation, which can be read in any order. Liberation Psychology is inspired by Gustavo Gutiérrez's (1973) *A Theology of Liberation*. However, as a secular critic, the works I consider influential in this study are Paulo Freire's (1970) *Pedagogy of the Oppressed* and Enrique Dussel's (1985) *Philosophy of Liberation*, in particular. Recent contributions that have also shaped my thinking include *Toward Psychologies of Liberation* (Watkins & Shulman, 2008) and *A People's History of Psychoanalysis* (Gaztambide, 2019). In other words, my conception of liberation psychoanalysis—as an anti-oppressive praxis—is premised upon my idiosyncratic interpretation of liberation psychology, pedagogy, and philosophy.

Ignacio Martín-Baró: Liberation Psychology

Ignacio Martín-Baró was a Salvadoran social psychologist and Jesuit priest. His work was not just theoretical; it was deeply embedded in a political reality, as his own life demonstrates. He was murdered in 1989 along with five other Jesuits by the Salvadoran Army. The context for this mythic violence was the Salvadoran Civil War (1979–1992), and the instrumental reason behind their brutal murder was that the Jesuits advocated for a ceasefire agreement between the government of El Salvador and the *Frente Farabundo Martí para la Liberación Nacional* (FMLN). This personal snapshot is necessary to frame the political stakes of Martín-Baró's research on liberation psychology in the face of the oppressive mechanisms that led to his untimely death. Martín-Baró's (1996) conception of oppression is informed by not only theology but also political economy, for he acknowledges the economic factors that contribute to oppression: "underdevelopment" and "dependency" (p. 17).

One of his most original contributions is his theory of *psychologization*, which functions "to strengthen the oppressive structures … by drawing attention away from them and toward individual and subjective factors" (p. 19). In essence, oppression is a psychosocial and material structure rather than a purely ideological or psychic phenomenon. Martín-Baró's understanding of oppressive structures is informed by dependency theory, which posits a structural inequality between the Global North (the core) and the Global South (the periphery). The latter is underdeveloped, overexploited, and thereby dependent as a function of neocolonialism—the last stage of imperialism, according to Nkrumah (1965).

For Martín-Baró, oppression is a social structure resulting from the material effects of dependency; it then gets internalized by the oppressed, and this is how it becomes a psychic mechanism of "conformist fatalism," which is "very convenient for the established order" (p. 30). The target of oppression is the psyche or the spirit, and the ideological purpose of oppression is to generate mass hopelessness so that nothing changes in the bourgeois order.

As such, Martín-Baró's antidote to this crushing of the spirit is liberation psychology, which he defines as "a praxis committed to the sufferings and hopes of the peoples of Latin America" (p. 32). Echoing the Marxian axiom that *social being determines consciousness*, Martín-Baró understands praxis as a form of practical knowledge that precedes consciousness:

> Consciousness is the knowing or not knowing of self, through the world and through others, with *praxis coming before mental knowledge*. Before it becomes thought, *knowledge as praxis is inscribed in the appropriateness of all behaviors to objective realities, becoming reflexive only conditionally, and only in part.*
> (p. 38, emphasis added)

Martín-Baró's conception of praxis is also aligned with the psychoanalytic notion of the unconscious, "From a psychological point of view, the knowledge that counts most is not explicit and formalized knowledge, but rather the *knowledge inherent in everyday praxis, usually implicit, structurally unconscious, and ideologically natural*" (p. 39, emphasis added). The point of praxis, in other words, is to produce critical consciousness, which arises from a revolutionary reflexivity *vis-à-vis* our social being. As such, we can frame liberation praxis as *critical unconsciousness*. Since the unconscious is the Other's discourse, the praxis of critical unconsciousness is none other than ideology critique, as *the critique of the Other's discourse*—that is, critically analyzing and reflecting on the socio-political forces that shape one's life.

In negating the oppressive structures resulting from bourgeois ideology, liberation praxis is both material and proletarian. Or to put it in the words of Otto Gross (1913): "The psychology of the unconscious is the philosophy of revolution." Gross (1919/1977) would later add, "*the demand for revolution as a result of the psychology of the unconscious becomes absolute as soon as it is demonstrated that the repression of these predisposed values* [i.e., our innate, inherent human qualities that exist in the unconscious] *means sacrificing the greatest human potential*" (p. 105, emphasis in original). Gross clearly qualifies the ethics of unconscious desire as a form of revolutionary thinking. For more on Gross, see Heuer (2016).

In contrast to psychologization, praxis is collective. It is an intervention at the level of social being. In ideology, the social link is fantasmatic or based on Imaginary identifications, typically with a charismatic leader or a social group. In praxis, the social link stems from the desire for collective liberation, a source of enjoyment driving comrades in solidarity (cf. Malherbe, 2024). As Martín-Baró argues, "it is difficult to conceive of a true historical consciousness developing or popular organizing taking place outside of the context of a popular practice, which must inevitably be *a class praxis*, that is, *one organized around popular interests*" (pp. 219–220, emphasis added).

Furthermore, praxis is related to the psychoanalytic concept of *hystericization* as a questioning of master-signifiers, which produces critical knowledge like psychoanalysis or Marxism. Martín-Baró writes, "Knowledge of reality follows social praxis" (p. 213). The capitalist ideology negates the materiality of social being. It presents us with an idealist conception of the world, which pits us against one another as isolated individuals with competing egos. We are not only oppressed by the ruling class; we also internalize oppression and blame ourselves for being oppressed. This explains Martín-Baró's emphasis on psychologization as a ruling idea that must be deconstructed.

Psychoanalysis becomes a liberation praxis when it is in service of the oppressed, particularly workers, racialized subjects, and women. Echoing Martín-Baró, "to achieve a [psychoanalysis] of liberation demands first that [psychoanalysis] be liberated" (p. 25). Martín-Baró identifies three essential elements, which we can consider as the building blocks of liberation psychoanalysis for the oppressed peoples of the world: (1) a new horizon, (2) a new epistemology, and (3) a new praxis. Martín-Baró focused on Latin America; my emphasis is on the oppressed in general, particularly in the Global South (i.e., the tricontinent of Latin America, Africa, and Asia). This is an ethico-political commitment to what is called Southern Theory (Connell, 2007), or Decoloniality, which can also be framed as *critical theory from the perspective of Exteriority*.

First, liberation psychoanalysis must break the ideological chains of psychosocial or material oppression through a sober analysis of "the intimate relationship between an unalienated personal existence and unalienated social existence" (p. 27). The liberation psychoanalyst, for example, must think about the relationship between a proletarian analysand's particular psychopathology *vis-à-vis* their distress as exploited workers. The purpose of liberation praxis is for the oppressed to overcome "their existential fatalism" (p. 27). In other words, liberation psychoanalysis envisions hope beyond alienation. Disalienation is theorized as a two-step process in psychoanalysis: first, separation; then, the traversal of fantasy.

Consequently, we must *separate* from bourgeois ideology in order to *traverse* the racial capitalist fantasy. As such, the new horizon is *socialism*–liberation as interdependency, fair labor, and structural equality. The new horizon is also *humanism*, given the historical and ongoing practices of dehumanization (through racism and sexism, for instance) within the apparatus of racial capitalism.

Second, liberation psychoanalysis presents a new epistemology: a human science of the unconscious, as practical knowledge. This human scientific and radical qualitative epistemology sheds light on the libidinal economy of the psyche and the political economy of the social. Together, these two economies—of surplus enjoyment and surplus value, respectively—are the material basis for *liberation praxis* qua *the reflection and action of our social being following the authority of historical reason.*

Martín-Baró writes, "The problem of a new praxis brings up the problem of power, and, therefore, the problem of the politicization of [psychoanalysis]" (1996, p. 29). Liberation psychoanalysis should never pretend to be neutral or unbiased:

> The fact that something is biased does not necessarily mean it is subjective; bias can be the consequence of interests, more or less conscious, but it can also be the result of an ethical choice. And while we are all affected by the class interests that bias our knowledge, not everybody makes conscious ethical choices consonant with those values.
>
> (p. 29)

The new praxis of liberation psychoanalysis entails "practical knowledge acquired through participatory research" and "should lead toward the people gaining power, a power that allows them to become the protagonists of their own history" (p. 30). Martín-Baró, like Michel Foucault, recognizes the dialectical relationship between knowledge and power at stake in any liberation praxis. The difference between the two thinkers, however, is that Foucault is Eurocentric in his theorizing through and through. Pavón-Cuéllar and González Equihua (2013) argue that Martín-Baró's liberation psychology, on the other hand, shares a commitment with Lacanian psychoanalysis to the subversion of so-called objective psychological knowledge, which tends to be ethnocentric and, thereby, oppressive. As such, the truth of subjective desire is foundational for what they term "subversive psychoanalysis."

Paulo Freire: Liberation Pedagogy

Similar to Martín-Baró's focus on praxis as a form of social and psychological liberation, Paulo Freire's work provides a pedagogical framework for understanding and dismantling oppression. Freire (1970) writes, "Oppression—overwhelming control—is necrophilic; it is nourished by love of death, not life. The banking concept of education, which serves the interests of oppression, is also necrophilic" (p. 77). Oppression can be a function of either instrumental reason—the use of reason for domination—or irrationalism. Modernization is sustained by oppression, and so is (anti)modernity. What Freire calls "the situation of oppression" is always accompanied by violence, potential or actual. For Freire, oppression—whether in society or the classroom—is dehumanizing and antidialogical.

Freire draws on several psychoanalytic concepts to make some of his key arguments. For example, he invokes the notion of *internalization*—a super-egoic function—to warn the oppressed against the problem of sub-oppression to which they have no immunity: "almost always, during the initial stage of the struggle, the oppressed, instead of striving for liberation, tend themselves to become oppressors, or 'sub-oppressors'" (p. 45). Later, Freire makes this internalization process explicit when he writes, "The oppressed, having internalized the image of the oppressor and adopted his [or her] guidelines, are fearful of freedom" (p. 47). Freire also indexes Frantz Fanon when discussing how the internalization of oppression leads to sub-oppression and manifests in the form of "horizontal violence" (p. 62).

For Freire, freedom is synonymous with humanization, which he regards to be "the people's vocation" (p. 43) and "the great humanistic and historical task of the oppressed: to liberate themselves and their oppressors as well" (p. 44). Freedom or humanization is a function of historical reason—the use of reason for liberation. This is a Hegelian and Marxist point about the logic of history being driven by the struggle toward freedom. For Freire, liberation is a humanizing struggle and a dialogical praxis, which is inherently revolutionary.

Liberation is a function of *conscientização*, often translated as critical consciousness. Still, I would argue that it is closer to *critical unconsciousness*, as practical knowledge or know-how (*savoir-faire*). Critical unconsciousness is essentially *critical meta-consciousness*, a *consciousness of consciousness*, because it is at the praxial level of social being, which involves reflection and action. What is consciousness of consciousness? I would argue it is the unconscious.

Critical pedagogy is the practice of liberation in the classroom—a microcosm of the social. Liberation praxis, for Freire, is a dialectical revolutionary process and "the very objective of organization" (p. 177). Liberation praxis is also a "dialogical cultural action which is prolonged in 'cultural revolution' once power is taken" (p. 160). In this context, he defines *conscientização* as a humanizing praxis, the purpose of which is for the oppressed to "leave behind the status of *objects* to assume the status of historical *Subjects*" (p. 160, emphasis in original). Becoming historical subjects is a dialectical revolutionary process, which is not possible within the dehumanizing situation of oppression—a violent and loveless situation. As such, liberation praxis constitutes, for Freire, "an act of love" (p. 45). Here, Freire seems to be echoing Walter Benjamin's (1921) thesis on *divine violence*:

> Consciously or unconsciously, the act of rebellion by the oppressed (an act which is always, or nearly always, as violent as the initial violence of the oppressors) can initiate love. Whereas the violence of the oppressors prevents the oppressed from being fully human, the response of the latter to this violence is grounded in the desire to pursue the right to be human.
>
> (Freire, 1970, p. 56)

The violence of oppressors is always mythic and unjust because it leads to nothing but dehumanization. However, the violence of the oppressed has the potential to be divine and just, particularly when its goal is "the humanization of all people" (p. 49). What came first, violence or oppression? Freire states, "There would be no oppressed had there been no prior situation of violence to establish their subjugation" (p. 55). I personally prefer the path of nonviolence, as stated before, but I also understand the practical necessity of revolutionary struggle in the face of oppression.

Love of life—which makes dialogue and dialectics possible—is at the core of liberation psychoanalysis. Love of learning (i.e., pedagogy) is "the practice of freedom" (p. 81). In 1906, Freud wrote to Jung that psychoanalysis is essentially a "cure ... effected by love" (as cited in McGuire, 1973, p. 13), which resonates with Freire's thesis on the centrality of love in liberation praxis:

> Love is at the same time the foundation of dialogue and dialogue itself. It is thus necessarily the task of responsible Subjects and cannot exist in a relation of domination. Domination reveals the pathology of love: sadism in the dominator and masochism in the dominated. Because love is an act of courage, not of fear, love is commitment to others. No matter where the oppressed are found, the act of love is commitment to their cause—the cause of liberation.
>
> (Freire, 1970, p. 89)

Liberation psychoanalysis is *a psychoanalysis of the oppressed*, a psychoanalysis "which must be forged *with*, not *for*, the oppressed (whether individuals or peoples) in the incessant struggle to regain their humanity" (p. 48, emphasis in original). Liberation psychoanalysis is a problem-posing practice that resolves the analyst–analysand contradiction. The analyst is not a master (*a subject supposed to know*); mastery is a falsity projected onto the analyst by the analysand as a function of the transference. The analyst, however, is the antithesis of a master, for they must assume the position of an object-cause of desire; this technique of operating as pure desirousness manifests as ethical listening and is the engine of analysis. To invoke a Zen Buddhist saying: "If you meet a psychoanalyst on the road, kill them."

To be a psychoanalyst is not to become enlightened, however; nor is it an ego identification with other psychoanalysts. Being a psychoanalyst is a paradoxical position that necessitates utter humility. It is a delicate role occupied by someone who has gone through years of (de)formation, or subjective destitution, to assume the ethical position of an analyst. Liberation psychoanalysis is dialogical, but most of the dialogue takes place in free association between the analysand and themself, a function of the psychic division between ego and unconscious—not mentioning the social division between the subject and the Other. The analyst's desire sustains analysis and facilitates the analysand's work. The analyst supports the analysand's own journey of subjective destitution as they navigate the symptomatic labyrinths of their unconscious desire, which are topologically distorted by the death drive. Following Freud and Lacan (or Lacan's return to Freud through structural linguistics, structural anthropology, phenomenology, and mathematics), liberation psychoanalysis is revolutionary love because it is the praxis of giving analysands what we do not have: *a pharmakon*. The desire of analysts fosters an analytic environment committed to a form of speech arising from curiosity about the unconscious: the unknown, the unknowable, the not-yet-known.

Does the analyst–analysand dialectic parallel the teacher–student contradiction? No. Because the analyst is not a teacher teaching the analysand about their unconscious. The analyst causes the analysand's desire to learn about their unconscious so that they may become aware that they are both the teacher/master (ego) and the student/slave (unconscious). Of course, the analyst–analysand relationship can potentially mirror the oppressor–oppressed contradiction in society, for the clinic is not an apolitical space (Altman, 2010; Dunker, 2011; Laubender, 2024).

Analysts can certainly act like oppressors when they slip in a position of mastery, which is a case of superposition. However, the central problem in liberation psychoanalysis is that of sub-oppression. Why do we (analysands) oppress ourselves and others, if we think we are the oppressed? And what are we to do about this internalization of oppression? Why do we internalize oppression in the first place, and how can we overcome sub-oppression? These are some of the questions that we must ask ourselves in self-analysis and psychoanalysis. Enrique Dussel's philosophy offers a foundational critique that helps us answer these questions, by tracing the historical and ontological roots of this oppression to the very beginning of modern thought.

Enrique Dussel: Liberation Philosophy

Like Martín-Baró, Dussel's (1985) understanding of oppression is informed primarily by dependency theory. Still, as a philosopher, he explains the roots of the politico-economic oppression of non-European cultures in the periphery in terms of an ontology of coloniality. For Dussel, Descartes's first principle (*cogito ergo sum*) is the foundation of modern philosophy and its colonial ontology. For him, the latter "arose from a previous experience of domination over other persons, of cultural oppression over other worlds" (p. 3). Dussel continues, "Before the *ego cogito* there is an *ego conquiro*; 'I conquer' is the practical foundation of 'I think.' The center has imposed itself on the periphery for more than five centuries" (p. 3, emphasis in original).

Dussel's philosophical critique of modernity is essential because, as we will see, it provides a crucial historical context for understanding the colonial underpinnings of psychoanalytic theory itself. Psychoanalysis inherits the Cartesian formulation: thinking → being. Liberation psychoanalysis acknowledges Dussel's intervention, which sheds light on a new formulation: conquering → thinking → being. In a sense, the unconscious of modern thinking/being is colonial: "I conquer." The negation of coloniality correlates with the negation of non-European ways of thinking and being. Of course, we must reject coloniality, but Dussel's point is that we cannot do so as long as coloniality is the negated logic of modernity. And because coloniality is negated (repressed, foreclosed, disavowed), the non-European Other is perceived from the center of Totality as "nonbeing, nothing, barbarity, non-sense" (p. 4).

Therefore, Dussel conceptualizes liberation through the concept of transmodernity, which affirms modernity and its alterity, while rejecting coloniality and (anti) modernity. Transmodernity is the sublation of Totality and Exteriority through historical reason. Transmodernity transcends the logic of alienation (either/or) and separation (neither/nor) by traversing colonial and (anti)modern fantasies. While the colonial fantasy is a function of instrumental reason, which conflates modernity with modernization, the (anti)modern fantasy is an effect of irrationalism.

For example, the logic of alienation is prominent in cultural discourses about East vs. West. The logic of separation is the logic of non-alignment: neither East nor West. The East–West dichotomy is replaced with geopolitical terms (i.e., Global South and Global North, or periphery and center) to emphasize the imperialism of global capital beyond cultural difference (Amin, 2010). Cultural difference has nothing to do with essentialism, but, rather, with "the structure of the signifier as difference" (Safouan, 2004, p. 18), for cultures are linguistically transmitted for the most part.

To accomplish the sublation of transmodernity, Dussel stretches dialectical materialism; I characterize his decolonial methodology as *analectical materialism*, which combines his theory of "authentic materialism" with what he terms "the analectical moment." For Dussel, an authentic materialist "interprets nature as matter for work. Things are relevant inasmuch as *with them* (that *with which* the artifact is manufactured is its materiality) are fabricated things needed by the other as such, beyond the present system of necessity" (Dussel, 1985, p. 103, emphasis in original).

Dussel situates dialectics within Totality. He affirms dialectics but considers analectics a decolonial sublation from the transmodern perspective of Exteriority (cf. Ciccariello-Maher, 2017). Dussel writes:

> The dialectical process as passage to a new totality cannot support itself only in the negative thrust of negation. It must also promote the affirmation of the alterity of the new system that arises from the manifestation of the exteriority of the other ... It is because of this that the analectical moment of dialectical movement is the origin and resolution of that same dialectics and its negativity.
>
> (1985, p. 137)

Any concrete historical praxis (e.g., liberation psychoanalysis) that ethically affirms the Exteriority of the non-European Other–whom I theorize as *the Other of the Other* (A^2)–is the *raison d'être* of the analectical moment. Dussel continues:

> The analectical refers to the real human fact by which every person, every group or people, is always situated "beyond" (*ano-*) the horizon of totality. Negative dialectic is no longer enough. The analectical moment is the support of new unfoldings. The analectical moment opens us to the metaphysical sphere (which is not the ontic one of the factual sciences or the ontological one of negative dialectic), referring us to the other. Its proper category is exteriority. The point of departure for its methodical discourse (a method that is more than scientific or dialectic) is the exteriority of the other. Its [principle] is not that of identity but of separation, distinction.
>
> (pp. 158–159, emphasis in original)

As such, liberation psychoanalysis, following Lacan and Dussel, may be framed as an analectical materialist praxis of liberation. Achille Mbembe (2001), for instance, contrapuntally links Africa's alter-modernity to Euromodernity using the following analectical argument:

> the peculiar 'historicity' of African societies, their own raisons d'être and their relation to solely themselves, are rooted in *a multiplicity of times, trajectories, and rationalities that, although particular and sometimes local, cannot be conceptualized outside a world that is, so to speak, globalized.*
>
> (p. 9, emphasis added)

This framing extends and clarifies the purpose of the contrapuntal methodology, particularly when applied to the question of radical or revolutionary politics.

Mary Watkins and Helene Shulman: Psychologies of Liberation

Mary Watkins and Helene Shulman (2008) provide a thorough overview of the psychologies of liberation—a pluriversal move that builds upon and complexifies Martín-Baró's singular vision of liberation psychology. For them, oppression is primarily a function of capital, but they also frame it as a "psychic wound" caused by colonial trauma (cf. Lazali, 2021).

Furthermore, they index the cultural work of Augusto Boal (1979), whose *Theater of the Oppressed* is conceived as "a rehearsal for the revolution" (p. 98) meant to liberate oppressed spectators. For Boal:

> The *poetics of the oppressed* [or the conquest of the means of theatrical production] is essentially the poetics of liberation: the spectator no longer delegates power to the characters either to think or to act in his [or her] place. The spectator frees himself [or herself]; he [or she] thinks and acts for himself [or herself]! Theatre is action!
>
> (p. 135, emphasis in original)

Watkins and Shulman problematize the term 'liberation' since it was invoked in the European colonial context of the civilizing mission. For them, liberation is

> a kind of jailbreak in which we find the fullness of ourselves and our communities ... In this scenario, what is imprisoned in silence, yearning, and marginalization, will have a chance to escape into image, language, symbol, performance, and action.
>
> (2008, p. 47)

The purpose of liberation, they argue, is the creation of "new commons" or "networks of renewed communities in dialogue and solidarity" (p. 48). I strongly agree with this argument, and I situate it in relation to what I term *divine jouissance* as *the collective enjoyment of the commons* (e.g., natural resources, healthcare, education, public transportation, worker cooperatives, open-source technologies, open-access knowledge, etc.); *divine jouissance* is the libidinal dimension of anarcho-communism (Goldman, 2017; Guérin, 2017; Kropotkin, 1995), which I say more about later on in the chapter.

Interestingly, in *The Question of Lay Analysis*, Freud's (1926) quasi-anarchist position is aligned with Benjamin's (1921) critique of violence. For example, Freud examines the arbitrariness of the Law or its status as mythic and unjust (1926, p. 79). In other words, Lawmaking and Law-preserving are the mythic dimension of *writing as a form of violence* (cf. Beshara, 2021a). Subsequently, given the status of Law, Freud believes that civil disobedience is warranted as a necessary cause of truth and justice: *rewriting as a form of nonviolence*, a Law-destroying divine violence in the words of Benjamin.

Since *the commons*—or *social relations of cooperation and reciprocity*—is a central concept in this project, I wish to take a moment and reference Silvia Federici's (2019) description of this radical politics. She essentially distinguishes the commons from public goods, which are controlled by the State; however, I consider both the commons and public goods to be important from the perspective of anarcho-communism.

The commons stand in opposition to the capitalist model of privatization and "enclosure." One way of understanding capitalism is as *the continuous expropriation of the commons* (e.g., land and natural resources, the body and reproductive work, as well as social wealth and knowledge), which are necessary for the reproduction of life (e.g., eating, sleeping, raising children, education, healthcare, etc.). Althusser (1970/2014) referred to reproduction under capitalism as the Ideological State Apparatuses. Therefore, capitalism's (C) *raison d'être* is transforming the reproduction of life (L) into the reproduction of labor power (P) through ideological interpellation: $C \Rightarrow (L \rightarrow P)$; however, socialism ($S$) is the reproduction of life (L) for its own sake: $S \Rightarrow L$. For Federici (2019):

> [C]ommons should be autonomous spaces and should aim to overcome the divisions existing among us and build the skills necessary for self-government … Commons are defined by the existence of a shared property, in the form of a shared natural or social wealth—lands, waters, forests, systems of knowledge, capacities for care—to be used by all commoners, without any distinction, but which are not for sale [e.g., Creative Commons] … Commons are not things but social relations [i.e., commoning].
>
> (pp. 93–94)

Consequently, liberation psychoanalysis is a praxis of commoning whose aim is the reproduction of life for its own sake. Watkins and Shulman invoke psychoanalysis as a tool for liberation along these lines when they write: "Psychologies of liberation sometimes draw on concepts developed by psychologies of the unconscious (depth psychologies), extending them to make links with historical and environmental conditions" (2008, p. 49). They cite Elizabeth Danto's (2005) *Freud's*

Free Clinics to make the case for the radical roots of psychoanalysis as a praxis oriented toward social justice. Furthermore, they also argue that psychoanalysis lost its radical potential once it "became whitened and myopic, often indifferent to racial and cultural issues, and unreflective of its own cultural location within a multicultural society" (2008, p. 57). Liberation psychoanalysis is committed to what Watkins and Shulman call its "night vision" or "its ability to critique society and to examine its intrapsychic implications from the position of an outsider and critic [cf. Dussel's Exteriority]" (p. 57).

For them,

> The most radical spirit of psychoanalysis requires that one follow symptoms across the boundaries of paradigms and familiar interpretations, if called; that one take note of what one begins to see that would ordinarily cause one to retreat to a narrower lens.
>
> (p. 62)

This is a Marxist argument about the primacy of distress under capitalism at the level of social being; this distress then materializes as particular symptoms for each singular subject. A subject's particular constellation of symptoms crystallizes in the form of a specific psychic structure (neurosis, psychosis, or perversion) depending on the subject's method of unconscious negation (repression, foreclosure, or disavowal). The liberation psychoanalyst interprets and reconstructs the analysand's speech with this racial capitalist context of distress in mind, without psychologizing.

Watkins and Shulman index numerous psychoanalytic concepts, which they consider essential tools in any liberation praxis. These concepts include anamnesis as "a process of reflecting on and emotionally working through one's relationship to past events with another" (p. 88), the traumatic Real, regression as "a stepping back from busy or manic doing toward a slower more reflective stance" (p. 135), dissociation or "the unconscious elimination of painful knowledge from conscious awareness" (p. 53), and complex or divided subjectivity.

The following, however, is perhaps their most illuminating and "subversive insight": "Renormalization [or "the constant refusal to explore what unexpectedly occurs in the environment through rupture, chance, accident, or contact with an unknown 'other'"] leads unconsciously to social narcissism, a complete identification with those perceived to be most like oneself, and an alienation and dissociation from those who appear different" (p. 138). Liberation psychoanalysis is not only dialectical, but also analectical; as such, it is the antithesis of "polarized identities," for even oppressors must be humanized!

Daniel José Gaztambide: Psychoanalysis of Liberation

Daniel José Gaztambide (2019) writes explicitly about Freud's "psychoanalysis of liberation" or his "psychoanalytic theory of the dynamics of oppressor and oppressed" (p. 175). Freud's theory sheds light on Freire's concept of internalized oppression. Gaztambide argues, following Freud, that the oppressed ideologically identify with their oppressors because this "neutralizes the envy and hostility the oppressed might otherwise feel and enact through rebellion against the powerful" (pp. 175–176). In other words, the guilt of the oppressed is a super-egoic function. Furthermore, "this illusory process of identification with the oppressor is maintained by splitting and projective identification of hatred toward another group of people which serves as an excluded third [i.e., the Other of the Other]" (p. 176).

The oppressed in Freud's (and Gaztambide's) analysis are working-class white people, while the oppressors are the white ruling class. In other words, the ideological function of oppression, at least in the context of Euromodernity, is *to produce whiteness as an ideological form of coloniality*. There is nothing pathological about being white; what is being critiqued here is the identification with the ideology of whiteness—a reification of the greatest degree, that is meant to cover over the materiality of class struggle. Whiteness is an ideological fantasy within the apparatus of racial capitalism that sutures the subject's desire for radical humanism, which is driven by historical reason. My invocation of historical reason and instrumental reason parallels Freud's distinction between the life drive and the death drive, but on a social level.

Liberation psychoanalysis is an analectical moment from the perspective of the "excluded third," a position within Exteriority that Freud identified with, as a "'Black' Jew" (p. 176)—or a non-European, to invoke Said's (2003) term. Jewishness and Blackness represent "an interesting dialectic" (p. 30) for Gaztambide, which is not to say that they are equal but isomorphic. In his *People's History of Psychoanalysis*, Gaztambide argues that "the question of race—especially the relationship between anti-Semitism and anti-Blackness" is "fundamental to our understanding of psychoanalysis" (p. 32). After all, "discourses of anti-Blackness" were "fundamental in forging not only psychoanalysis, but the centrality of social justice to the psychoanalytic project" (p. 50).

Gaztambide states, "Freud had a vision of social justice in which we renounce our aggressive instincts and desires to make space for the other, a space created out of a libidinal and affectionate tie" (p. 177). This renunciation of the death drive is the psychoanalytic path of sublimation, that is, "putting the object in the place of the Thing" (Safouan, 2002, p. 100), which can take many liberatory forms, such as poetics (Boal) or pedagogy (Freire), but in this book I am mainly concerned with the following liberatory forms of sublimation: ethics, politics, and aesthetics. Nevertheless, divine violence (e.g., the general strike) against any oppressive ideology is justified, if the goal is the humanization of all. To rephrase Fanon, decolonization, *qua* traversal of fantasy, is always a violent phenomenon. Decolonization is not a metaphor, it is ideology-destroying. I will argue later in the book that *decolonization is a metonym.*

Why Psychoanalysis?

Why not? The real question is: Why Freudo–Lacanian psychoanalysis, in particular? Here, I agree with Filip Kovačević (2007) that "a critical perspective grounded in a Lacanian interpretation of Marx and Freud is the best model for theoretical and practical engagement in changing existing social and political realities" (p. ix) and with Jeffrey Abramson (1984) that "Freud can be seen as contributing to a more communitarian vision of liberation and well-being" (p. 2). As such, I write about psychoanalysis as a heretic, or as a heterodox Freudo–Lacanian leftist (cf. Robinson, 1969; Stavrakakis, 2007), who acknowledges that

> central to psychoanalysis is a libertarian ethos, by which the subject seeks to gain a greater autonomy (from authoritarian leaders and the groups constituted around them), and where the subject is encouraged, through the rules of 'free association', to speak the truth of the unconscious.
>
> (Newman, 2010, p. 61)

In other words, I am against both orthodox Freudo–Lacanians and Leftists who are dismissive of Freudo–Lacanian psychoanalysis. To put it differently, I am concerned with the problem of institutional failure in relation to the authoritarianism of charismatic leaders—such as Freud and Lacan, who were both founders and legislators—which, for Jacqueline Rose, following Hannah Arendt, stems from confusing *people power* with *legislative authority* (as cited in Safouan, 2000, p. 33). In simple terms, institutions, like subjects, are divided between the unconscious power of the people and the egoic authority of leaders; therefore, institutions fail when they act ideologically, as if they are undivided, which paradoxically creates more division under the guise of fantasy. On the other hand, institutions are more likely to not fail when, in the dialectic between power and authority, they are able guarantee *lack as a third space*, not reducible to any one or any thing. This is the third space of desire as a source of life-driven enjoyment. In either case, the questions of transference and identification are always at work in any group structure or process.

François Tosquelles (2024), the Catalan Marxist, who founded institutional psychotherapy, inspired the anti-psychiatry movement, and influenced Frantz Fanon, Jean Oury, and Félix Guattari; he had the following to say about Lacan: his "doctoral thesis sets out a concrete, social-historical conception of personality that seems to reflect the essential ideas of dialectical materialism. We have recently taken up his concept of the 'complex' and his phenomenology of the doctor/patient relationship" (p. 79) and "Lacan has given the most complete description and analysis of the phenomena of transference and the successive identifications of which the doctor is the 'provocative-support' during the process of a psychoanalysis" (p. 81). I write this for the schizoanalytic naysayers, who wish to dismiss Lacan or reduce him to the status of an oppressive master, for anti-Oedipus means not only anti-Lacan (pro-Foucault) or anti-Freud (pro-Nietzsche), but also anti-neurosis (pro-psychosis): "A schizophrenic out for a walk is a better model than a neurotic lying on the analyst's couch" (Deleuze & Guattari, 1983, p. 2).

Deleuze and Guattari (1983) characterize the neurotic—which is the most common psychical structure in a given society—as "a pitiful creature who eternally consumes daddy-and-mommy and nothing else whatsoever" (p. 20). On the other hand, one of the goals of psychoanalysis, for Freud, as early as *Studies in Hysteria*, is turning "hysterical misery into common unhappiness" (Freud & Breuer, 1895/2004, p. 378), which I read as a statement about how liberation praxis will always include pain, but does not have to include suffering, because to be human is to have a body, that is, to experience pain (and pleasure) and to ultimately die; however, psychological suffering is optional because of the potential for healing—analytically or otherwise—without projecting our suffering onto the world.

The following is a statement regarding Freud's conception of liberation psychoanalysis, which is distinct from two mistaken projects of liberation within psychoanalysis: Reichian therapy and ego psychology. According to Abramson (1984), Freud warns of

> two mistaken projects of liberation. The first identifies ourselves too completely with instinctual expression, thereby confusing freedom with determinism and leaving unexplained the very fact of repression, that we are not harmonious with our desires, that we do strive to idealize our own nature. The second mistaken path identifies ourselves too purely with reason, thereby seeking to deny the constraints of nature that are not open to us to deny. *A truer account of liberation thus waits on a reconciliation of reason and desire*, a reconciliation which we have seen Freud gesture toward in his concept of sublimation and in his practice of therapy but which he does not complete.
>
> (p. 137, emphasis added)

This reconciliation of reason and desire is what my project is about. Would psychoanalysis be necessary or relevant in a truthful and just society? The short answer is no. A truthful and just society is acephalous: free from exploitation, racism, sexism, and other forms of oppression, according to the ancient Egyptian Maatian principle (Karenga, 2003)—I say more about the relationship between science (truth) and politics (justice) in the concluding chapter of the book, but also see Chapter 4 of *Freud and Said* (Beshara, 2021a). To ask the first question differently: Would there be repression without oppression (Oliver, 2004)? This second question historicizes the unconscious, the product of a certain time and place. The third question poses itself: What can we do now, at least as far as psychoanalysis is concerned, to prefigure a truthful and just society? Is it possible to prefigure this society-to-come in our clinics, institutions, and beyond?

This is the socialist and humanist challenge to psychoanalysis as it exists today since, in most cases, the talking cure is not revolutionary but, on the contrary, is about adapting to a liberal-conservative (i.e., untruthful and unjust) order. Therefore, a radical anti-oppressive logic must inform our relations as practitioners, scholars, and activists. This logic can only be thought from the perspective of analysts–analysands, particularly oppressed ones. In other words, we must hystericize the field to extinction because the unconscious would most likely be irrelevant in a society built on a kincentric ecology, or kinship among humans as well as between humans and the non-human world (Cajete, 2000; Estes, 2019; Kimmerer, 2013). Enrique Salmón (2000), for example, equates kincentric ecology with the Rarámuri concept of *iwígara*, which signifies "the total interconnectedness of all life … physical and spiritual" (p. 1328).

To become a psychoanalyst, the modern subject must undergo analysis for a period of time in an effort for them to listen to their own unconscious in a new way and to come to terms with their particular psychic structure and their singular form of symptomatic enjoyment, that is, their unique navigation of the threshold between pleasure and pain. The point of this rite of passage is not to necessarily get rid of one's symptoms, as is the assumption in psychiatry; rather, the aim of working through our symptoms toward the end of analysis is *subjective destitution* or *traversing the fantasy*, which is the opposite of both acting out and the *passage à l'acte*.

To be a modern subject is to have colonial fantasies, which when acted out via group identification lead to catastrophic results in the form of colonial practices, which can range from genocide and enslavement to (post)modern varieties of racism. Traversing the fantasy signifies analyzing the unconscious desires covered over by ideological fantasies (colonial or otherwise) in order to have an ethical fidelity to the open-ended act of desiring itself. Similarly, to be a transmodern subject is to have decolonial fantasies, which, when acted out, may lead to (anti)modern practices. As such, *traversing (de)colonial fantasies through the discourse of (trans)modernity is the goal of liberation psychoanalysis*, which is not only the end of analysis, but also the end of psychoanalysis, as we know it.

Psychoanalysis was invented in Vienna in the late 19th century in the context of New Imperialism, particularly the Scramble of Africa. Because it was invented by an oppressed subject, a Jew in an anti-Semitic environment, it contains within itself the radical seeds of its liberation; this is the Otherness of psychoanalysis, which makes immanent critique possible. The less liberatory aspects of psychoanalysis are a function of Freud's assimilation, or his identification with Europeanness; bearing in mind that Freud's Europe was immersed in a white supremacist ideology *vis-à-vis* the non-European world. The ego of psychoanalysis, then, is tethered to a master's discourse that posits civilization against savagery, which Freud effortlessly indexed in some of his works, notably *Totem and Taboo* and *The Uneasiness in Culture*—my preferred translation for *Das Unbehagen in der Kultur*. This is the normative dimension of psychoanalysis, wherein the modern subject of the unconscious is presumed to be civilized (i.e., European, male, and bourgeois). When I write about rethinking the field from the perspective of oppressed analysts–analysands, it is meant as a direct challenge to 'civilized' analysts *qua* masters and 'civilized' institutions *qua* universities. Lacan (1991/2007) shows that the university is always subservient to the master.

According to Freud (1930/1961):

> what we call our civilization is largely responsible for our misery, and that we should be much happier if we gave it up and returned to primitive conditions. I call this contention astonishing because, in whatever way we may define the

> concept of civilization, it is a certain fact that all the things with which we seek to protect ourselves against the threats that emanate from the sources of suffering are part of that very civilization.
>
> (p. 38)

In 1930, James Strachey, the editor of *The Standard Edition of the Complete Psychological Works of Sigmund Freud*, translated the German title of Freud's *Das Unbehagen in der Kultur* to the English *Civilization and Its Discontents*. The literal translation of the German title is *The Uneasiness in the Culture [of Euromodernity]*; so, one must raise an uneasy question about the displacement from culture to civilization, which entails a theoretical leap from the particular to the universal. The indexing of civilization as a signifier on the part of Strachey suggests something about what he thinks is the place of psychoanalysis within the civilizing mission of Euromodernity—an ethnocentric culture whose rhetoric is sustained by a colonial logic. Freud was correct to point out that culture is both a source of suffering and a defense against this suffering. However, he was absolutely wrong to assume that non-Europeans lack culture and, therefore, are uncivilized.

Freud sees our misery as human subjects to be mainly a function of the Symbolic, or the superegoic demands of culture—a welcome view that constitutes a psychosocial framework for distress and as such is more critical than current notions of psychic disease that reduce it to the level of the individual, typically in the form of their behavior, cognition, or neurochemistry. However, juxtaposed to this radical Freudian reading of Euromodern capitalist culture—as a source of disease or distress—is a reactionary fantasy of plenitude, which is the basis for any nationalist ideology, wherein the premodern primitive subject is framed paradoxically as both superior and inferior to the modern civilized subject (i.e., the miserable neurotic): superior in terms of her happiness because she is supposedly *natural* as a function of her being uncivilized or uncultured; inferior in terms of her psychosexual development, which posits a universal temporality or linear trajectory, from the perspective of Euromodernity.

In the culture of Euromodernity, Europe figures as both the center of the world and the zero point of time. The non-European world, subsequently, is framed as barbaric because it is Exterior to the culture of Euromodernity, that is, 'civilization.' Similarly, non-linear temporality is considered primitive because of its circadian rhythm. The barbaric and primitive dimensions of non-European space and time constitute the figure of the 'savage' in Euromodern ideological fantasies. It is worth noting here, as Said (2003) points out, that Freud, of course, was both a Euromodern scientist and a non-European Jew. So, what then is the relationship between culture and civilization?

For Freud (1930/1961),

> the word "civilization" describes the whole sum of the achievements and the regulations which distinguish our lives from those of our animal ancestors and which serve two purposes—namely to protect men against nature and to adjust their mutual relations.
>
> (p. 42)

Following Freud's definition of culture, the logic of Euromodernity's civilizing mission is clearly at work when Freud is writing about "the victory of Christendom over the heathen religions" (p. 38). Freud's assimilation, in the manifest form of his Euromodern ego, exhibits what Sándor Ferenczi (1949) termed *the identification with the aggressor*. The radical, or antifascist, potential of psychoanalysis stems from the split-off part of Freud's subjectivity, his Jewish unconscious—a latent Otherness. As such, while psychoanalysis is certainly a radical modern discourse, a hermeneutics of suspicion, it also wrestles with its own shadow, a colonial logic.

The point of my critique is to shed light on this colonial logic in order to replace it with an Other logic, a decolonial logic grounded in the Exteriority and futurity of the (non)European. What is Exterior is not outside, but rather extimate, which implies an ana-dialectical relationship between the Global North and the Global South. This relationship is not only structured by the exploitative logic of capitalism, but also sutured via racist forms of surplus-enjoyment. In other words, economic development is linked with psychosexual development. The developmental discourse is not a scientific description of reality; it is a political and libidinal tool of managing human difference.

To put it differently, in the apparatus of racial capitalism, subjects are positioned as points on a hierarchical Cartesian coordinate system along two axes: sexual difference and colonial difference. The former is the hetero-patriarchal regime, which distinguishes Man from Woman. The latter is the colonial regime, which differentiates human (Man and Woman) from non-human (~~Woman~~ and ~~Man~~). The question of sexual difference is central for psychoanalysis, but the field is mute on this Other question—a silence constituting the unconscious of psychoanalysis *qua* the negation of Exteriority. Following Freud, it is also the negation of nature (as opposed to culture) *vis-à-vis* the figure of the happy 'savage,' who is in contradistinction to the miserable but 'civilized' neurotic. What explains this colonial silence or racist negation? Cohn (2010) writes about the "anarchist unconscious" *qua* Eros, and perhaps one explanation has to do with the authoritarian unconscious *qua* Thanatos?

The decolonial argument is not to reject modernity wholesale, but, rather, to delink the colonial unconscious, as a structuring logic, from psychoanalysis as a modern discourse. The product of this delinking is what Dussel (1985) terms transmodernity, which synthesizes modernity along with its negated alterity. What renders this synthesis decolonial is the fact that it is enacted from the perspective of Exteriority, which is the perspective of the damned (Fanon) or the oppressed (Freire). In other words, the so-called savagery of the savage is nothing but the projected savagery of the 'civilized,' which is the savagery of colonialism that makes capitalism, as a Euromodern world-system, possible. I speak of the savagery of civilization because we would not be facing climate change or the possibility of a nuclear apocalypse today, if it were not for 'civilization.' The alternative to this narrow notion of 'civilization' *qua* Euromodern culture is Wahba's (2022) radical humanist axiom: *one civilization, many cultures*.

The civilizing logic at the heart of psychoanalysis can only be truly challenged from the perspective of 'savage' analysts–analysands, be they primitives or barbarians. Following Freire, we can call it *Psychoanalysis of the Oppressed* or *Liberation Psychoanalysis*. Simply put, we continue to see ethical breaches committed by abusive analysts today as a result of a colonial logic at the heart of the theory and the practice of psychoanalysis. This colonial logic prevents analysts from ethically listening to analysands and leads institutions to silence the victims when they should be facilitating an ethics of free association. The two key principles of psychoanalysis, which I regard as comprising its radical potential, are: *ethical listening* and *free association*.

Ethical listening is listening to the speaker's unconscious without judgment or over-interpretation but with practical know-how, which develops with practice. This kind of listening can eventually transform the speaker (analysand), who does most of the work of analysis, hence why they are often the leaders when it comes to liberation praxis. Free association has at least two equally important meanings: a political one as the basis of anarchist relations and a psychoanalytic commitment to speaking freely. Both meanings revolve around an ethics of unconscious desire as a life-driven source of *jouissance*. To live is to desire, and to desire is to be alive. I characterize death-driven—or violent and oppressive—forms of enjoyment as *mythic jouissance*.

At this point, I want to clarify that analysts are not oppressors. However, the clinic may replicate some oppressive dynamics within a given society, since clinics do not exist in a political vacuum (Powell, 2018). The clinic, after all, is a psychosocial space; in other words, there is a dialectical relationship between what is psychically repressed and who is socially oppressed—what Bollas (2015), Lau (2021), and others call "the return of the oppressed." Having said that, analysts can be comrades, and many of them are. The problem with oppression, however, is that it is a function of material and ideological structures that have accumulated and sedimented over time, which is why they are hard to change. This is why I define *coloniality as the psychic remainder of colonialism*—an oppressive afterlife. My argument here is to reflect on psychoanalysis *vis-à-vis* these oppressive structures, not to replicate them in the clinic or analytic institutions. However, a more radical wager would be to change these oppressive structures through liberation psychoanalysis by pre-figuring non-oppressive relations between analysts–analysands, within analytic institutions, and beyond.

The principal thesis of liberation psychoanalysis is that sexual difference is structured by colonial difference. Colonial difference is a function of the asymmetrical power/knowledge relationship between Totality and Exteriority. Transmodernity signifies the end of colonial difference, when the decolonial unconscious has displaced the colonial unconscious of modernity. Transmodernity affirms the modernity of psychoanalysis but rejects its colonial unconscious. Transmodernity also negates the (anti)modern unconscious, which is occasionally conflated with decoloniality. Liberation psychoanalysis is an analectical materialist praxis driven by historical reason, and it entails affirming the two Others: the Other of Totality and the Other of Exteriority–the latter is what I refer to as *the Other of the Other* (A^2). Pavón Cuéllar (2010) has written about the Exteriority of the unconscious in contrast to the interiority of consciousness; however, this fact is further complicated by the historical materialist reality of colonial difference, which resulted in the double-unconsciousness of Exteriority itself.

In summary, *decolonial psychoanalysis* is the theoretical project of critiquing and reimagining psychoanalysis to account for colonialism, *contrapuntal psychoanalysis* is the methodological tool for carrying out this project by reading texts and histories in a way that reveals colonial power dynamics, and *liberation psychoanalysis* is the emancipatory goal and practical application of these concepts in the service of socio-political change.

Anarchist Power: Pre-Figuring an Impossible Republic

In *Freud and Said* (Beshara, 2021a), I alluded to the legitimacy of "anarchist power," which is people power or the power of free association (cf. Newman, 2017). Free association is the central technique in psychoanalysis, which Freud developed in lieu of hypnosis. In liberation psychoanalysis, free association acquires a more explicit political meaning, one that is grounded in the libertarian socialist tradition. Noam Chomsky (2005) defines anarchist power as "a community of free association without coercion by the state or other authoritarian institutions, in which free men [and women] can create and inquire, and achieve the highest development of their power" (p. 112). For Chomsky, "free association and democratic control" are the foundations of "a rational social order" (p. 114).

Saul Newman (2004) spells out the theoretical correspondence between anarchism and Lacanian psychoanalysis when he writes, "both the anarchists and Lacan would see power and authority in terms of a specific *structural logic* of self-perpetuation, pointing to the dangers of revolutionary endeavors that do not deal directly with this question" (p. 305, emphasis in original). Therefore, my indexing of the paradoxical phrase "anarchist power" is a provocation against the self-perpetuation of new masters.

Free association is the democratic control of workers over the means of production. It is the anarcho-syndicalist alternative to capitalist exploitation and socialist state bureaucracy (Chomsky, 2005, p. 124). This model of anarchist power is not necessarily anti-statist, for it supports confederal and internationalist forms of organization (cf. De Geus, 2014; DeLeon, 1994; Hartung, 1983; Ward, 1966); rather, it is anti-authoritarian. Anarchy or *an-arché* means lacking a central ruler, leader, or authority. The 'ruler' in an anarchist society is not a person or a class but *the collective will of the people*, expressed through voluntary cooperation and self-management. We can also posit the leadership of the oppressed as a *collective leadership*. Authority is a relevant question, too (cf. Chapter 2 in *Freud and Said*), and we can think, for instance, about *the authority of historical reason* as driving liberation praxis. Nevertheless, power always requires legitimation. Anarchist power is material in a dual sense: *the analysand's unconscious power to associate freely* (i.e., practical knowledge) and *the workers' democratic power through free associations* (i.e., practical power).

The concrete utopia prefigured by liberation psychoanalysis is what I term an *impossible republic* (cf. Clark, 2022; Hallaq, 2012; Lundström, 2023). I would even explicitly call it an *anarcho-communist republic* to index a key contradiction within socialism. Anarchism and communism both aim for liberation through socialist economics, but they focus on different aspects: anarchism on political liberation and communism on economic liberation. Their inherent antagonism can serve as a check, preventing a return to individualism or authoritarianism, respectively. So, what of ethical or sexual liberation? And why this attachment to the republican form of governance? Louis Adeane (1945) would argue that the last question, in particular, signifies an attachment to "the government within."

Both Frederick Engels and Errico Malatesta argue, from different perspectives, for the reconstruction of the family as opposed to its abolition (cf. Tutt, 2022), which is the trend today (e.g., Lewis, 2022). The problem for Engels (2004) is not the family *per se*, but how the logic of private property within the capitalist apparatus perverts family dynamics and renders them oppressive to women, in particular:

> Thus, full freedom in marriage can become generally operative only when *the abolition of capitalist production, and of the property relations created by it*, has removed all those secondary economic considerations which still exert so powerful an influence on the choice of a partner. Then, no other motive remains than mutual affection.
>
> (p. 86, emphasis added)

In other words, Engels is arguing for the abolition of private property since he views it as the main cause behind the patriarchal or sexist oppression of women (p. 21). Freud (2021), however, was skeptical about the communist hypothesis and regarded the abolition of private property to be an illusion that will not resolve the problem of the death drive. My theoretical position integrates Engels's critique of capitalism with Freud's skepticism. I argue that sexual difference is not merely a difference in sexual enjoyment within modernity, as psychoanalysis would have us believe, but, rather, that it is marked by a colonial logic, which takes many violent and oppressive forms, such as exploitation, racism, and/or sexism. Is the abolition of capitalism, racism, and sexism equivalent then to the end of the death drive? No, the death drive will remain as a self-destructive structural possibility within transmodernity that must be creatively fused and redirected into life-driven forms of enjoyment at psychic, social, cultural, and political levels, which are the RSI dimensions of ethics, politics, and aesthetics.

The transmodern world-system, like any Symbolic order, is a tube torus comprising a Real hole at its center, the traumatic site of both Eros (divine *jouissance*) and Thanatos (mythic *jouissance*). As Kovačević (2007) argues:

> Eros binds the aggression of Thanatos, and, in a dialectical fashion, raises the tangled bundle to a higher level, a level where unjust social antagonisms are

> transcended, where a work-democracy [cf. Bennett, 2010], a non-repressive civilization, or a Dionysian play become guiding principles.
>
> (p. 99)

Kovačević qualifies death-driven mythic *jouissance* as the "rock of jouissance" and here is his antidote:

> The only way to disturb and dissolve this "rock of *jouissance*" is by liberating (sexual) desire, which brings into being the lack of satisfaction with the status quo. As I see it, this is best accomplished by the discourse of the hysteric, and that is why I have designated the hysteric as the most appropriate agent of sociopolitical change. The hysteric, motivated by presence of the precious object *a*, demands of the Other to produce new bodies of signifiers to satisfy his or her desire and, in doing so, makes possible the re-articulation of the relations between the symbolic and the real in the history of humanity.
>
> (p. 219, emphasis in original)

Echoing Engels but from the perspective of anarchism, Malatesta (2015) maintains: "Reconstruction of the family, as will emerge from *the practice of love*, freed from every legal tie, from every economic and physical oppression, from every religious prejudice" (p. 20, emphasis added). Reconstructing the family, for Malatesta, involves the practice of love, the aim of which is the realization of diverse family structures that emphasize individual autonomy, community involvement through mutual support and cooperation, and social and economic justice. To materialize this idea of the family as a secular and non-dogmatic institution free from coercion and characterized by voluntary relationships and economic independence, entails an analectical materialist praxis grounded in an ethic of radical humanism.

The family is an important nodal point in our analysis because it is intricately linked with the State, according to Engels (2004). The patriarchal family is a means for the bourgeoisie to control inheritance and wealth, and the State is the primary tool for protecting private property and maintaining the social order through its endorsement of the patriarchal family structure. The historical and ongoing tension between communists and anarchists at times seems like a narcissism of minor differences, particularly in light of the following words from Engels (2004) about the possibility of a classless society:

> The state, then, has not existed from all eternity. There have been societies that did without it, that had no idea of the state and state power … the state will inevitably fall. Society, which will reorganise production on the basis of a free and equal association of the producers, will put the whole machinery of state where it will then belong: into the museum of antiquities, by the side of the spinning wheel and the bronze axe.
>
> (p. 160)

I agree with the necessity of abolishing capitalist production and private property, but I wish to re-envision—and reconstruct as opposed to abolish—the family and the State as holarchical institutions characterized by self-organization (i.e., free association). My analysis extends to other organizations, such as psychoanalytic institutions and clinics. Here, my thinking is informed by the connections between psychoanalysis, anarchism, complexity science or complex systems science (cf. Cohn, 2010; Cudworth & Hobden, 2010; Fox, 2011; Galatzer-Levy, 2017; Hourigan, 2012; Krakauer, 2024; Lees & Cleminson, 2015; Lenti, 2014; Maldonado & Mezza-Garcia, 2014; Newman, 2017; Workers Solidarity Movement, 2009). Aside from Plato's (2000) argument for the republic as the most just and stable form of governance, it is essentially difficult to dismiss the radical and revolutionary origins of republicanism (Hayat, 2023; Leipold, 2024). However, the point is not to be nostalgic about that form of governance, but, rather, the question becomes: how can we radicalize or revolutionize the republic using anarcho-communist principles that align with liberation psychoanalysis *qua* complexity science?

An impossible republic-to-come would be structured holarchically like fractals, through (a) local communities or neighborhood councils (e.g., worker cooperatives and community land trusts), (b) regional networks, and (c) a decentralized confederation of regional networks. This holarchical structure would accentuate local autonomy, decentralization, and participatory decision making (Kadalie, 2019; Öcalan, 2022). The republican form would function as a minimal safeguard against democracy's eventual deterioration into tyranny, as Plato (2000) warned.

Historical and ongoing examples of micro or mezzo scale impossible republics include the Zapatistas in the Chiapas region of Mexico, Rojava in northeastern Syria, and the CNT-FAI during the Spanish Revolution. These cases are inspiring; however, we are yet to see macro level impossible republics scaled up for actualizing proletarian internationalism, which I would think requires the State form in some capacity (Bamyeh, 2009). As such, an impossible republic, conceived of as a complex form of organization, would be characterized by interconnectedness, nonlinearity, emergence, self-organization, feedback loops, dynamic behavior, uncertainty and unpredictability, and holism (cf. Nappalos, 2019). How, then, can liberation psychoanalysts facilitate the emergence of impossible republics? Liberation psychoanalysts are tasked to engage in a radical form of intellectual labor, becoming "epistemic toolmakers," whose function is to analyze

> the emergent dynamics of social systems that produce either hierarchical or egalitarian relations and, instead of trying to solve the problem of hierarchy themselves, translates their analysis into terms that anyone can use, to aid people in their own efforts to mitigate hierarchy and strengthen equality. The goal of this labour is to facilitate the broadest possible distribution of intellectual labour, what in computer science is called a distributed system, and thereby facilitate a radically democratic deliberation over the productive forces of human society.
>
> (Powell, 2023, p. 35)

Sheehi and Sheehi (2024) critique what they term the "colonial republic of psychoanalysis," which I read ana-dialectically as opening up the possibility for reconstructing liberation psychoanalysis as *a decolonial republic*, along the lines of anarcho-communism, radical humanism, and complexity science. To put it in formal or mathematical terms, following set theory, I would argue that liberation psychoanalysis is a complex science, which aligns with anarcho-communism—when considering the praxis of free association and free clinics—and affirms the ethic of radical humanism through its commitment to collective liberation via an internationalist politics of difference driven by historical reason.

Liberation psychoanalysis, as a complex science of the unconscious, is capable of not only critiquing ideology, but also deconstructing the racial capitalist apparatus housing said ideology. The subject of psychoanalysis is a set comprising ego and unconscious: S = {ego, \$}. Similarly, the Other is a set comprised of the *objet a* and the barred Other: O = {*a*, Ⱥ}. In the case of transmodernity, there would be a squaring of these elements as a function of relationship between Totality and Exteriority, which is characterized by colonial difference; however, throughout this book, I am attempting to analectically deconstruct this asymmetrical power/knowledge relationship via *decolonial difference*, from the perspective of Exteriority.

Fantasy describes the relationship between the unconscious and the *objet a*: $F = (\$ \Diamond a)$. Discourse chronicles the relationship between the ego (*qua* master-signifer or S_1) and the ~~Other~~ (*qua* knowledge or S_2): $D = (S_1 \rightarrow S_2)$. Ideology is a process whereby a function of discourse and fantasy is materialized by the apparatus, while a Real remainder is always present.

In other words, ideology is a set that is produced from the interaction of discourse and fantasy: $I = \phi(D \cup F)$. This formula expresses that ideology is the product of a function that operates on the union of discourse and fantasy. The function ϕ is what conceals the inherent contradiction between D and F. It presents them as a single, coherent whole. The Real is not part of this union, but is the unrepresentable void that the ideological process attempts to conceal.

The apparatus is the materialization of ideology, a process that accounts for the Real. The apparatus (α) takes ideology and materializes it, but its function is always incomplete because it cannot fully account for the Real. The material output of the apparatus is a duo of political economy (*PE*) and libidinal economy (*LE*): $(PE, LE) = \alpha\ (I) \setminus R$. This formula shows that the apparatus acts on ideology to produce a material reality, which is always marked by a void, represented by the subtraction of the Real, as the unmaterializable remainder, the very limit of the apparatus's ability to create a seamless, unified reality.

Whereas the political economy is the mode of production, or the forces and relations of production, the libidinal economy is the mode of enjoyment. A capitalist mode of production is characterized by the profit motive, private property, and wage labor. Conversely, a socialist mode of production is typified by production for use, social ownership of the means of production, and a free association of producers. The political economy's purpose is to satisfy the people's hierarchy of needs, which is a spectrum from physiological and safety needs to demands for love, esteem, and self-actualization (Maslow, 1943). The capitalist mode of production fails to satisfy these popular needs and demands, except for the 1%—to index a master-signifier from the Occupy Movement. This is why a concept like "luxury communism" (Bastani, 2019) is an attractive alternative to austerity capitalism.

Furthermore, *mythic jouissance* is the death-driven (i.e., self-destructive) capitalist mode of enjoyment. It is the collective enjoyment of oppression and violence, which is then ideologically justified. On the other hand, *divine jouissance* is the collective enjoyment of liberation and (non)violence, that is, the commons—be they material or cultural resources. Commoning is grounded in what Said (1983) terms "affiliation" and what Day (2005) labels "affinity." For Saidiya Hartman (1997):

> the "community" or the networks of affiliation constructed in practice are not reducible to race—as if race a priori gave meaning to community or as if community was the expression of race—but are to be understood in terms of the possibilities of resistance conditioned by relations of power and the very purposeful and self-conscious effort to build community.
>
> (p. 59)

Community is the collective of subjects engaged in a praxis of commoning. My notion of non-identity politics finds resonance in Hartman's argument about community:

> The commonality constituted in practice depends less on presence or sameness than upon desired change—the abolition of bondage. Thus, *contrary to identity providing the ground of community, identity is figured as the desired negation of the very set of constraints that create commonality*—that is, the yearning to be liberated from the condition of enslavement facilitates the networks of affiliation and identification.
>
> (p. 59, emphasis added)

Following from the Lacanian axiom that $Desire = Demand - Need$ (Lacan, 2006, p. 580), the socialist mode of enjoyment is scientific in a psychoanalytic sense; it is not premised on obtaining objects of desire that would satisfy us through mindless consumption within a market economy grounded in planned obsolescence. To put it differently, the socialist mode of enjoyment recognizes the indeterminacy of desiring as a process, which is experienced as a creative source of enjoyment in and of itself; the enjoyable process of desiring is life-driven or driven by historical reason.

The complete formula is as follows: $(PE, LE) = \alpha(\phi(D \cup F)\backslash R)$. This formula encapsulates the entire theory of liberation psychoanalysis: the apparatus of racial capitalism materializes a seemingly unified ideology (e.g., patriarchy, exploitation, racism, sexist oppression, etc.) into a physical reality: a profit-driven political economy centered on private property and a libidinal economy driven by *mythic jouissance*. However, this materialization is never complete because it is always marked by the impossible remainder of the Real, which acts as a fundamental limit to the ideological process. This Real, being the unrepresentable truth of ideological fantasy, is what I term *colonial difference* as the onto-epistemic foundation of sexual difference, 'racial' difference, and class struggle.

The Structure of the Book

The book is structured in 15 chapters, wherein I address liberation psychoanalysis from different perspectives while focusing on a variety of salient topics. There is a political emphasis on relevant current events throughout the book, from the Gaza genocide to pop cultural references (e.g., wokeism, "cultural Marxism," Ye, *Anora*, etc.). After this Introduction, Chapter 2 is on Djehuty, Ibn Rushd, and the question of esoteric writing. In Chapter 3, I think about what a decolonial palimpsest might look like, given that (post)colonial psychoanalysis is a form of over-writing. Chapter 4 is an addendum to *Freud and Said*, wherein I show the theoretical links between Lacan and Said. In Chapter 5, I argue for the importance of Freudo–Lacanian psychoanalysis for liberation praxis by explicating central concepts, such as the unconscious and the Gaze. In Chapter 6, I offer a liberation psychoanalytic account of racism, whereby I historicize racism and analyze it through a dialectical materialist lens. In Chapter 7, I unpack not only the psychoanalysis of racism but also the racism of psychoanalysis. In Chapter 8, I try to imagine post-abyssal (or liberation) psychoanalysis through the thinking of Boaventura de Sousa Santos, who is a controversial figure now after reports by seven women accusing him of harassment became public. In Chapter 9, I explore analectical psychology as a transmodern praxis. In Chapter 10, I critique the ideology of liberal wokeism as a form of postcolonial unreason. In Chapter 11, I perform a Lacanian Discourse Analysis of the conservative anti-CRT ideology. Chapter 12 is an addendum to my book *A Psychoanalytic Biography of Ye*, wherein I theorize Ye's fascist turn to aestheticizing politics with the release of *Vultures*. Chapter 13 is a psychoanalytic reading of the film *Anora*, which homes in on the impossibility of sexual rapport, particularly under capitalism. In Chapter 14, I provide three clarifications on *Freud and Said* in response to a critic. Chapter 15 addresses the psychoanalytic significance of ethically representing Gazans during the war. In the Conclusion, I revisit the question of transmodernity in relation to liberation psychoanalysis.

Chapter 2

Djehuty, Ibn Rushd, and the Question of Esoteric Writing

Writing is history, history is writing, and "the history of writing suggests that there is no sexual relationship" (Lacan, 1977–1978, p. 6). There is no political, economic, or sexual liberation without writing and no writing is outside of history. To write is to historicize, and vice versa. In essence, writing traverses the registers of the Real, the Symbolic, and the Imaginary on the level of the subject and also cuts through the realms of ethics, politics, and aesthetics on the level of the Other. I agree with Jacques Derrida's (1997) critique that philosophy (and, by extension, psychoanalysis) is a *metaphysics of presence* that privileges speech over writing. At the heart of logocentrism, phonocentrism is an assumption about "the absolute proximity of voice and being" (p. 11). For example, Plato wrote about what Socrates said/thought.

Lacan's Seminars are supposedly a return to Freud's thinking through speech. Writing necessitates the spoken authority and material historicity of a master. Death, of course, is the absolute master; hence, the prominence of the death drive in the politico-libidinal economy. However, for Derrida (1997), *thinking is a form of writing*. This is also implicit in psychoanalysis, as I will show. So, we can argue that this latent position—negating the primacy of writing *qua* thinking—functions as the unconscious of psychoanalysis itself. In essence, I will argue that liberation psychoanalysis is a *pharmakon*, a writing cure (cf. Lieber, 2020).

For Derrida (1997), writing is extimate; it is "at the same time more exterior to speech … and more interior to speech, which is already in itself a writing" (p. 46). For me, writing is to speech what the unconscious is to the ego. As such, I conceive of *unconscious thinking as a form of writing* in tension with the *speaking being* (*parlêtre*). Writing signifies *differànce* because it presupposes an Other, who writes through us and for whom we write. We defer to the Other, that is, to difference. This Other is Logos, as in discourse and reason or logic.

According to Raymond Tallis (2018), the concept of Logos can be traced back to Ancient Egyptian esoteric philosophy, particularly "the Pyramid Texts of Heliopolis" (p. 33), but Logos was rendered exoteric by Ancient Greek philosophers, including the Presocratics (e.g., Heraclitus), Plato, Aristotle, and the Stoics (e.g., Philo of Alexandria). Nevertheless, Logos became popular in its Christian iteration through the Gospel of John: "In the beginning was the Word (Logos), and the

DOI: 10.4324/9781003768104-2

Word (Logos) was with God, and the Word (Logos) was God … the Word (Logos) became flesh" (John, 1:1, 14).

This famous quote from the Bible describes the logical sequence of the incarnation of Logos from a transcendental signified (or concept) to the materiality of the signifier: (1) Logos as the Name-of-the-Father (YHVH, God, or Allāh), i.e., the Symbolic order as an ideal concept or a transcendental signified; (2) Logos as the desire of the mOther, i.e., the Holy Spirit as the vanishing mediator (or community of believers) standing in for the traumatic Real; and (3) Logos as the materiality of the signifier or as the Letter: Jesus, the Imaginary son, as the immanence of the Father.

The Real incarnation of Logos occurs in writing through what Lacan (2013) terms "the gullying of the signified." Lacan adds, "Writing does not copy the signifier, but its language effects." In Seminar XX, Lacan (1998) echoes Derrida when he says, "Writing is thus a trace in which an effect of language can be read" (p. 121). Writing can be schematized as follows: *a* (writing *qua* trace of language effects from A) → $ (the written symptom to be read or interpreted). In short, writing = analysis. The effect of writing/analysis is an encounter with our Otherness through the unconscious, which is what Lacan (1998) calls "para-being" (p. 45). Para-being within Totality opens the transmodern possibility for *para-becoming* in Exteriority.

Psychology is *the Logos of psyche*, often translated, in a scientistic way, as the study of human behavior and neuro-cognitive functions, which can be experimentally and objectively verified. However, I understand psychology, from a critical psychological—or human scientific—perspective, as *the discourse of psyche*, which can be empirically and (inter)subjectively verified. Freud's move away from Logos and toward analysis—or from psychology to psychoanalysis—coincides with his decentering of the subject from ego to unconscious—a Copernican revolution of sorts. The Logos of psyche is the ego: the body of Christ. But what of the unconscious of Christ *qua* God's discourse? I ask this question with Lacan's (1977/2004) reformulation of Nietzsche's "God is dead" in mind: "the true formula of atheism is *God is unconscious*" (p. 59, emphasis in original).

Logos—in its mythic form—is not only the Word but also Reason (cf. Tallis, 2018), a totalizing (and, perhaps, totalitarian) reason: *the totalizing reason of the I*. As such, Logos is the foundation of instrumental reason (modernization/colonization), that is, the use of reason for the purpose of domination. Logos—the mythic discourse of instrumental reason—is addictive because it is also a *pharmakon* (cf. Cassin, 2019). Logos is both a cure and a poison; hence, the problematic of modernity/coloniality that we continue to wrestle with.

Whereas modernity (and, by extension, psychoanalysis) is a cure through love, coloniality is a hateful poison. This is why I believe in *the passion of learned ignorance* as the key to actualizing transmodernity. In my view, learned ignorance is the central decolonial method of analectical materialism. I label it as *critique from a place of love* to capture the paradoxical nature of critiquing Totality from the perspective of Exteriority, which includes modernity as much as it excludes coloniality. There are two other critical positions, which I am less convinced by: *rejection from a place of ignorance* and *disruption from a place of hate*. My position is that of a critique characterized by ambivalence and resistance, the second critical position is a rejection or foreclosure of psychoanalysis, and the third critical position is a performance meant to disrupt and derive a certain enjoyment from unmasking the 'masters' (e.g., Freud and Lacan) by proving that they are frauds.

I have addressed the question of modernity in depth elsewhere (Beshara, 2024b); however, I wish to underline specific arguments here. Whereas Dussel (1985) views modernity as an event that originates in 1492, I view that date as the beginning of modernity/coloniality specifically—the ghost in the racial capitalist machine. Modernity itself is much older and can be traced back to ancient philosophy because it has to do with *the search for pluriversal truth*, which continues to drive our *philos* (love) of *sophia* (wisdom). It is no coincidence then that the Renaissance—the precursor to modernity—was the rebirth of ancient art, science, and spirituality. In essence, modernity was a traversal of the antimodernity of the Dark Ages—the millennia of Christian dogmatism since the brutal murder of Hypatia.

What modernity failed to traverse is its own shadow (coloniality). This is the task of transmodernity, to shift gears from instrumental reason and irrationalism to historical reason. There are many examples of transmodernity on the level of culture, such as *Handel's Messiah: A Soulful Celebration* (1992), which interprets the 1741 oratorio through the rich tapestry of African American music, *Mozart l'Égyptien* (1997), the brainchild of Ahmed al-Maghreby, which reconstructs some of Mozart's compositions through traditional Egyptian and Arabic music, or the TV show *Reservation Dogs* (2021), the first American series to feature all Indigenous writers and directors who attempt to reimagine what it means to be Indigenous on Turtle Island today. These are, of course, important counter-ideological interventions, but the task of analectical materialism is to overcome racial capitalism—the apparatus within which modernity/coloniality is housed. Critique is the first step in any liberation praxis.

If instrumental reason is a function of Logos, then historical reason can be revealed through analysis, which involves the loosening up of Logos. Through analysis, we encounter the *objet a* of Logos in the Other's discourse. However, analysis is not exclusive to Totality, so we find the same prefix "ana-" in analectical materialism, which implies a materialist critique of Totality from Exteriority: breaking up the modern/colonial Other to set free the transmodern Other of the Other. Whereas the colonial unconscious is the negation of Exteriority, the decolonial unconscious is the negation of coloniality. When modernity is negated in the name of decoloniality, we are in the realm of antimodern fantasy, contrary to colonial fantasy and implicating transmodernity.

Jesus represents the divided subject ($\$$), while God represents the barred Other (Ⱥ). Their non-sexual rapport is framed by the logic of fantasy ($\$ \lozenge a$), wherein the Holy Spirit represents the object-cause of desire (a), that enjoyable bit of the traumatic Real. In other words, the Holy Spirit, or the community of believers necessary for sustaining the dialectical journey of Logos from spirit to flesh and back, is a surplus or supplement. This community is, of course, led by mOther Mary. As such, we can say that *in the beginning was Logos (God* qua *the Name-of-the-Father, as the Symbolic order of language and Law), and Logos (Holy Spirit* qua *the desire of the mOther, as the Real order of the community of believers) was with God, and Logos (Jesus* qua *divided subject) was God.*

What is mythic is Logos's false universality (i.e., Totality), which Lacan (1975/1998) would term *the phallic logic of the All*. This is the mythic logic behind colonialism, racism, nationalism, ethnocentrism, etc.—what Derrida (1997) terms *phallogocentrism*. This is how Christianity was put in the service of European colonialism and imperialism at the forefront of its civilizing mission. Logos becomes divine through the analectic jump from the singular to the pluriversal. The analectic is *the post-phallic logic of the non-All*, which Freud (1939) identifies with Maat (truth and justice)—cf. Karenga (2003). Here, we find a radical interpretation of Christianity as a singular/pluriversal project of liberation, which leads African American philosopher Cornel West to call himself "a follower of a Palestinian Jew named Jesus" (as cited in Needleman, 2021). This is a case for the non-European-ness or Exteriority of Jesus and Christianity. Just like Moses was an Egyptian for Freud, Jesus is a Jew for West.

Interestingly, in John Huston's (1962) *Freud: The Secret Passion*—which Jean-Paul Sartre worked on as a screenwriter but for which he was never credited—there is a scene between Freud and his mother (Amalia), wherein he is remembering a traumatic experience from his childhood, and he asks, "Mother, when we were in Breslau [Wrocław, Poland] in our hotel, where did I sleep?" Amalia, "In my bed. To comfort you for your first day away from home." Freud, "Uh-huh. And father?" Amalia, "He was in the next room. He also had heard your crying, got up, and he came in." Freud, "Hmm. Heard me crying, at night, in a hotel." Amalia, "Yes. I gave you this to play with." Amalia references her serpent bracelet. Freud, "Yes, I remember! And what was it you called me? My little …" Amalia (joyously), "Arab." Freud, "Arab." Amalia, "Because your hair was so black." Freud, "Mother, may I have that?" Amalia takes off her serpent bracelet and hands it to Freud, thereby repeating an earlier soothing memory. Amalia, "Yes." Freud, "For a few days." Amalia smiles.

That night, Freud has an eerie dream, wherein he is a mountaineer entering a cave—regressing back into the womb—while holding a Polish ciupaga (a condensated object): a walking stick, which is also a mountain axe. In the dream, Freud is being pulled by a little Arab through a rope wrapped around his waist and which seems to be coming out of his navel like an umbilical cord. In *The Interpretation of Dreams*, Freud (1899) describes *the navel of the dream* as "the spot where it reaches down into the unknown" (p. 528). Inside the cave, Amalia is seated on an elevated rock formation like the High Priestess, the second card of the Major Arcana of the Tarot. The High Priestess symbolizes the unconscious, particularly as the "dark continent" of feminine *jouissance* (Freud, 1926). The little Arab brings Freud face to face with his mother and then begins to vigorously enjoy the breast while Freud is watching in horror this traumatic staging of the Oedipal fantasy by his unconscious through the dream-work. Amalia is gazing at Freud while this is happening, provoking his anxiety while causing his desire. Meanwhile, Freud covers his face with one hand, but leaves one eye uncovered, which speaks to the division of subjectivity *vis-à-vis* unconscious desire. The egoic eye is censored, but the unconscious I is not.

Finally, Amalia hands over a Real serpent to Freud, a phallic object *par excellence*, particularly as the ouroboros (a serpent eating its own tail)—a variation on the Möbius strip—which signifies the subject-as-drive's infinite (i.e., symptomatic or repetitive) *jouissance* in relation to the *objet a* (the breast). Freud famously had an oral fixation, as he was known to smoke around twenty cigars per day. The dream ends when a superegoic militaristic father figure appears from nowhere like *deus ex machina* and chastises Freud, thereby, prohibiting his transgressive incestuous fantasy. Frustrated, Freud raises the serpent (phallus) above his head signifying his Symbolic castration and subsequent submission to the phallic order of privation, wherein the mother *is* the phallus, the father *has* the phallus, so Freud must accept his lack of being.

I wish to juxtapose's Freud's "little Arab" dream—"a kind of writing that is mainly a rebus" (Safouan, 2002, p. 40)—with Said's (2001) statement about himself being "the last Jewish intellectual." These metonymic displacements signify the groundless ground of non-identity, or Otherness, for subjectivity in general and the productive libidinal investments behind the 'cousin' metaphor, in particular, as the condensatory link between Arabs and Jews—both being (non)European subjects, who have so much Abrahamic *jouissance* in common beyond the narcissism of minor differences.

The unconscious (like the proletariat) has a revolutionary potential because it signifies that truth is *that which is unjustly negated but which can still be affirmed through science*. Logos exploits the unconscious the way the bourgeoisie exploits the proletariat. Coloniality is the unconscious of modernity, the negation of Exteriority. However, this negation alludes to the possibility of transmodernity: integrating Totality with Exteriority through the traversal of colonial and antimodern fantasies, which structure the (non)European unconscious. This racial capitalist structure is characterized by colonial difference: *there is no such thing as a colonial relationship*. Mythic *jouissance* is premised on a phallic logic of exception: *all humans are civilized, except this group of savages (i.e., non-Europeans)*. According to divine *jouissance*, *not all humans are civilized, and there are no exceptions*.

Not all humans are civilized because not all humans *act* civilized. Civilization is not an ontological privilege of a particular social group–this is the universalizing error of Totality *qua* Logos. Rather, civilization is a politico-libidinal praxis of liberation realized through Maat (truth and justice), a function of historical reason. The death drive affects all human subjects to the extent that human civilization, and any culture, is an open-ended praxis characterized by failure more than success, which is why we write and historicize—this is what led Freud (1930/1961) to write about the uneasiness (*das unbehagen*) of being in culture. Culture is a particular response to the Real in the form of a demand. We should strive to *act* civilized, by being truthful and just, while knowing that we will likely fail, so the lesson is to follow Samuel Beckett's advice: *to fail again but to fail better*. Liberation psychoanalysis is one way of failing better. We enjoy listening to unconscious truths to do justice to desire.

The Logos (the sign) becomes, in the words of Maurice Merleau-Ponty (1968), not only *the flesh of the world* (God as the transcendental signified) but also *the flesh of the body* (Jesus as the materiality of the signifier). The fantasmatic relationship between Jesus and God is not without conflict, which sheds light on the dimension of the traumatic Real (i.e., the community of believers). Derrida (1981) writes, "The seed must thus submit to *logos*. And in so doing, it must do violence to itself, since the natural tendency of sperm is opposed to the law of *logos*" (p. 154, emphasis in original). Hence, dissemination or deconstruction entails psychosocial fidelity to the dialecticization of desire, the play of signifiers, which is not a nihilistic discursive exercise but a material praxis at the intersection between *the flesh of the body* (subject) and *the flesh of the world* (Other) enacted through *the flesh of the word.*

Submitting to Logos—*qua* metaphor of the One—signifies alienation or being subjected to the universal (i.e., cultural) demands of the Other: "Thou shalt ..." However, our unconscious tendency as subjects is to separate from these demands to figure out our singular form of desiring and enjoying, which is idiosyncratic, as in symptomatic or metonymic: $a \rightarrow \$ \rightarrow S_1 \rightarrow S_2$. In essence, deconstruction is a traversal of fantasy, which displaces Logos (the Other or the transcendental signified). Instead of fantasizing about the object-cause of desire, we become driven by it and enjoy this desirous experience. This is the politico-libidinal telos of decolonial subjectification.

Nevertheless, the condensation of the Word (Logos) as Jesus (Being) illustrates what Derrida (1997) terms logocentrism, "the metaphysics of phonetic writing," which for him is "nothing but the most original and powerful ethnocentrism" (p. 3). Phonetic writing systems, which privilege speech (the Word *qua* Being), have historically displaced logographic writing systems (e.g., Egyptian hieroglyphs, Sumerian cuneiforms, and Chinese characters) through colonialism. This led Derrida (1997) to claim, "It is not by chance that in mythology, the Egyptian in particular [i.e., Djehuty], the god of sciences and technologies is also the god of writing" (p. 313).

The logographic writing of the non-European Other is absent because its Exteriority was seen as a dangerous supplement to the Totality of Euromodernity, a surplus-*jouissance* that European archeologists had to tame by decoding it and confining this form of writing to Orientalist experts. Is this the destination of the Letter? The lesson from deciphering the Rosetta stone—thanks to Napoleon's instantiation of the Orientalist archive—is that the Greek signifier materialized the death of the Hieroglyphic Letter. Is it a coincidence that Greek was the ruling class's language after Egypt was colonized?

For the longest time, the Sumerians were assumed to be the inventors of writing. However, Joann Fletcher (2016) argues that Ancient Egyptian tax labels are "the earliest evidence for writing found anywhere in the world, apparently pre-dating that of Mesopotamia, and proving that Egypt had a 'phonetically readable' written script by around 3250 BC" (p. 35). This ancient link between writing and taxation illustrates the inscription of the Symbolic order through language and Law, and how the material dimension of the political economy (i.e., the history of class struggles) sustains the ideological and fantasmatic dimension of the libidinal economy (i.e., the life and death struggle—or the desire–for recognition). These seemingly insignificant tax labels mark "the beginning of Egypt's historical period" (p. 35).

The ruling class invented writing as an administrative tool, an extension of power. Moustapha Safouan (2007) affirms this thesis when he divulges the secret of writing, "*it sees without an eye and it speaks without a voice … writing is the silent place of Truth*" (p. 75, emphasis in original). This implies that writing always takes a symptomatic toll on the body of the subject, or, as Lacan (2006) puts it, "if symptoms can be read, it is because they themselves are already inscribed in a writing process" (p. 371). The written (the subject of the statement) is the product of writing, but there is also the unwritten (the enunciating subject), as loss/lack or surplus-*jouissance*. Writing taxes the unwritten, which may as well be unwritable and unreadable (cf. Gutermann-Jacquet, 2015). Moving from being written over by the Other to (re)writing our unconscious desire is one of the liberating effects of analysis.

Jamieson Webster (2018) explores these liberating effects by concretely linking somatic/symptomatic writing to psychoanalytic change, particularly when she argues that the unconscious is an organizing script for the human subject as a sexed body; in other words, the unconscious is "a kind of writing that organizes both the field of representation and the surface of the body together, that is, what we might call the sexual" (p. 119). For Webster, following Freud and Lacan, writing ruptures knowledge and speech (p. 21); it is an "absolute materiality" because it is embodied, a "writing of the body" (p. 59). Furthermore, writing is a conversion of symptoms, a "somatic upheaval," a form of "writing that only bodily possession can do" (p. 109). Finally, analytic writing, as a writing of the body "from the place of a loss or knot in one's libido" (p. 115), both transmits and disorders psychoanalytic knowledge, which is an "erotic experience" from the perspective of a reader (p. 254).

If the mind speaks using signifiers, then the body writes using symptoms. The logical movement from the signifier to the symptom is what Breuer and Freud (Freud & Breuer, 1895/2004) call conversion, which they define as "the transformation of psychical excitation into chronic physical symptoms" (p. 135). Accordingly, hystericization—a critical form of knowledge that arises through the analysand's questions—is the inverse of conversion, for it is a movement from the symptom to the signifier. Conversion is a movement not only from body to mind, but also from ego to unconscious. In my view, conversion is one of the most elegant solutions to the mind–body problem. I show this by retranslating the Cartesian axiom *cogito ergo sum*: I (the body) think through symptoms that I write; therefore, I (the mind) am a speaking being.

In seeking relief from the pain of physical symptoms through, let us say, stretching or yoga, the subject may experience psychological relief. Similarly, in working through a psychological disorder—that is, suffering at the level of the signifier—through, let us say, psychoanalysis or writing, the subject may experience pain relief. The dialectical relationship between the mind and the body is complex because it is characterized by not only positive correlation, but also negative correlation. In a sense, *jouissance* describes the subject's unique way of correlating pleasure and pain.

Psychoanalysis may increase or decrease pain just as yoga may increase or decrease suffering and vice versa. There is no guarantee either for the relief of symptoms to bring about the end of suffering or for free association to extinguish symptoms. This "no guarantee" is lack itself, and the psychoanalytic resolution entails embracing this lack (of guarantee) and working with both signifiers and symptoms in a variety of ways, for signifiers/symptoms may be experienced simultaneously or *not*. The 'not,' of course, may point to a knot, a symptom holding together the subject's division. In psychoanalysis, the cause of desire is championed as the free associative method for modifying the subject's libidinal economy, or how they enjoy their symptomatic knots through the *not*-said.

In this context, Safouan (2007) distinguishes between the "ideal writing" of the ruling class, which is premised on the superegoic (or ideological) function of unconscious self-censorship, and what we may term *Real writing* (p. 77). Real writing, a material legacy of linguistic humanism, is a praxis of (re)writing/translating, which can bring about revolutionary change. For example, the Protestant Reformation was an effect of Martin Luther's translation of the Bible from Latin to German, thereby, secularizing a sacred text by making it accessible to the masses and open to the hermeneutics of interpretation. Safouan assigns a "double obligation" to Real writers: "to write in the language people speak *and* to call for a democracy that truly expresses the people's sentiments and the differences between its classes" (p. 81, emphasis in original). Real writing is *(re)writing the unwritable, translating the untranslatable.*

In Ancient Egypt, literacy was limited to the ruling class: royalty and nobility, priests, scribes, and some merchants and artisans. Hieroglyphs were considered a sacred language primarily used in religious texts. The signifier 'hieroglyph' means sacred carving. This reveals the ideological function of hieroglyphs, which were considered to hold magical power. Therefore, the expansion of literacy is a counter-ideological function of historical reason. Literacy is the means of liberation, and it is more than the ability to read and write effectively. Literacy is a liberation praxis through which we can change ourselves and the world.

As Paulo Freire and Donaldo Macedo (1987) suggest, critical literacy is about reading not only the word but also the world; by extension, *critical literacy is about writing not only the word but also the world.* There is a magical (i.e., revolutionary) power to literacy, which is not exclusive to the ruling class. The working class or the oppressed have the capacity to write the world they desire. This is the life-driven enjoyment of critical literacy, which I term *divine jouissance*. Nonetheless, writing this world-to-come is a heuristic that depends on how we read our current world. Therefore, critical literacy entails *reading as a critique of ideology* and *writing as a revolutionary praxis*.

Psychoanalysis is, after all, a talking cure, wherein talking or speaking is a form of symptomatic writing (cf. Hanrahan, 2013). Oppression is a symptom of instrumental reason or modernization. As such, oppression is a palimpsest, a form of overwriting, wherein oppressed cultures and peoples are written off or erased *literally* through genocidal extermination and over-exploitation (i.e., enslavement) or *metaphorically* through marginalization. Liberation, on the other hand, is a symptom of historical reason, which is the use of reason for the sake of liberation. In other words, *liberation is a form of collective writing with Others*.

Free association is nothing but a (re)writing of one's symptoms; we can liberate ourselves as singular subjects through *speechifying as a writerly act*. Still, the question of liberation on the collective level is not that different either, for it is also a question of free association. Said's (1983) term for free association is *affiliation*, and he was interested in questions not of origin but of beginning. Questions of origin tend to be dogmatic, for they seek the Absolute Truth (Wahba, 2022). However, questions of beginning are historical and material questions. How do we begin a transmodern world system premised on Maat (truth and justice)?

Similarly, Fanon (1952/1967) wrote about the distinction between ontogeny and phylogeny, the former being concerned with the psychosexual development of the subject and the latter having to do with our evolution as speaking beings. However, Fanon was interested in the question of sociogeny, which is the dimension of historical materialism. According to the sociogenic principle, we should think about the material history of the divided subject, if we are interested in the question of liberation (cf. Turner & Neville, 2020). Here, I also follow Lacan (1966/2006) in terms of his thinking about the Letter, or *the materiality of the signifier*. Liberation is not an ideology but a collective praxis: the historical materialist writing of a democracy-to-come: *the democracy of the proletariat*. What does being liberated as an individual or a collective mean? To think about answers to this question entails writing (i.e., historicizing).

For the remainder of this chapter, I wish to answer this question indirectly by exploring two non-European beginnings of psychoanalysis. These are neither the origins of psychoanalysis nor the only non-European beginnings. They are two relevant beginnings to me for theoretical and personal reasons. Theoretically, I appreciate the ambiguity of the term 'non-European,' which negates the European through the prefix 'non' while also affirming the 'European.' I qualify this sublation as transmodern, my interpretation of *the negation of the negation*. In other words, *transmodernity negates Totality's negation of Exteriority*. Eurocentrism and coloniality are being negated to actualize an expanded version of modernity, one that is aligned with historical reason.

Personally, the 'non' concretely means Egyptian (and, by extension, Coptic), Islamicate, and Arabic—I am using adjectives (e.g., Arabic) instead of nouns (e.g., Arab) to emphasize the linguistic over the ethnic. However, I have always felt like *a minority in the minority*, even in Egypt, because I was baptized Catholic—when the official minority is Coptic. My Catholicism has to do with the m(O)ther's desire because my mother is Polish–European, yes, but more specifically, Eastern European or Slavic. As such, I see myself as (non)European: both European and non. However, I have never lived in Europe. I was born and grew up in Egypt until my mid-20s. My father is Copt, so the Name-of-the-Father signifies Egyptian indigeneity, perhaps a fantasmatic regression to Ancient Egypt. To recap, I am ethnically Copt and Polish, yet my cultural identity is Egyptian, which is, by extension, Arab-Islamic. Following Said (1983), while I am not *filiated* with Arabs and Muslims, at least as far as my nuclear family is concerned, I am certainly *affiliated* with them.

In other words, while we are not the same ethnically or religiously, there is solidarity because of our cultural affiliation, which is threaded by the Arabic language. I write in English from the U.S. but think in Arabic as an Egyptian. I think about Ancient Egyptian aesthetics, medieval Islamic ethics, and modern Arab politics. This is why I am seduced politico-libidinally by not only *Arab internationalism* but also pan-Africanism and, by extension, the non-alignment movement of the Global South. These are my free associations on the *'non' du père* question.

To be alienated is to think that *I am either Egyptian or Polish*. To separate from this alienation is to realize that *I am neither Egyptian nor Polish*. In other words, a human being. To traverse the (anti)humanist fantasy, I write: *I am both Egyptian and Polish*: a (non)European. My Polishness is my unconscious. I repress my Polishness, therefore, I have a Slavic unconscious. Is it a European unconscious? The Eastern European represents the Other of the Western European subject. In other words, Eastern Europe is the unconscious of Western Europe. My ego is Egyptian; this is the Imaginary fantasy I identify with.

However, my desire is elsewhere. I desire as a Slav (i.e., as a slave). I am a slave to love, like Bryan Ferry. My illusions of mastery stem from my Egyptian ego, but I am driven to enjoy through my Slavic unconscious. This is why I usually write out what is unwritable. My unconscious was the 'non' in Egypt, but now–in the U.S.—*my subjectivity is the 'non.'* My being is in question. Strangely, my mother tongue is Arabic, yet my mother is Polish. This is evidence of the Otherness of language. In Arabic, I desire what the Other desires for me, and I desire through this Other. Not to mention that I desire to be desired by the Other, and I also desire this Other. I speak neither Coptic nor Polish, and yet a Polish unconscious sustains my Coptic identity. This is the problem of the (non)European, which concerned Said greatly as a Palestinian Christian, who grew up in Egypt yet ended up living and working in the U.S. like me.

Said (1993) also framed this problem as the question of "exilic marginality." He identified this condition in numerous (non)European intellectuals, including Freud, and as a result, his Exterior sense of affiliation led him to dub himself "the last Jewish intellectual" (Said, 2001). I use transmodernity interchangeably with the (non)European because it signifies the dimension of pluriversality: European and non-European universalities regarding truth and justice. Europe is a universe, a Totality. Its understanding of modernity is tied to the question of coloniality. The tricontinent of Africa, Asia, and Latin America is a parallel universe, an Exteriority. Its explication of transmodernity is informed by the question of decoloniality. We must traverse both *the colonial fantasy* and *the antimodern fantasy*.

The colonial fantasy is that Europeans have the right to subjugate non-European cultures and peoples in the name of modernization or civilization. The antimodern fantasy is that non-Europeans can simply reject (Euro)modernity and build a new world from scratch or return to an old world that never really existed, but is romantically imagined from today's perspective. So far, I have illustrated an instance of self-analysis, which entailed the sublimation of my symptomatic or divided subjectivity through writing and historicization—and, by extension, hystericization. I think; therefore, I write. I write; therefore, I historicize. I historicize; therefore, I hystericize. I hystericize; therefore, I am. In this context, I wish to introduce two master signifiers (Djehuty and Ibn Rushd), which will provide me with an opportunity for Exterior self-criticism.

Djehuty

I trace the beginning of psychoanalysis to Djehuty. Robert Rieber (2012) argues "that ancient Egyptian mythology and art shaped [Freud's] theories of the unconscious and sexuality in a much more profound way than he was willing to admit" (p. 10). I regard Djehuty as the *nṯr* of psychoanalysis, even though psychoanalysis is supposed to be methodologically atheistic. Rieber considers Djehuty to be the basis for Freud's concept of the superego, which aligns with my claim.

What do I mean by calling Djehuty the *nṯr* (or superego) of psychoanalysis? If the unconscious is the discourse of the Other, then *psychoanalysis is the discourse of the Other of the Other*. There is no metalanguage, but there is an ur-language—an Other language. By creating hieroglyphs, Djehuty invented the unconscious (and, by extension, psychoanalysis), thereby affording us *the possibility of writing the unconscious* (cf. Hecq, 2008), that is, *the impossibility of writing the Real* (Greenshields, 2017). Safouan (2002) argues that "the technique of structuring language through writing is the technique used by the unconscious [i.e., primary process] in order to get something signified" (p. 29). Similarly, in "The claims of psycho-analysis to scientific interest," Freud (1913b) posits:

> the interpretation of dreams is completely analogous to the decipherment of an ancient pictographic script such as Egyptian hieroglyphs. In both cases there are certain elements which are not intended to be interpreted (or read, as the case may be) but are only designed to serve as 'determinatives', that is to establish the meaning of some other element. The ambiguity of various elements of dreams finds a parallel in these ancient systems of writing; and so too does the omission of various relations, which have in both cases to be supplied from the context.
>
> (p. 177)

Building on Freud's analogy, Lacan (1975/1988) explicitly links hieroglyphs with the unconscious in Seminar I: "The dream is constructed like hieroglyphics" (p. 245). So, if Djehuty invented hieroglyphs according to Ancient Egyptian mythology, and dreams are constructed like hieroglyphs, then Djehuty is the *nṯr* of the unconscious and, by extension, psychoanalysis. If we agree with Prospero (and Shakespeare) that "we are such stuff as dreams are made on," then how come the language of our dreams (hieroglyphs) is minimized and eclipsed by later ancient Greek myths, whether Oedipus or Antigone?

The Djehuty complex refers to *the negation of non-Europeanness*, which can also manifest as the assimilation of non-Europeanness (in this case, Egyptianness) into the Totality of Euromodernity. Assimilation is one of the main effects of Orientalism in general and Egyptology in particular (Hanna, 2025). In this context, it is worth considering Martin Bernal's thesis that this negation of non-Europeanness–i.e., the Djehuty complex–is specifically a function of 19th-century historical revisionism. Bernal (1987) writes:

> The 'Ancient Model' was the conventional view among Greeks in the Classical and Hellenistic ages. According to it, Greek culture had arisen as the result of colonization, around 1500 BC, by Egyptians and Phoenicians who had civilized the native inhabitants. Furthermore, Greeks had continued to borrow heavily from Near Eastern cultures.
>
> Most people are surprised to learn that the Aryan Model, which most of us have been brought up to believe, developed only during the first half of the 19th century. In its earlier or 'Broad' form, the new model denied the truth of the Egyptian settlements and questioned those of the Phoenicians. What I call the 'Extreme' Aryan Model, which flourished during the twin peaks of anti-Semitism in the 1890s and again in the 1920s and 30s, denied even the Phoenician cultural influence. According to the Aryan Model, there had been an invasion from the north—unreported in ancient tradition—which had overwhelmed the local 'Aegean' or 'Pre-Hellenic' culture. Greek civilization is seen as the result of the mixture of the Indo-European-speaking Hellenes and their indigenous subjects.
>
> (pp. 29–30)

Bernal (1987) argues that the Ancient Model had to be overthrown and replaced by the Aryan Model because for "*19th-century Romantics and racists it was simply intolerable for Greece, which was seen not merely as the epitome of Europe but also as its pure childhood, to have been the result of the mixture of native Europeans and colonizing Africans and Semites*" (pp. 30–31, emphasis in original). In other words, the Djehuty complex refers to a modern symptom of historical amnesia, which continues to divide our world today through colonial difference.

Analectical materialism resolves this historical amnesia by (re)writing/historicizing the 'non' in (non)European. Suppose the Oedipus complex is about the ontogenic desire to kill the father and marry the mother. In that case, the Djehuty complex is about the sociogenic desire to kill coloniality/antimodernity and marry modernity with its alterity. Resolving the Djehuty complex entails recognizing the Other of the Other in its Exteriority: Djehuty is close to the ancient Egyptian pronunciation of *Ḏḥwtj* and translates 𓅞𓏏𓏭 as *He Who is Like the Ibis*. Djehuty becomes assimilated as Thoth, even though the Greek Θώθ (Thṓth) is borrowed from the Coptic θωογτ (Thōout). He is known as تحوت in Arabic.

I am not attempting to replace one myth with another one. I am neither pro-Oedipus (like an orthodox psychoanalyst) nor anti-Oedipus (like an anti-psychoanalytic schizoanalyst). I am non-Oedipus; I am open to psychohistorical or heterodox arguments for Freud's seduction theory (cf. DeMause, 1982; Masson, 1984). Furthermore, I wonder about the pluriversal applicability of Oedipus, since Safouan (1981), for example, does not think that Oedipus is universal and Lacan (2016), too, acknowledges that: "The Oedipus complex is, as such, a symptom" (p. 13). Lacan is suggesting that Oedipus is a particular construction—a way for the modern subject to deal with the Real of their existence within Totality. Furthermore, Ortigues and Ortigues (1966) argue that Oedipus is irrelevant in the African context, based on their empirical studies in Senegal—see also *The Arab Oedipus* (Carlson, 2005). Nevertheless, Iwuanyanwu (2015) argues, "Africa is obviously important to Lacan's analytic especially as it relates to the phenomenology of writing, history, and what the analyst describes as the 'complex of cultural encirclement'" (p. 90). As such, I agree with Kovačević (2007) that Oedipus must be liberated, and maybe the key to his liberation is that we must move beyond Oedipus Rex to consider Oedipus at Colonus, as Fernanda Magallanes (2018) suggests. For Kovačević, liberating Oedipus "stands for making a metonymy out of a metaphor, a displacement out of condensation, the emergence of desire out of the rock of congealed *jouissance*" (p. x, emphasis in original).

By invoking ancient Greek mythology, Freud authorizes psychoanalysis as a European discipline following the Aryan model. However, an ambivalence remains. Freud himself is not Aryan; he is Afro-Asiatic like myself: a (non)European. Furthermore, Freud's office was full of Ancient Egyptian artifacts. According to the Freud Museum London (2019), "One of Freud's favorite objects was a statuette of Thoth as a baboon. His housekeeper Paula Fichtl noted his habit of stroking the marble baboon, as he did his own pet dogs" (p. 39).

The representation of Djehuty as either an ibis or a baboon mirrors the division of the subject, for the Other is divided as well. Djehuty may be a *nṯr*, yet he is divided between *a* (ibis) and Ⱥ (baboon). The ibis-headed Djehuty is like the analyst who causes our desire: *Che vuoi?* But since the unconscious is structured like hieroglyphs, the baboon form of Djehuty signifies that even *nṯrw* are lacking. This lack drives Djehuty to write and to enjoy his lack through writing/desiring. As a messenger of the *nṯrw*, Djehuty acts as a vanishing mediator between humans and the *nṯrw*. As such, he has a fantasmatic function and embodies the social link between the subject and the Other.

Djehuty is also a record keeper of the unconscious, that hieroglyphic discourse of the *nṯrw*. In *The Book of Going Forth by Day*, a scene depicts Anubis weighing scribe Hunefer's heart on the scale of Maat (Djehuty's wife) against the feather of truth. Djehuty is seen standing while documenting the outcome. If the heart's weight equals exactly the weight of the feather, then Hunefer is allowed to pass into the afterlife. However, if his heart is heavier, then he will get devoured by the crocodile-headed Ammit. Ancient Egyptians believed the heart (not the mind) to be the core of subjectivity; in other words, the heart represents the unconscious.

In the Papyrus Ebers, which is one of the earliest and most significant medical papyri of Ancient Egypt dating back to 1550 BCE, there is a section on psychology that is often referred to as the "book of hearts," "treatise on the heart," or simply "the heart and the circulatory system" (Bryan, 1931). The heart, and not the mind, was regarded by Ancient Egyptians as the seat of consciousness, and I would go further and argue that *the heart is the seat of the unconscious*, too. Here are some passages from the *Papyrus Ebers* on psychosomatic ailments as varied as sadness, aversion, oppression, and anger—the reader should note, in particular, the reference to the anal drive when it comes to the affect of aversion, which is one of the three Lacanian passions:

> When the Heart is sad, behold it is the moroseness of the Heart, or the vessels of the Heart are closed up in so far as they are not recognizable under thy hand... When the Heart feels an aversion, behold it is the Bitterness of the Heart because of *Inflammation in the Anus*...When the Heart is sick, behold Oppression of the Heart...When his Heart is afflicted and has tasted sadness, behold his Heart is closed in and darkness is in his body because of anger which is eating up his Heart.
>
> (Bryan, 1931, pp. 127–129, emphasis added)

Ancient Egyptian psychology prefigured not only psychoanalysis (the first force), but also transpersonal psychology (the fourth force). According to Kathleen Pike (2022):

> Sigmund Freud, the father of psychoanalysis, published *The Interpretation of Dreams* in 1899 ... The ancient Egyptians had their own version of dream interpretation many centuries earlier. In ancient Egypt, a person suffering from psychological distress would be sent to a sanatorium, a sleep temple dedicated to healing. In the sanatorium, they would enter a dark cell and prepare for a "therapeutic dream." A hypnotic sleep state was induced by lamps and burning perfumed wood. Priests interpreted the dreams and consulted the "Egyptian Dream Book" to find cures. Unlike Freud who believed that dreams represent an individual's unconscious and internal psychic conflict, the ancient Egyptians understood dreams to be supernatural, where gods were responsible for shaping dream content and protecting against bad dreams.

The sleep temple was a healing site of *dream incubation*, "a practice in which a person performs a ritual act and then sleeps in a sacred place, with the deliberate intention of receiving a dream" (El-Kilany & Elgammal, 2019, p. 98), for "the

Egyptians believed that dreams could serve as oracles, bringing messages from the gods" (Asaad, 2015, p. 14). According to Tarek Asaad (2015):

> To incubate dreams, Egyptians would travel to a sanctuary or shrine, where they slept overnight on a special dream bed in the hope of receiving divine advice, comfort, or healing from their dreams. There were dream or sleep temples built specifically for this reason. The temples were open to everyone who believed in the god the temple was dedicated to, as long as they were considered pure. To achieve this, the person often went through a ritual of cleansing that included fasting and abstinence for several days prior to entering the temple to assure their purity. The name of the god the person hoped to contact at the temple was written on a piece of linen and that linen cloth was burned in a lamp while at the temple. To help call the god, the dreamer would often recite a special prayer to him or her. Once they visited the ancient Egyptian dream temple, the person would often go to a priest or dream interpreter for dream analysis.
>
> (p. 14)

In other words, the sleep temple is the prototype for the psychoanalytic clinic. Dream incubation was complemented by dream interpretation, which was carried out by an expert—the equivalent of today's psychoanalyst—who was "a mixture of priest, physician, and magician" (p. 96). The title of such an expert reminds one of the analyst as the subject supposed to know: *sesh per-ankh rekhet* (Scribe in the House of Life, Knower of Things).

The contemporary analyst is also a scribe, attentive to the Letter of the analysand's speech. The house of life is the analyst's discourse, which is grounded in psychoanalytic know-how about the unconscious. The analyst's discourse produces new master-signifiers through free association (i.e., the hystericization of old master-signifiers); as such, interpretation is a process of dialectization *vis-à-vis* the subject's unconscious desire.

What Pike (2022) refers to as the "Egyptian Dream Book" is a series of fragments from the Hieratic papyri of the Ramesside Period (c. 1292–1077 BCE). The Dream-book follows what Alan Gardiner (1935) calls a "general scheme," which looks like this: "*If a man see himself in a dream doing so-and-so, good (or bad); it means such-and-such a thing will happen*" (p. 9, emphasis in original). Furthermore, the Dream-book is structured around a central dichotomy between Horian dreams and Sethian dreams.

Therefore, the Dream-book, like the dreaming-subject, is essentially divided. *The Contendings of Horus and Seth* is a mythical account of the decades-long struggle between Horus and his uncle Seth for the throne of Egypt, which was ultimately decided by the divine council (the Ennead) in favor of the legitimate heir, Horus, to restore Maat. *The Contendings of Horus and Seth* is the mythical framework that splits the Dream-book into two (*The Interpretation of Dreams of the Followers of Horus* and *The Interpretation of Dreams of the Followers of Seth*)—a division mirroring the conflict between the two fundamental drives: Eros and Thanatos.

Millennia later, when Freud decided to call his magnum opus *The Interpretation of Dreams*, it was a dialectical effort on his part at epistemologically sublating this mythical and driven conflict between Horus/Eros and Seth/Thanatos by integrating magic and religion under psychoanalysis (the science of the unconscious).

The supernatural dimension of dreams, according to Ancient Egyptians, was a function of *heka* or magic, which existed side-by-side with medicine and religion. As such, Erika Kelley (2022) argues, "it is clear that the ancient Egyptians were using transpersonal psychology to cope with the mental trauma of giving birth" (p. 57). Therefore, Ancient Egyptians not only had a conception of trauma almost five millennia before the invention of psychology as a scientific discipline, but also developed tools for coping with trauma through *heka* that centered around using "different objects, texts, spells, rituals, and imagery [that] were purposefully made, said, or conducted to ensure that the mother and child were safe during the process and protected by their deities" and "to stimulate poignant moments, peak experiences, and mystical encounters" (p. 57).

The weighing of the heart ceremony resonates with the ethics of psychoanalysis. A heavy heart is typically a function of guilt or any of the negative affects stemming from alienation. A light heart, on the other hand, signifies the outcome of being life-driven, having traversed destructive fantasies. Oppressors may rationalize their dehumanizing actions through various defense mechanisms; however, there is no way of tricking the heart or the unconscious, for it keeps an archive of our speech acts, and an accumulation of guilt results in a heavy heart or what we may call fixations. Freud (1939) went further in *Moses and Monotheism* and argued that this guilt-ridden unconscious archive of the heart is transmitted transgenerationally in the form of historical trauma through what he calls "archaic inheritance."

The first test that the deceased must go through to achieve eternity or become an *akh*, which happens to mean brother in Arabic, according to *The Book of Going Forth by Day*, is the passage through the *duat* (underworld)—a challenge of knowledge and navigation *à la* the Lacanian Pass. The second test is what is called the negative confessions, which are forty-two sins that must be negated in front of Osiris, Anubis, Djehuty, and a host of other divine judges, who may or may not grant one passage to the next stage: the weighing of the heart ceremony.

The forty-two negative confessions are the basis for the ten commandments; in other words, the mythical and historical foundation of the world's hegemonic Symbolic order is the monotheisteic Atenic order, which has been, and continues to be, disseminated through Semitic languages and Abrahamic Law. The key distinction between the forty-two negative confessions and the ten commandments is grammatical—an affirmative statement about the past vs. an imperative statement about the future—which translates as the structural difference between ritual purity and societal law.

The linguistic structure of the Maatian confessions, as a ritualistic ethical system, is first person singular + perfect tense + negative in the form of "I have not done X." In contrast, the linguistic structure of the ten commandments, as a theological legal system, is second person singular + imperfect/jussive/prohibitive in the form of "You shall not do X." The former is a retrospective magico-religious affidavit, wherein the deceased is an autonomous subject testifying on their own behalf about their past conduct to a tribunal of gods, the latter is a prescriptive Law, wherein the divine sovereign is commanding a living subject what they must not do going forward.

Whereas the negative confessions are a tool designed to magically protect the heart from testifying against the deceased during judgment, the ten commandments are a legal mandate or a covenant, whose emphasis is on obedience to a single transcendent deity (YHVH). In essence, this grammatical shift from "I have not killed" to "You shall not kill" strips away the ritual and polytheistic elements of the Egyptian code to establish a divinely sanctioned set of universal laws for הלגס ם (am segulah) "a peculiar people," as God's private, treasured possession.

The judgement of the dead in Ancient Egypt took place in the Hall of Two Truths, which is a reference to the objective truth of Maat (i.e., the 42 Laws) and the subjective truth of *ib* (the heart or the unconscious), which is the dimension of justice *vis-à-vis* the ethics of desire, hence, the weighing of the heart against the feather of Maat. The Socratics translated this Ancient Egyptian Maatian notion of ethics in terms of the equation: the good life = the analyzed life, an equation that grounds the ethics of psychoanalysis as that of creatively speaking truth to one's unconscious desire.

The scale signifies the movement from the balance of order (Maat) to the imbalance of chaos (Isfet), which I read through the dialectics of the drive: the creative balance of the sex/life drive vs. the destructive imbalance of the ego/death drive. If balance leads to eternity, then the outcome of imbalance is a second death, which brings to mind Antigone, whose ethics of desire took her to the limit between the Symbolic world of the living and the Real world of the dead. In other words, whereas the first death is the Symbolic death of the body *qua* the ego, the second death is the Real death of the heart *qua* the unconscious.

Like Antigone, we continue to invoke Freud's and Lacan's names because they have survived this second death, thus avoiding being devoured by Ammit and becoming immortal 'brothers,' thereby replacing the murdered primal father, who survived his second death through the totemic form. Freud and Lacan—as a band of immortal *akhu*—were true to their desire and just to the cause of psychoanalysis. They survived their second death by laying down the fundamental rule of psychoanalysis, for there would be no psychoanalysis without taboos: free association = no censorship.

In *Freud and Said* (Beshara, 2021a), I wrote about the ethico-political significance of Maat (truth and justice) for Freud in *Moses and Monotheism* (1939); Carol Lipson (2004) argues that Maat functioned as "a Superaddressee in the [Ancient Egyptian] letters … an ultimate addressee beyond the writer and the immediate reciver" (p. 79). To put it differently, Djehuty invented (unconscious) writing for Maat (the Other). According to Freud (1939), Moses was an Egyptian, so non-identity (i.e., Otherness) is foundational to subjectivity. There is the ego identification with Moses as the founder of Judaism alongside his Egyptian unconscious as a follower of Akhenaten (cf. Abraham, 1941). Interestingly, the poet H.D. (2012), who was Freud's analysand, links Moses to Djehuty when she writes in her *Tribute to Freud*:

> it was in the desert that Moses raised the standard, the old T or Tau-cross of Thoth of the Egyptians. The Professor [i.e., Freud] had been working on a continuation of his "Moses, the Egyptian" theme, though we had not actually discussed this when I had my "real" dream of the Egyptian Princess.
>
> (p. 100)

Furthermore, Maat represents historical reason *qua* the renunciation of the drives, for truth without justice is essentially instrumental reason. In other words, Maat is the fusion and redirection of death-driven oppressive fantasies, which are neither true nor just. To accomplish this sublimation, we need the tools of Djehuty, which include writing and wisdom. Then we can work through our oppressive fantasies in automatic writing while being guided by the wisdom of the heart, that is, the unconscious wisdom of the *nṯrw*—the ancestors in many ancient or Indigenous traditions.

The Ancient Egyptian *nṯrw* represent the principle of Exteriority: the Other of the Other. Freud (1939) called this dimension "archaic inheritance," which I understand as a transgenerational traumatic legacy. In the *longue durée* between us in the present and our ancestors in the past, there is a Real traumatic gap, which is covered over by all sorts of Imaginary fantasies about the future related primarily to ideological notions of identity that fix the subject and render them undialectical.

Dialectics and analectics, on the other hand, are counter-ideological methods concerned with revealing truth and actualizing justice. Truth being not only objective, but also subjective—and, more specifically, unconscious. In other words, truth as knowledge and wisdom—the latter is sometimes referred to as intuitive knowing or practical know-how. There is no justice without Law, but which Law? Perhaps, the Law of Thelema? "Do what thou wilt shall be the whole of the Law … Love is the law, love under will … There is no law beyond Do what thou wilt" (Crowley, 1909).

Derrida (1981) invokes Plato's *Phaedrus*, wherein Socrates discusses why Djehuty invented writing:

> Socrates: All right. The story I heard is set in Naucratis in Egypt, where there was one of the ancient gods of Egypt—the one to whom the bird they call the 'ibis' is sacred, whose name is Theuth. This deity was the inventor of number, arithmetic, geometry, and astronomy, of games involving draughts and dice—and especially of writing. At the time, the king of the whole of Egypt around the capital city of the inland region (the city the Greeks call 'Egyptian Thebes'), was Thamous, or Amon, as the Greeks call him. Theuth came to Thamous and showed him the branches of expertise he had invented, and suggested that they should be spread throughout Egypt. Thamous asked him what good each one would do, and subjected Theuth's explanations to criticism if he thought he was

going wrong and praise if thought he was right. The story goes that Thamous expressed himself at length to Theuth about each of the branches of expertise, both for and against them. It would take a long time to go through all Thamous' views, but when it was the turn of writing, Theuth said, 'Your highness, this science will increase the intelligence of the people of Egypt and improve their memories. For *this invention is a potion for memory and intelligence.*' But Thamous replied, 'You are most ingenious, Theuth. But one person has the ability to bring branches of expertise into existence, another to assess the extent to which they will harm or benefit those who use them. The loyalty you feel to writing, as its originator, has just led you to tell me the opposite of its true effect. It will atrophy people's memories. Trust in writing will make them remember things by relying on marks made by others, from outside themselves, not on their own inner resources, and so writing will make the things they have learnt disappear from their minds. Your invention is a potion for jogging the memory, not for remembering. You provide your students with the appearance of intelligence, not real intelligence. Because your students will be widely read, though without any contact with a teacher, they will seem to be men of wide knowledge, when they will usually be ignorant. And this spurious appearance of intelligence will make them difficult company.'

(Plato, 2002, pp. 68–69, emphasis added)

In a sense, this passage reflects the position of Socrates, who understood philosophy as a living praxis, an open-ended dialogue, a series of speech acts between a teacher and a student. In other words, Plato's writings can be regarded as a betrayal of philosophy. The essence of philosophy is philosophizing through speaking, according to Socrates. Once philosophy is written down, it becomes fixed and undialectical, a *semblance* of wisdom but not essential wisdom.

In Lacan's (1977–1978) words, "Writing is an artifice … linked to the fact that there is speech and even saying" but "one cannot say the truth" (p. 3), so can one write the truth? Lacan adds, "What is most real is writing and writing is confused" (p. 4). In sum, writing deceives because it solidifies and crystallizes wisdom (*aletheia*), which is inherently amorphous. Édouard Glissant (1997) recognizes this indeterminate essence of truth from a poetic perspective through his insistence on *the oppressed's right to opacity*, his antidote for reductive transparency, which he associates with violence against the Other.

Derrida (1981) explains the ambivalence of writing by highlighting Djehuty's equivalence between writing and *pharmakon. Pharmakon* is translated as 'potion' above; however, it is often translated as either 'remedy' or 'poison,' which speaks to the undecidability of writing, rewriting, translating, etc. The ambiguity of *pharmakon* sheds light on the *jouis-sense* (enjoy-meant) of writing, for signification entails both pain and pleasure—the pain of deferral and the pleasure of difference.

Writing (like psychoanalysis) is an enjoyable antidote. Writing is a toxin that stimulates an immune response, producing antibodies against the toxin. The method of deconstruction is premised on this paradoxical effect of writing (i.e., that it undoes itself). This is how writing or psychoanalysis becomes a cure. Writing, as a supplement, atrophies our memory, but in doing so, it can also improve our memory. This analysis can be extended to the effects of algorithmic writing, too.

Smartphones and social media extend our minds; what we do with that extension is up to us, so the question of undecidability remains, for algorithmic writing is also a *pharmakon* (poison/remedy). We must go through *semblance* to get to the *essence* of truth. To use a popular metaphor, we must dream through the matrix before waking up in the desert of the Real. The virtual and the actual are parts of an analectic. Modernity/coloniality is the matrix, and transmodernity/decoloniality is the desert of the Real. To actualize transmodernity through analectical materialism, we must traverse the virtual specters of coloniality and antimodernity. They are ghosts driving the racial capitalist machine through instrumental reason and irrationalism. The analectical materialist union of Totality and Exteriority (i.e., pluriversal internationalism) is the telos of historical reason.

J. M. Coetzee said, "all writing is autobiography." I write; therefore, I am. Our social being, how we were materially written by the Other, determines how we write our subjectivity. However, there is still freedom in our alienation; in the face of his miserable fate, Sisyphus chose to be happy. How we write our subjectivity entails unconscious thinking *qua* writing, historicizing, and hystericizing.

For Derrida (1987), writing is not only autobiographical but also autothanatographical; it is not a *graphía* of the self or the author, but of "life death." *Autós* is in reference to the drive. Derrida (1987) frames Freud's speculative writing style as an "autobiography of *the writing*," which "posits and deposits simultaneously, in the same movement, the psychoanalytic movement" (p. 303, emphasis in original). In other words, writing is not just about what an author (e.g., Freud) consciously intends to say but also about what is unconsciously left behind in the text, much like how a psychoanalyst listens not only to what is said but also to what is left unsaid or what slips out as a trace of the unconscious. Furthermore, Derrida (1987) alleges:

> speculation is not only a mode of research named by Freud, not only the oblique object of his discourse, but also the operation of his writing, the scene (of that) which he makes by writing what he writes here, that which makes him do it, and that which he makes to do, that which makes him write and that which he makes—or lets—write.
>
> (p. 284)

To put it differently, speculation is the *objet a* causing Freud's (and our) desire, that is, speculation drives the enjoyment of writing (about psychoanalysis). The irony, of course, is that Freud's speculative research method—cf. Kant's (1781/1998) "speculative reason"—was, in regards to the death drive or *jouissance*, beyond the pleasure principle. Safouan (2002) argues that Freud's speculative turn, in *Beyond the Pleasure Principle*, is a dialectical move inspired by ancient Greek philosophy (p. 83).

Speculation is simultaneously a specular act because it involves observing a scene that reflects back on oneself through the mirror of one's theoretical framework.

Therefore, self-writing is the writing of one's own death, which is always already a writing for the Other. The very act of writing, which seems so personal and self-contained, is fundamentally structured by its destination and its potential to be read and interpreted by others. This echoes, of course, Lacan's (2006) statement: "a letter always arrives at its destination" (p. 30). But this arrival occurs through a Real structure of abeyance, which speaks to our subjection to the Letter *vis-à-vis* self-representation (*Vorstellungsrepräsentanz qua* the signifier)—a subjection that arises from Symbolic castration and which gives rise to a lack of understanding, as far as Imaginary others are concerned.

This is what Paul De Man (1979) means by "Autobiography as De-facement." Self-representation is a paradoxical act, which entails both self-annihilation and self-creation, effacement (erasing one's face) and de-facement (constructing a mask). We submit ourselves to the masochistic pleasure of language through writing to resignify the alienating reality of our castration: "a signifier [S_1] represents a subject [\$] to another signifier [S_2]" (Lacan, 2006, p. 713). Therefore, writing is striving to represent ourselves, while knowing that self-representation is doomed to fail because it will always be overdetermined by non-self elements. So why not give up?

We can write our subjectivity in an ideological or bourgeois way by reinforcing oppressive master-signifiers (e.g., capitalism, modernity/coloniality, universality, etc.) and instrumental forms of knowledge, or we can write our subjectivity in a critical or proletarian way by analyzing our historico-material or psychosocial distress through psychoanalysis and producing liberatory master-signifiers (e.g., socialism, transmodernity/decoloniality, pluriversality, etc.). Writing is both a bourgeois poison and a proletarian remedy. Is modernity the same? Can we separate the remedy of modernity from the poison of coloniality? Is transmodernity another *pharmakon*? In other words, is decoloniality a new poison? To put it differently, how does liberation psychoanalysis treat the poisons of coloniality and antimodernity?

Djehuty is an Ancient Egyptian *neter* (divine force) who is more known by his Ancient Greek name, Thoth, which is a homonym for *thought*. In psychoanalysis, thinking is equated with the unconscious. Was there thinking before writing, or does writing prove the actuality of thinking? This is the historical dimension of the unconscious, which is also a material dimension. The unconscious materialized through the historical invention of writing, which made negation and critical reflexivity possible. To write something means to negate many things, which then become traces that inform what we have chosen to affirm. Writing also affords critical reflexivity, reflecting on the act and the form or style of writing, not just the manifest content. What is written or *maktub* has to do with fate, but writing is destiny. Writing is both the journey and the destination. Writing is a choice, an unconscious one. Writing is desiring/enjoying.

What is the unconscious but a meta-consciousness (a consciousness of consciousness)? For Julian Jaynes (1976), divided subjectivity begins after the breakdown of the bicameral mind in the ancient period—which is an alternative to the Freudo-Lacanian thesis that traces the origin of the divided subject to the modern period, particularly as a function of Cartesian dualism. In a sense, Jaynes's argument is that our original psychical structure in the ancient world was more psychotic; however, after the invention of writing we became more neurotic.

The tripartite structure of the psychic apparatus (id, superego, and ego) theorized by Freud, and later conceptualized by Lacan as orders or registers (Real, Symbolic, and Imaginary), was prefigured in Ancient Egyptian psychology, thousands of years ago, as *Ka* (double), *Akh* (intellect), and *Ba* (personality). The Ancient Egyptian psychological model of the psyche is as sophisticated as psychoanalysis in its account of complex subjectivity; it included other psychic dimensions, too, like *Ren* (name), *Ib* (heart), and *Sheut* (shadow), which can map onto the Other, Being, and the unconscious, respectively.

Ren, in particular, is an impressive concept, which shows that Ancient Egyptians recognized the magical power of the signifier, for it affords one immortality through the imperishability of the Letter—the materiality of one's true name, as inscribed on a cartouche, for example. This recognition of the magical power of the signifier is clear especially in the following Ancient Egyptian proverb: "To speak the name of the dead is to make them live again." Freud was heavily influenced by Ancient Egyptian wisdom and our incessant invocations of his name attest to the immortality of his ideas, as a function of his *magic writing*—that is, *the power of psychoanalytic signifiers*.

I read *Moses and Monotheism*, specifically, not as a minor or eccentric text in Freud's oeuvre; rather, I interpret it through the concept of *Nachträglichkeit*, wherein the psychoanalytic project is retroactively constructed *après-coup* from the end to the beginning through a non-linear lens. Moses is not a true name, but a partial name, which means "to be born" or "child of" in the Ancient Egyptian language. The name Thutmose (the third pharaoh of the 18th Dynasty), for example, signifies "Djehuty is born."

Therefore, Moses is a part-object, psychoanalytically speaking, orbited by the partial drive of monotheism. Here, monotheism is viewed not as a unified belief system, but as a partial drive that fragments the world, evident not only in the endless divisions of the Abrahamic faiths into Judaism, Christianity, Islam, and countless sects, but also in the violence and holy wars waged in the name of a single, indivisible God. Monotheism strips away the pantheon of nṯrw (e.g., Ra, Isis, Osiris, Horus, Anubis, Djehuty, Maat, and Amun-Ra) and reduces them to a single and abstract signifier (Aten → YHVH → God → Allāh).

Lacan (2018) characterized our symptomatic attachment to a master-signifier (S_1) using the concept of *Yad'lun* (there is something of the One). The subject's singularity of being is the Real One (1), which is a specific formation of the barred subject ($), as a signifier of a lack in the ~~Other~~ [S(Ⱥ)]; however, that singularity is often sacrificed for the Symbolic One [I(A)] and/or the Imaginary One [i(a)]. The Symbolic One is the Law one aspires to follow, while the Imaginary One is the perfect self one imagines oneself to be. Both the Symbolic One and the Imaginary One are attempts at resolving or managing the trauma of *jouissance*.

By removing the divine name from Moses, the new monotheistic tradition symbolically severed the subject's link to a polytheistic past of polymorphous perversity. The name Moses thus becomes a stand-in for this abstract drive toward a single deity—a drive that can never be satisfied, except in the mythic form of fundamentalism, that is, *thinking of what is relative in absolute terms* (Wahba, 2022). The partiality of both Moses and monotheism reflects a shared process of fragmentation and abstraction. Moses's incomplete name is not a flaw but a feature, embodying the very nature of a new set of religions (the Abrahamic faiths) that operate through a partial object-cause of desire—*Ephnuti*, the Coptic word for God, which is derived from Demotic, and literally means: the one of the *nṯr*.

As Rieber (2012) shows,

> In the concepts of Ba, defined variously as the soul or self, and of Ka, a spirit that served as its doppelganger in life and as a guardian of the individual in the afterworld, Freud found a fertile source for his own theories of personality.
>
> (p. x)

Unlike psychoanalysis, Ancient Egyptian psychology theorized the bicameral mind. According to Jaynes (1976):

> In funerary scenes, the ba is usually depicted as a small humanoid bird, probably because visual hallucinations often have flitting and birdlike movements. It is usually drawn attendant on or in relationship to the actual corpse or to statues of the person. That after the fall of the more king-dominated Old Kingdom, the ba takes on some of the bicameral functions of the ka is indicated by a change in its hieroglyph from a small bird to one beside a lamp (to lead the way), and by its auditory hallucinatory role in the famous Papyrus Berlin 3024, which dates about 1900 B.C. All translations of this astounding text are full of modern mental impositions, in eluding the most recent, otherwise a fascinating chore of scholarship. And no commentator has dared to take this "Dispute of a man with his Ba" at face value, as a dialogue with an auditory hallucination, much like that of a contemporary schizophrenic.
>
> (pp. 193–194)

Whereas Jaynes believes that humans went from being psychotic to becoming neurotic through writing, Marshall McLuhan (1962) makes the exact opposite argument; however, McLuhan confuses subjective division with schizophrenia and his analysis of the impact of literacy is undergirded by a colonial logic, which confirms my thesis about *coloniality as a psychic remainder*; regardless of his intention, his method is racist. McLuhan (1962) asserts:

> No pictographic or ideogrammic or hieroglyphic mode of writing has the detribalizing power of the phonetic alphabet. No other kind of writing save the phonetic has ever translated man [sic] out of the possessive world of total interdependence and interrelation that is the auditory network. From that magical resonating world of simultaneous relations that is the oral and acoustic space

> there is only one route to the freedom and independence of detribalized man [sic]. That route is *via* the phonetic alphabet, which lands men at once in varying degrees of dualistic schizophrenia.
>
> (p. 22)

For McLuhan, phonetic writing detribalizes and therefore civilizes. McLuhan argues that "detribalization, individualization, and pictorialization are all one" (p. 52). According to McLuhan, "Schizophrenia may be a necessary consequence of literacy" because "phonetic writing split apart thought and action" (p. 22). Building on the work of J. C. Carothers, McLuhan posits that the invention of phonetic writing led to "the breaking apart of the magical world of the ear and the neutral world of the eye, and to the emergence of the detribalized individual from this split [Spaltung?]" (p. 22).

McLuhan essentially believes that phonetic writing is a sign of civilization, particularly in relation to non-alphabetic forms of writing, and he states, "Civilization gives the barbarian or tribal man [sic] an eye for an ear" (p. 25). Similar to how Freud compared the civilized neurotic to the noble savage, McLuhan wishes to neutralize his racist analysis by contending that the civilized psychotic is in the process of "retribalization" (p. 7), as a function of the electronic age or (post)modern world, that is, the "global village" (p. 21). McLuhan's problematic model makes specific epistemological claims about non-alphabetic cultures:

> the ideograph even more than the hieroglyph is a complex *Gestalt* involving all of the senses at once. The ideogram affords none of the separation and specialization of sense, none of the breaking apart of sight and sound and meaning which is the key to the phonetic alphabet. So that the numerous specializations and separations of function inherent in industry and applied knowledge simply were not accessible to the Chinese.
>
> (pp. 34–35)

Furthermore, these epistemological claims reveal the colonial logic of power that the claims aim to justify. This is clear when McLuhan writes, "any society possessing the alphabet can translate any adjacent cultures into its alphabetic mode. But this is a one-way process. No non-alphabetic culture can take over an alphabetic one; because the alphabet cannot be assimilated; it can only liquidate or reduce" (p. 50). The translation of Exteriority and its assimilation into Totality produces colonial difference. When McLuhan is referring to the power of translation, he is explaining how colonialism works:

> Only the phonetic alphabet makes a break between eye and ear, between semantic meaning and visual code; and thus *only phonetic writing has the power to translate man from the tribal to the civilized sphere, to give him an eye for an ear*. The Chinese culture is considerably more refined and perceptive than the Western world has ever been. But the Chinese are tribal, people of the ear.

> "Civilization" must now be used technically to mean detribalized man [sic] for whom the visual values have priority in the organization of thought and action.
> (p. 27, emphasis added)

Some of McLuhan's statements support my thesis in this chapter and prefigure Derrida's *Of Grammatology* in a way, such as: "writing affects speech directly, not only its accidence and syntax but also its enunciation and social uses" (p. 35). However, I cannot, in general, agree with McLuhan, not only because of the colonial logic informing his racist analysis, but also because he thinks Chinese ideograms and Egyptian hieroglyphs are only useful "as a means of enhancing [Euro-American children's] appreciation of [the Latin] alphabet" (p. 47). Unlike McLuhan, I believe non-Europeans have the right to opacity, which aligns with the unknowability of the unconscious itself. The transparency of alphabetic or phonetic writing can be used to justify colonialism and racism, and this is why I argue that *writing is a form of killing* in *Freud and Said* (Beshara, 2021a). While it is true that literacy is a sign of civilization, it is not reducible to *phōnḗ* (sound or voice); literacy must engage all of the senses, that is how *writing (and reading) can become a form of living.*

In Ancient Egyptian mythology, Djehuty is the god of art, science, and wisdom, and he is also credited for inventing writing, among other things. The Greeks worshipped him in the form of Hermes, and the Romans revered him as Mercury. An esoteric tradition by the name of Hermeticism arose around the mysterious figure of Hermes Trismegistus, or Hermes the Thrice-Greatest. I shall interpret this Thrice-Greatness through a Lacanian lens and claim that Djehuty is the god of psychoanalysis because he is the god of the unconscious *qua* writing or history, that is, the god of RSI (the Real, the Symbolic, and the Imaginary).

Consequently, Djehuty can teach us about the ethics, politics, and aesthetics of esoteric writing, which can take four forms: defensive esotericism, protective esotericism, pedagogical esotericism, and political esotericism (Melzer, 2014). The pedagogical and political esotericism of liberation psychoanalysis stem from the impossibility of colonial difference, "which cannot be said, yet must equally be communicated" (Valentini & Tourage, 2019, p. 4). To put it differently, "Everything that is written stems from the fact that it will forever be impossible to write, as such, [the colonial] relationship" (Lacan, 1998, p. 35). Therefore, the esoteric writing of liberation psychoanalysis is an attempt at pluriversal writing "to say different things to different people" (Melzer, 2014, p. 74).

Pluriversal writing aligns with Glissant's (1997) argument for the "right to opacity." Even if colonial difference is resolved by transmodernity and replaced by what Bhabha (1994) terms "cultural difference," the latter will continue to function as *the untranslatable Real.* The dimension of the death drive will always be there, and it can only be represented in an obscure way or anamorphically. I would argue, for instance, that the esotericism of deconstruction is an effect of deconstruction being through and through "a deconstruction of racism" (Derrida, 2003), for racism essentially is an unconscious ideological fantasy about the Other. Barnor Hesse (2023) further claims that deconstruction is a decolonial methodology. For this reason, I see deconstruction as a crucial method in liberation psychoanalysis.

Ibn Rushd

Mourad Wahba (2004) ends his book, "The Paradox of Ibn Rushd" (in Arabic, untranslated into English), with two questions requiring psychoanalytic answers (p. 143). (1) "What are the unconscious reasons for persecuting Ibn Rushd?" Wahba claims that Ibn Rushd was persecuted in the Arab-Islamic world and excluded from its culture, which amounts to the corruption of reason. By Arab-Islamic, I mean the 22 Arab states that form the Arab League in addition to non-Arab Muslim-majority countries (e.g., Turkey, Iran, and Pakistan). (2) "Is the human subject afraid of exposing deeply rooted illusions, which may disturb their alleged psychic stability?" Two more questions follow these and require epistemological answers: (3) "What are the epistemic factors for excluding Ibn Rushd?" (4) "Is the human subject afraid of descending to relative thinking instead of ascending to absolute thinking?"

The last question has to do with Wahba's neo-Kantian distinction between secularization and fundamentalism. Wahba (2022) defines secularization as *thinking of what is relative in relative terms* and fundamentalism as *thinking of what is relative in absolute terms*. As to the epistemic factors for excluding Ibn Rushd, they are numerous and include (a) the intellectual tension between philosophy and theology when it comes to *fiqh* (Islamic jurisprudence), (b) political transformations within the Almohad Caliphate during the reign of Yaqub al-Mansur (1184–1199), (c) changes in the authority's cognitive map, (d) a literalist turn to traditional religious texts following the Ẓāhirī school, and (e) the later charges of apostasy or heresy, popularized by the proto-Salafi theologian Ibn Taymiyya, which were leveled against the Commentator (i.e., Ibn Rushd) for his metaphorical approach to jurisprudence. For a thorough account of Ibn Rushd and his philosophy, see Beshara (2024b).

Ibn Rushd viewed philosophers (and not theologians) as closer to Allāh because they valued *the authority of reason*. Whereas the theologians were sophists, the philosophers were logicians, who approached religious texts through a hermeneutical methodology of allegorical interpretation, which allowed for two potential readings: a latent reading and a manifest one. This was later understood by the Scholastics as the Double Truth Theory and was foundational for the secular separation of Church and State. In other words, Ibn Rushd was interested in the unconscious of the Qur'ān since it revealed Allāh's desire. After all, *the unconscious is the Other's discourse*, and what is the Qur'ān but Allāh's discourse? Recall that God is the unconscious, for Lacan.

Ibn Rushd's translations of, and commentaries on, Aristotle were partly responsible for the Renaissance, so there would not have been Descartes without Ibn Rushd, and there is no Freud without Descartes. However, more importantly, Franz Brentano lectured on Ibn Rushd at the University of Vienna (cf. Brentano, 1977). Brentano's Aristotelianism/Averroism, or his empirical approach to psychology as a human science, influenced his students tremendously, leading Edmund Husserl to establish phenomenology and Sigmund Freud to invent psychoanalysis. Ellie Ragland (2004) develops an erudite account of the Aristotelian foundations of

Freudo–Lacanian psychoanalysis, but John Hendrix (2015) underlines the theoretical lineage from Ibn Rushd to Freud through Brentano:

> According to Franz Brentano, Averroes' active intellect makes "images intelligible in unconscious thought," and the material intellect "receives from the images the concepts of sensible things." Perhaps Brentano's attribution of unconscious thought to Averroes was discussed in his philosophy seminars at the University of Vienna, attended by Sigmund Freud.
>
> (p. 12)

According to Wahba (1980), the paradox of Ibn Rushd is that there is a strong intellectual tradition of Latin Averroism in Europe with no equivalent Rushdiyya (Arab Averroism) in the Arab-Islamic world. There have been numerous political attempts at reviving Ibn Rushd in the modern Arab world by diverse intellectual figures such as Mohamed Abduh, Farah Antun, Mahmoud Qasim, Mohamad Ammara, and Mohamed Abdel al-Jabri. Some scholars of medieval Islam, such as Anke von Kügelgen (1996), do not seem to be impressed with these attempts. She regards these "revivals" to be misreadings that serve the modern Arab intellectual's political agenda, which can range from causes as disparate as secularization and fundamentalism.

Having said that, I find von Kügelgen's (1996) harsh dismissal of modern Arab intellectuals to be Eurocentric, if not outright racist, particularly when she writes,

> it seems to me that the decisive inducement to actualize and instrumentalize Ibn Rushd is the desire to prove that Islamic culture is equal in value to Western culture. As long as this proof has not been furnished, Arabs can neither feel themselves to be equal in rank, nor will they be accepted by the West as equal partners.
>
> (p. 117)

In addition to the thinkers that von Kügelgen (1996) critiques in depth, we can add a list of other contemporary Arab philosophers, who have contributed positively to the project of Rushdiyya: Mourad Wahba, Mona Abousenna, Mohammed Arkoun, Nasr Hamid Abu Zayd, George Tarabishi, and Hassan Hanafi.

Wahba (2006) uses another metaphor for Ibn Rushd, which is helpful in our application of transmodernity *qua* liberation psychoanalysis. The *paradox* of Ibn Rushd can be resolved by using Ibn Rushd as a *bridge* between Totality and Exteriority. There is no clash of civilizations because human civilization is singular with many particular cultures; this is why we must write about the pluriverse, that is, civilization. However, there is indeed a clash of fantasies, which led to the ideological division between Totality and Exteriority along the material lines of colonial difference.

Non-European modernity was negated as savage, barbaric, or primitive. This is the colonial fantasy. However, there is also the fantasy of antimodernity, which is often conflated with decoloniality and entails rejecting anything originating from the Totality of Euromodernity. Sayyid Qutb, for example, who continues to inspire Salafi jihadists, believed that Euromodernity was nothing but crass ignorance (*jahiliyyah*), which is a codeword for pre-Islamic, wherein *Islam = the Absolute Truth.*

Terrorism (Islamic or otherwise) is not decolonial. Decoloniality is the rejection of coloniality, not modernity. Antimodernity is a regressive and reactionary fantasy of a return to a blissful time of organic harmony, which never existed and never will. Still, this time of the Pious Predecessors (*al-salaf al-ṣāliḥ*) is idealized and romanticized from today's perspective following the teachings of Ibn Taymiyya and Muhammad Ibn Abdul-Wahhaab. The fundamentalist's mythic relationship with their past actualizes as *the return of the repressed*, such as the sexual enslavement of Yazidis by members of the Islamic State of Iraq and the Levant (ISIL). Both colonial and antimodern fantasies manifest as mythic violence, an Exterior source of *mythic jouissance.* Adam Curtis (2004) analyzed the dialectical relationship between American neoconservatives and Muslim fundamentalists in *The Power of Nightmares. Divine jouissance*, on the other hand, has to do with *the knowledge of dreams*—i.e., dream interpretation or analysis.

On the surface, American neoconservatives and Muslim fundamentalists are official enemies in the "war on terror"; however, they are more similar than different because they share a nightmarish vision of the world, which stems from an unjust and false truth: the kernel of their respective death-driven fantasies. As such, both groups reject historical reason in favor of modernization (instrumental reason) or antimodernity (irrationalism), respectively.

Divine jouissance is a function of historical reason. Ibn Rushd believed that there should be no conflict between philosophy and religion. Still, if a conflict arose between philosophers and theologians, as a function of Imaginary aggressivity, one should resort to *the authority of reason.* This logical solution affirms the dialectical tension between rationalism and mysticism, which is resolvable through dialogue and interpretation on the line of Symbolic, while negating literalism as undialectical or dogmatic.

It is worth noting that Lacan's invocation of the Letter is not to be confused with dogmatic literalism. The Letter refers to *the materiality of the signifier vis-à-vis* chains of signification and figurative linguistic structures that necessitate interpretation. However, dogmatic literalism fixes the sign at the level of the signified, as a transparent and direct meaning, which happens to be the only correct one. This is why Wahba (2022) calls literalists, dogmatists, or fundamentalists as "the bearers of the Absolute Truth." They believe to have direct access to the Absolute Truth, and anyone speaking on behalf of the Truth without any sense of doubt is more likely to justify all sorts of unjust political actions. However, the secular path—as the ethical path of desire—recognizes the uncertainty of scientific knowledge, hence, the preference for epistemic relativism and allegorical interpretation.

Psychoanalytic accounts of Islam (e.g., Copjec, 2025; El Shakry, 2017; Pandolfo, 2018) have tended to assume that there is an isomorphic relationship between *aṣ-Ṣūfiyya* and psychoanalysis, implying that the unconscious is somehow mystical or irrational; this is clear, for example, in El Shakry's (2017) book on Egyptian psychologist Yusuf Murad, whom she dubs as "the Arabic Freud," when Egyptian psychoanalyst Mustafa Zewar actually deserves the title (cf. Ben Slama & Beshara, 2024; Kader & Beshara, 2023). El Shakry (2017) writes:

> I explore Islamic mysticism, or Sufism, as a particularly fruitful point of entry for thinking about the relationship between Islam and psychoanalysis in terms of the theorization of the relations among ethics, eros, and the unconscious. Like Michel de Certeau, I find that mystical religious literature often shared an epistemological alignment with psychoanalysis.
>
> (p. 8)

However, I read the unconscious, through a rationalist lens, as following an Other logic, which does not contradict historical reason. For example, my preference for Ibn Rushd, as a representative of Islamic rationalism, stems from an attempt to challenge the dominant trend of psychoanalytic Sufism or Sufi psychoanalysis. The unconscious is the discourse of the Other, and this discourse is part of an apparatus (racial capitalism), and can be historicized as such, particularly in relation to libidinal fantasies that drive the political economy. This does not mean that I do not appreciate what *aṣ-Ṣūfiyya* has to offer because one of my favorite texts, *Ḥayy ibn Yaqẓān*, is a classic Sufi text, which is considered to be the first philosophical novel; also, it happens to be authored by Ibn Rushd's mentor: Ibn Tufayl. Therefore, my challenge is in the spirit of opening up a new reading of Islamic psychoanalysis and psychoanalytic Islam (cf. Beshara, 2019a; Parker & Siddiqui, 2018). Having said that, I think that rationalists and mystics—the latter being empiricists of sorts, given their fidelity to direct experience—should band together against *the irrationalism of the literalists*, who are not able to see through their dogmatism because they take their nightmarish fantasies too literally instead of traversing them through Eros: sublimation, free association, etc.

(Counter)terrorism is acting out, whether it is state terrorism or religious terrorism. We must traverse (counter)terrorist fantasies. Transmodernity is a name for this traversal, which orients liberation psychoanalysis. We must liberate ourselves from colonial and antimodern fantasies by subjectifying the cause of analectical materialism. Transmodernity is the sublation of Totality and Exteriority, but it is "not one, not two," as the Zen saying goes. The paradox of modernity is that while it unquestionably unified the world, it did so through the divisive Totality of a colonial system: the apparatus of racial capitalism. Fanon (1961) was the first to write about colonial difference in *The Wretched of the Earth* (which should, technically, be titled *The Damned of the Earth*), "The colonial world is a Manichaean world."

Transmodernity is *not one* because the (un)translatability of cultural difference is a function of not only sexual difference but also colonial difference. In other words, the difference between the west and the rest (or the North and the South) is a question of the politico-libidinal economy. To put it differently, there is an isomorphism between the modern oppression of women and sexual minorities in the zone of being and the colonial violence against racialized peoples in the zone of nonbeing. The reader is encouraged in this context to juxtapose Tommy J. Curry's (2017) *The Man-Not* to Paul B. Preciado's (2021) *Can the Monster Speak?*

Curry's analysis of anti-Black misandry as the racial–sexual negation of the "Man-Not" and Preciado's interrogation of the "patriarchal–colonial" regime of sexual difference are demands for us to recognize that the (post)modern oppression of racialized/politicized women-not and men-not, though constitutive of Europatriarchy's binary logic, fails utterly to account for non-European and non-patriarchal experiences of sexuation, which are violently repressed yet return in the form of colonial difference. This colonial difference often manifests violently as either settler colonialism or franchise colonialism—the first type is also called internal colonialism or endo-colonization. However, colonial difference is experienced, too, as an oppressive specter in the form of coloniality—a psychic remainder of colonialism. In sum, sexuation, like capitalism, has always been racial. And, yes, the subaltern/monster can speak (and write)!

Curry's (2018) notion of *phallicism* or "the condition by which males of a subordinated racialized or ethnicized group are simultaneously imagined to be a sexual threat and predatory, and libidinally constituted as sexually desirous by the fantasies or fetishes of the dominant racial group" (p. 31), in particular, complexifies the Lacanian account of sexual difference and indicates the direction of what I have been writing about as *colonial difference* (cf. Derrida's critique of phallogocentrism). In my view, sexual difference–because of its location in the zone of being–is embedded in what I term *mythic jouissance*, which is the dominant form of enjoyment within Totality. Sexual difference describes the difference between masculine (phallic) *jouissance* and feminine (Other) *jouissance*. Sexual difference is ontogenic—and, to some extent, phylogenic.

Colonial difference, however, is sociogenic, and it unsettles the question of sexual difference from the zones of nonbeing and becoming, which include the perspectives of the colonized, the racialized, the politicized, the subaltern, the proletariat, the sexually oppressed, etc. As such, I claim that *divine jouissance* is a subversive form of enjoyment within Totality, which is tethered to Exteriority. I say *subversive* because many sub-oppressors internalize the hegemonic model of *mythic jouissance*. Therefore, traversing the phallic (and colonial) fantasy of *mythic jouissance* requires the transmodern subject to confront their lack of being, moving beyond the hysterical pursuit of a new master-signifier to find enjoyment in the life drive.

However, Derrida's deconstruction of phallogocentrism suggests that Lacan remains trapped in the very Aristotelian structure he attempts to transcend, since elevating lack to a central truth still anchors the world in a masculine logic of presence and absence: *having* the phallus vs. *being* the phallus. Curry further complicates this debate by arguing that these psychoanalytic and deconstructive frameworks are often Eurocentric, since they fail to account for *phallicism* within the structure of chattel slavery and beyond. Phallicism describes the racial–sexual process of *(un)genderization* that transforms the Black man into a ~~Man~~ characterized as a *hyper-masculine* sexual predator to justify their lethal oppression while remaining *hyper-vulnerable* to sexual violence and erotics that are ideologically denied under white patriarchy and "faux feminism" (Khader, 2024). Because Black males were historically excluded from the category of Man (as defined by a white supremacist patriarchy), they cannot be patriarchs in the same sense as white men, for they were positioned as objects of a totalizing projection, fungible commodities to be over-exploited. Coloniality, as a psychic remainder of colonialism, explains how the dehumanizing logic of phallicism functions as a colonial tool of social death, even after the end of slavery.

Curry's analysis does not deny the existence of horizontal violence among the oppressed, instead he is calling for an empirical approach that can account for complexity without uncritically employing reductive categories as self-evident explanations. For him, reductive categories such as patriarchy are essentially ideological and not scientific. I would even argue that these categories exhibit an Aristotelian or masculine logic of universality, as in *all men are patriarchs*. And this is exactly what I mean by faux feminism.

One antidote to faux feminism is Serene Khader's (2018) notion of "nonideal universalism," wherein "anti-imperialist feminism" comes to be defined negatively as "opposition to sexist oppression" (p. 8). Furthermore, for Khader, "transnational feminist praxis is a justice-enhancing exercise whose practical implementation requires actively attempting to offset imperialist idealizations" (p. 8). However, Curry (2021b) argues that non-ideal theory, which aims to provide a more accurate account of the real world than ideal theory, fails because it relies on "*abstractions of* social groups rather than *empirically informed theories about* social groups" (p. 22, emphasis in original). Pluriversality, then, is one alternative to nonideal universalism, which allows for multiple, empirically grounded ways of interpreting and reconstructing the world, as defined by the marginalized themselves.

For Curry, phallicism is not a universal fantasy structure to be traversed but a colonial tool to be dismantled for its negation or dehumanization of the Black male—i.e., Black boys and men. The same analysis applies to the Black female as ~~Woman~~; however, whereas the ~~Man~~ is in a contradictory relationship to white patriarchy, the ~~Woman~~ is in a contradictory relationship to faux feminism. For Curry (2021a), intersectionality is an example of faux feminism since it often renders the specific sexual vulnerabilities of Black males invisible because it assumes the male category always implies privilege, thereby reinforcing the phallic myth that Black men cannot be victims. Consequently, the apparatus of racial capitalism exploits the contrary relationship between ~~Woman~~ and ~~Man~~ to divide and conquer the oppressed. My perspective stretches Curry's analysis to the racialized and the politicized in general to include the experiences of political, ethnic, and/or sexual minorities around the world.

Curry's epistemological solution to the phallic fantasy is to stop interpreting the Black male through Eurocentric theories and start listening ethically to their lived experience with oppression and violence. As such, he proposes Black Male Studies as a sociogenic method of empirical analysis, a *genre* study of how the ~~Man~~ was dehumanized and excluded from the category of *gender*. Preciado's (2021) somatic revolution, on the other hand, is to "escape the serfdom of the binary system of sexual difference" (p. 13) through becoming queer, trans, or nonbinary. In sum, the transmodern subject does not seek to *be* or *have* the phallus, but works through the material conditions that make the phallus a colonial tool of necropolitics. I agree with Curry's and Preciado's critiques of the coloniality of sexual difference; however, we probably disagree on the liberatory potential of psychoanalysis as a radical politics of eros.

If the ideologies of secularism and fundamentalism are essentially mythic (as colonial and antimodern fantasies, respectively), then the praxis of *decolonial secularization* must be divine. What is philosophy—this love of wisdom—if not a form of secular spirituality (cf. Solomon, 2002)? In a similar vein, psychoanalysis can also be considered as a form of secular spirituality (Miller, 2010). Humanism—the most concrete practice of secular spirituality—restores the divinity of the subject *vis-à-vis* the Other in the here and the now through an emphasis on unconscious truth and social justice, that is, on scientific politics and an ethics of desire.

The mythic subject prefers idealizing the past or imagining their future self in heaven, but what of the earth now? The instrumental reason of coloniality and the irrationalism of antimodernity are both dehumanizing in their ideal detachment from *the materiality of the Other*. In the former, one is either colonizer or colonized. In the latter, one is either decolonizer or decolonized. However, decoloniality is not a sadomasochistic game of role reversal. Decoloniality is (dis)alienation as in *the humanization of all*. Does that mean that radical humanism exhibits a phallic function in its universalizing logic? Perhaps, which is why we must also insist on *decoloniality as the not-all* that affords us pluriversal forms of humanity.

Transmodernity is *not two* because it is the cultural pluriverse we call human civilization; to put it differently, the singular *is* pluriversal and vice versa. As above above, so below. As such, there is a parallel to be drawn between *the division of the subject* between ego and unconscious after the invention of writing/history and *the division of the world* between Totality and Exteriority after the overwriting of modernity/coloniality. Furthermore, there is a necessity for rewriting/translating the division of sexual difference and its relationship to colonial difference.

Writing is often a form of mythic violence, or Law-making, which confirms the proverb that "history is written by the victors." Claude Lévi-Strauss (1961) explicitly identifies these victors as enslavers or colonizers, asserting that "the primary function of writing, as a means of communication, is to facilitate the enslavement of other human beings" (p. 292). Derrida (1977) terms this mythic dimension of writing identified by Lévi-Strauss as "the violence of the letter," a concept Melanie McMahon (2023) historicizes by arguing that "the imposition of alphabetic writing entails a violent intrusion, one which is more or less synonymous with, and indeed inextricable from, European colonization" (p. 4).

Furthermore, McMahon posits that Athenian philosophy, emerging from the invention of the alphabet, served as both the ideological foundation of Western civilization and the material base of European colonization, which was premised on "the idea that oral cultures are *ipso facto* unworthy, and it begins with Plato—one of the first alphabetic thinkers" (p. 76). This foundational prejudice highlights why the Greek alphabet, as McMahon shows, was not just another writing system among many; rather, it became "the code of all codes." She concludes: "A code that begets all other such codes is 'universal' and universalizing. Its uniquely decontextualizing function features heavily in the movements and transplantations that characterize settler colonialisms" (p. 23).

While Djehuty is credited with inventing writing, the actual development of Egyptian hieroglyphs was certainly driven by the needs of the ruling, administrative class. Crucially, since hieroglyphs are a complex, non-alphabetic writing system that remained highly specialized and difficult to master, literacy was restricted to a small, elite scribal class rather than being widely disseminated. One can argue that although the Ancient Egyptian political structure was highly centralized and authoritarian—focused inwardly on maintaining cosmic order (Maat) and exploiting the Nile Valley's resources—its three-millennia span as a civilization was primarily premised on resource control and internal stability, not on the kind of large-scale, systematic, and universalizing colonialism associated with later alphabetic Western powers.

Writing fundamentally served as a method for establishing and maintaining the politico-economic power of the ruling class. This ideological dimension is the imperialist side of writing—its legal role in justifying the building and preserving of empire. The colonialist side, however, is what I term *palimpsestic overwriting*: the deliberate erasure of the colonized, the writing off of Other cultures, histories, and languages. Historically, as state-sponsored literacy expanded, it paradoxically introduced the conditions for its own inversion.

Tragedy, McMahon (2023) argues, was a response to what she terms "the trauma of literacy." The trauma of literacy was a function of the literal arbitrariness of any Law; an arbitratiness that renders Law senseless or irrational. McMahon writes, "Oedipus loves the Letter and the Law. He cannot fail to bear its incisions" (p. 43). As the embodiment of the State's legal and epistemic order, Oedipus represents the ultimate self-infliction of the trauma of literacy. His devotion to uncovering the truth inscribed in the prophetic text (the Oracle's Letter) turns the arbitrary and destructive power of the Law against him, so the lawmaker and sovereign that sought to uphold the Law was hoisted by its own petard. Therefore, the "divine violence" or Law-destroying capability of tragedy affords us a liberatory form of *counter-writing* or *counter-historicizing* (cf. Trouillot, 1995), which, in the hands of the oppressed, can entail turning the master's tools against the master.

The tragic form, by exposing the inherent contradictions and destructiveness of the Law, provides a counter-space, wherefrom the established legal order can be conceptually dismantled. Essentially, liberation, as counter-writing, enters into an analectical relationship with the Law, *viz.* fixed prophecy, or that which is written. This relationship is not merely a dialectical negation, but an ethical transcendence from the Exterior perspective of the traumatized, who aspire to actively rewrite their symptoms against all odds.

Foucault (1977) considers counter-writing to be a form of "counter-memory," which he defines as "a transformation of history into a totally different form of time" (p. 160). Indeed, there is *the linear time of historicism*, which organizes human history along a progressivist timeline defined from the perspective of Totality: prehistory → history (ancient → medieval → modern → postmodern). We can translate this timeline as such: orality → alphabetic writing (agricultural revolution → industrial revolution → digital revolution). Linear historicism stems from the dichotomy between orality and literacy, wherein orality signifies non-alphabetic (non-European) writing, and literacy means alphabetic writing, or the beginning of European history.

Then there is *the nonlinear time of historical materialism*, which can be framed following Bruno Latour's (1991) argument that "we have never been modern," which I would reframe as *we have always been modern*: present → past → future. I say this because the Renaissance, which came to define modernity, is the *rebirth* of modernity through a return to ancient philosophy, which synthesized science, art, and spirituality in a wholistic way. Europeanness (and, by extension, whiteness) was then constructed retroactively as a fixed ideological identity that always was, when the ancient world was not actually divided between 'Europe' and its Other.

In *Ethics of Liberation*, Dussel (2013) identifies three interregional systems (Egyptian-Mesopotamian, Indo-European, and Asiastic-Afro-Mediterranean) that preceded the establishment of the modern world system. For Dussel (1985), *modernity* began in 1492 with the *colonization* of the Americas, which is why decolonial scholars write about this tragic event as *modernity/coloniality*.

Ibn Rushd returned to Aristotle, but it was not a fantasmatic return to solidify a fixed ideological identity (e.g., Europeanness). Ibn Rushd admired Aristotle's scientific approach, which evinced a cosmopolitan move beyond ethnocentrism. It was not a question of liking Aristotle because Ibn Rushd identified with him as a 'European.' The context of the flourishing of Islamic philosophy was, of course, the Islamic Golden Age, which does not fit within medieval historiography. How can there be a Golden Age during the Dark Age? Unless the function of the Dark Age, as a theoretical construct, is to undermine (and cover over) the historical importance of Islamic philosophy, the paradoxical bridge between the ancient and modern worlds?

The historicist timeline of linear progress makes no sense unless we acknowledge the vanishing mediator of what Jim al-Khalili (2011) terms "Arabic science." The phrase "Arabic science" is meant to capture the history of a time when mainstream science was communicated primarily in Arabic, as opposed to English nowadays. Any signifier associated with Islam must be negated, however. Europe is Christian, or—as any historical revisionist would argue—Judeo-Christian. Or maybe Europe was always secular? Whatever the case may be, Europe never was and can never be Islamic.

After all, the "war on terror," as Bush (2001) tells us, is a continuation of the Crusades. We are also told that there is *a clash of civilizations*. The Cold War was a distraction. Forget about the red scare. The green peril is the enemy of Western

(Judeo-Christian) civilization. Never mind the historical materiality of al-Andalus, wherein Muslims ruled over the Iberian peninsula for nearly 800 years. Is it a coincidence that the Reconquista's success, or the Spanish crown's victory, resulted in the colonization of the Americas in 1492? Yes and no.

Christopher Columbus was trying to chart a new navigation route to India when he stumbled across Guanahaní (San Salvador Island) in the Bahamas. This is why the Indigenous peoples of the Americas were labeled 'Indians,' which also speaks to the Orientalism of the Spanish Conquistadors *vis-à-vis* the 'New World.' Is it a coincidence, too, that the Spanish Conquistadors perceived the Indigenous peoples of Turtle Island and beyond through the racializing lens of religious racism (anti-Semitism and Islamophobia, in particular)? The Spanish Crown's victory led to a racist policy against Jews and Muslims, who were forced to choose between two forms of alienation: either convert or be expelled! Conversion did not signify equal status in the new Spanish racial state, for converted Jews and Muslims were not considered to have "purity of blood" like Christians.

As such, the event of 1492 marks the beginning of religious racism on a mass scale, particularly since this imperial policy in the Spanish metropole informed the colonial policy against the Indigenous peoples of the Americas, who were the subjects of the Valladolid debate (1550–1551), a theological and legal debate between Juan Ginés de Sepúlveda and Bartolomé de las Casas about the humanity of Indigenous peoples and whether they possessed souls, to begin with; in other words, the argument centered on whether Indigenous peoples were even redeemable through conversion to Christianity, or whether they were no different from non-human animals, objects or things that can only be treated as commodities. This racial capitalist logic drove the civilizing—and, I would add, totalizing—mission of Euro-modernization, which was effectively accomplished through Christian colonization, primarily via the instrumental techniques of genocide and enslavement. But mythic violence was not the only means of oppression.

In addition to the literal (material) extermination of non-European peoples, there was also the metaphorical (ideological) erasure of their cultures and languages through the invention of whiteness, cultural assimilation, boarding schools, missionary work, scientific racism, etc. This is the dimension of overwriting, for *colonialism is a palimpsest.* Writing → Unconscious → History. Overwriting → Exteriority → ~~History~~.

To counter the ego, which fantasizes about mastering mythic writing, we must engage in unconscious writing, counter-writing, divine writing, arche-writing, automatic writing. To counter Totality, we must overwrite our Exteriority, not in the spirit of narcissistic self-assurance, but in service of historical reason, which recognizes *the humanism of not-all* (i.e., any one oppressed by the all). Overwriting our Exteriority will manifest as counter-palimpsests about our alter-modernity. In my case, I (over)wrote about the modernity of an ancient Egyptian god, a medieval Muslim philosopher, and a modern Arab intellectual.

Now, let us turn to Wahba's (2004) second question regarding Ibn Rushd: "Is the human subject afraid of exposing deeply rooted illusions, which may disturb their alleged psychic stability?" This is a leading question that echoes Freud's assertion that religion is an illusion or a fantasy that ideologically sustains reality. However, I would rephrase Wahba's question as: What was the unconscious desire behind the persecution of Ibn Rushd? This is also a variation on Wahba's first question.

First, we can identify a fundamentalist desire for religious purity and control, which was enacted defensively as the repression of intellectual freedom, for heresy (*zandaqa*) is impurity *par excellence* and is considered blasphemy (*kufr*) and apostasy (*ridda*). Ibn Rushd was exiled, and his books were burned despite his status as grand jurist of Córdoba.

The Persian Sufi poet al-Hallaj, for example, was executed for claiming, "I am the Truth," which was heard as "I am Logos." al-Hallaj's point was that he reached a point of *fanaa* (ego-annihilation), wherein Allāh (the Other of the Other) could unconsciously speak through him—psychoanalysts today would probably consider al-Hallaj to have a psychotic psychic structure. The persecution of heretics (rationalists and mystics alike) signifies a negation of the unconscious, which amounts to a foreclosure of the Name-of-the-Father, or metaphoricity as such. Unlike Christianity, Allāh in Islam is not a Father. That metaphor is not permitted. Metaphorization *vis-à-vis* Allāh, in general, is not allowed.

Nevertheless, there are the 99 names of Allāh, and these Beautiful Names (*Asma'ul Husna*) signify His divine qualities or attributes. Two of these names, for example, are included in the *Bismillah*, which begins every chapter in the Qur'ān: *Bismillah al-Rahman al-Raheem* (In the name of Allāh, the Most Gracious, the Most Merciful). The 99 names function as metonyms because the attributes are parts that refer to a whole that is greater than the sum of its parts. This gestalt can be translated in terms of the desire of the Other. The Muslim subject desires through Allāh or via the Qur'ānic unconscious. The problem with fundamentalism is the dogmatic belief that one *knows* Allāh's desire (i.e., the Absolute Truth) and, therefore, one is justified in judging others on His behalf. However, desire is unconscious, which can hypothetically drive the enjoyment of interpretation.

Conversely, philosophers like Ibn Rushd are curious about Allāh's desire, but their relationship to knowledge is not paranoiac. As such, they are humble about their relative understanding, even as advanced scholars, and what they offer or produce is not unlike psychoanalytic interpretation. Philosophers share the humility of analysts—a humility that is necessary to face the abyss of freedom. The literalism of the fundamentalist—a lack of humility—explains their psychotic symptomatology or their delusions of persecution. Fundamentalists feel perpetually persecuted, so—in their victim mentality or slave morality—they defensively project this insecurity by actually persecuting heretics like Ibn Rushd. This is the unconscious logic driving the practice of *takfīr*, which was championed by Ibn Taymiyya (1263–1328), the *grandfather* of Salafiyya. The title of *father* belongs to Muḥammad ibn ʿAbd al-Wahhāb (1703–1792).

al-Hallaj, on the other hand, represents the subjective destitution experienced after the end of analysis, wherein one can no longer conflate the truth of desire with the falsity of fantasy. al-Hallaj's enunciation, "I am the Truth" signifies his traversal from the singularity of being to the pluriversality of knowing, which I explore further in the concluding chapter to this book. al-Hallaj's enlightenment stems from his recognition of the falsity of being, as the egoic or Imaginary dimension of smokes and mirrors. This recognition allowed him to surrender to a direct experience with the Real unconscious *qua* Truth or Logos. His error was translating this untranslatable experience Symbolically using the signifier, "I am the Truth," which betrayed the materiality of his experience and ultimately led to his execution.

What is the Islamic unconscious, except the discourse of the Qur'ānic Other (i.e., Allāh)? al-Hallaj neither lied nor claimed to *represent* the Absolute Truth, like fundamentalists; rather, he spoke too truthfully about a spiritual encounter, which fell on traumatized ears. His execution symbolizes what I call *writing as a form of killing*, the Lawmaking and Law-preserving dimension of mythic violence (Benjamin, 1921). The Letter of the Law killed al-Hallaj because his body uttered the whole truth beyond the limit of mythic jouissance, something which Lacan (1998) warned about: "the whole truth is what cannot be told. It is what can only be told on the condition that one doesn't push it to the edge, that one only half-tells (*mi-dire*) it" (p. 92, emphasis in original).

It is worth invoking Peter L. Berger (1979) here, who argues that modernity is "the universalization of heresy." To be a heretic means to make a choice in the face of alienation, which implies unconscious thinking, as that which is *maktub*. After all, alienation is the first moment of metaphorization in our constitution as divided subjects. *Transmodernity then is nothing but the pluriversalization of heresy.*

The rationalism of Ibn Rushd's philosophical approach was considered heterodox; thereby, it was seen as a political challenge to the orthodox literalism of theologians. As such, dogmatic desire is the negation of critical thinking. Psychoanalytically, persecution is often a delusional symptom experienced by a psychotic subject. Is fundamentalism then a form of psychosis? After all, we know about the strong relationship between paranoia and knowledge, and the fundamentalist believes that *he*—and rarely *she*—*knows* because they have an *exclusive* access to the Absolute Truth. But why does the fundamentalist feel threatened by epistemic relativism? Perhaps their belief is on shaky grounds, to begin with?

Ibn Rushd's attempts to reconcile philosophy with theology triggered *a fear of Otherness*. Ancient Greek philosophy was Exterior to Islam, and in its Exteriority, it unraveled a latent question within Islamicate culture: *the question of the Other of the Other*. This is a question that eventually led to the double-Otherness of Islam. We can also think of Ibn Rushd's persecution in terms of superegoic censorship (cf. Strauss, 1988). As such, his persecution was the result of a projection stemming not only from psychic instability but also from social uncertainty. Superegoic censorship is not a sign of political strength. Rather, it signifies a teetering Symbolic order. Anoush Ganjipour (2021) frames this instability in terms of the political ambivalence of Islam:

> Islam has internalized two heterogeneous paradigms of authority: on the one hand, the monarchical paradigm and, on the other hand, the pastoral paradigm

> which is based on the idea of guidance. Monotheism, the divine government of the world, the relationship of God to men, prophecy: the Islamic tradition, from its genesis, has wanted to think and systematize all this from both the monarchical and the pastoral paradigms. It is thus the telescoping of the two paradigms that has structured the theological-political relationship of Islam as an ambiguous image.

In other words, the tension between reason and faith, exemplified by the work of Ibn Rushd, is essentially a Real tension within Islamicate culture (or any culture), which is not resolvable. In sum, the persecution of Ibn Rushd was a defense mechanism. We have yet to work through the paradox of Ibn Rushd in the Arab-Islamic world, particularly given that Giorgio Agamben (2000) argues that "modern political philosophy does not begin with classical thought [e.g., Aristotle] … but rather only with Averroism, that is, with the thought of the one and only possible intellect common to all human beings" (p. 10). Avveroism is the bridge, as Wahba reminds us.

For Agamben (2000), "the true political meaning of Averroism" lies in how Ibn Rushd "links the political vocation of man [or woman] to the potentiality of the intellect" (p. 141). Agamben recognizes the function of historical reason in Ibn Rushd's philosophical project, which prefigures modernity by centuries. In a sense, Ibn Rushd's model of the Active Intellect, a development of Aristotle's account, is a precursor to the Freudian unconscious *qua* psychopolitical potentiality. As Hendrix (2015) also argues:

> Averroes (1126–98) developed a concept of what can be called "unconscious thought" in the theory of active intellect … Union with the active intellect, the final entelechy, is the highest bliss in life. The suggestion of unconscious thought in Averroes' philosophy of intellect, was pointed out by Franz Brentano. Perhaps this was discussed in a seminar taught by Brentano and attended by Sigmund Freud at the University of Vienna.
>
> (p. 105)

If Djehuty inadvertently invented the historical unconscious, a surplus product of his invention of writing, then Ibn Rushd reinvented the unconscious by translating and rewriting Aristotle through the matrix of Islamic philosophy. Rewriting or translating breaks open the political field through the generative potentialities of interpretation and (re)construction. The historical reason of analysis—i.e., analectical materialism—is union with the Active Intellect, which is the telos or final cause of liberation praxis. Transmodernity signifies this union, a sublation that tarries with the negative.

Politics corresponds to the fifth and final stage (the genital stage) of Freud's model of psychosexual development. This is the discursive dimension of revolutionary love: *giving what one does not have*. Pre-Oedipal fixations, or regression in general, often manifest in the hateful form of reactionary politics because authoritarian tendencies within the subject are typically death-driven. Other jouissance signifies *non-phallic jouissance*, which refers to post-phallic forms of jouissance (e.g., genital, invocatory, and scopic). Whereas pre-phallic jouissance is mythic and reactionary, post-phallic jouissance has a divine and revolutionary potential. Conversely, latency corresponds to the passion of ignorance, which can be either crass or learned. As such, latency functions as a transitional phase between death-driven hate (authoritarianism) and life-driven love (libertarianism).

The oral drive is cannibalistic (because it is about incorporation), and the anal drive is sadomasochistic (because it is about controlling waste); these pre-Oedipal drives inform mythic forms of enjoyment: *eating the Other* or *treating the Other like sh*t*. The phallic drive is, of course, fantasmatic, which is why Lacan (1998) qualified this form of jouissance as masturbatory, for it is solipsistic, yet central in ideology, for fantasy is the Imaginary foundation of the social link between the subject and the Other.

On the other hand, the genital drive is about reproduction, which is polysemous and can signify everything from sexual reproduction to the social reproduction of life (childbearing and childrearing) and labor-power (Bhattacharya, 2017). Post-genital jouissance–through the Gaze and the Voice, for instance—tends to manifest as sublimation or the renunciation of the drives. Post-genital jouissance is cultural jouissance, a complex development of latent jouissance, that relies on hieroglyphic codes. One of the tasks of analectical materialism is to translate post-genital jouissance, through the pluriversal lens of transmodernity, as divine jouissance—*the collective enjoyment of historical reason* in its material manifestation as *the desire for the commons* in the Real, Symbolic, and Imaginary realms of ethics, politics, and aesthetics.

Chapter 3

A Decolonial Palimpsest

This chapter is a modified text of a talk (palimpsest) I gave for the 2022 Days of Assembly of the Lacan School of Psychoanalysis (LSP). The palimpsest was part of my formation as a research psychoanalyst. It marks my transition from being a pre-candidate of the School to becoming a candidate analyst. The purpose of the palimpsest was to express my desire to become a candidate analyst by writing over two foundational texts of the School written by André Patsalides and Nathan Adler. In the process, I attempted to deconstruct the palimpsest methodology through a decolonial meta-reflection.

When a colleague, who happens to be a well-respected Lacanian analyst, learned that I was applying to the Lacan School to become a research psychoanalyst, their advice was, "Don't hystericize them too much!" Of course, the unconscious translation of their advice is precisely *to hystericize the School*! Moreover, another analyst recently told me, "jouissance has nothing to do with culture." I immediately disagreed with them but was curious about what others thought, so I posted the quote on Twitter (X), and there was unanimous disagreement.

Therefore, I plan to hystericize you (the reader) by arguing that *jouissance has everything to do with culture* (cf. Klein & Vieira, 2024). That will be the thesis of my decolonial palimpsest. I wish to begin with André Patsalides (1992), not because Lacan analyzed him or because he was one of the founders of LSP, but because he speaks Arabic (my mother tongue, even though my mother is not an Arab) and, consequently, he has access to Arab culture—a culture to which I belong in an affiliative sense.

For Freud (1927), "culture is something which was imposed on a resisting majority by a minority that understood how to possess itself of the means of power and coercion" (p. 9). Freud specifies two cultural means of power and coercion: compulsory labor and the renunciations of the drives (p. 14). These means are essentially cultural demands that produce alienation in the subject, who is "virtually an enemy of culture" (p. 9), according to Freud. Compulsory labor is a function of the capitalist mode of production, but the renunciation of the drives points to the dimension of libidinal economy, about which Freud has a number of things to say.

Freud also writes about cultural chauvinism—which is how cultural difference becomes colonial difference—as the narcisstic enjoyment of a "cultural ideal" that

DOI: 10.4324/9781003768104-3

resolves "the hostility to culture within the cultural group" (p. 18). In other words, the enjoyment of one's culture is premised on the hatred of other cultures. Furthermore, this enjoyment sutures class struggle through the "identification of the suppressed with the class that governs and exploits them" (p. 18). This is how whiteness, as an ideology, functions, for instance, when the white proletariat is seduced to identify with the white bourgeoisie on the basis of an ideological fantasy (whiteness), thereby suturing the Real of class struggle and the Symbolic potential for working-class solidarity, regardless of 'race' or ethnicity. To enter into culture, like entering into language, implies becoming barred or losing something, which Freud qualifies as a *frustration* resulting from cultural *prohibitions* that produce an overall condition of *privation* (p. 14); the proletariat, in particular, struggle with a "surplus of privation" (p. 16), according to Freud. Surplus privation is the central contradiction within the capitalist mode of production that grounds our cultural uneasiness (*das unbehagen in der kultur*).

Our life-driven desire for liberation is sacrificed for cultural membership. Culture, however, is a double-edged sword, for it also prohibits the death-driven desire to oppress, since the State has sole monopoly over violence. In exchange for our sacrifices, Freud argues, "art offers substitutive gratifications for the oldest cultural renunciations" (pp. 18–19), which reveals the ideological function of art; however, art can be a subversive form of renunciation, too, an immanent critique of ideology, and a radical praxis. Freud does not reject this possibility when he claims:

> One might suppose that *a reorganization of human relations should be possible*, which, by abandoning coercion and the suppression of the [drives], would remove the sources of dissatisfaction with culture, so that undisturbed by inner conflict men [and women] might devote themselves to the acquisition of natural resources and to the enjoyment of the same.
>
> (p. 10, emphasis added)

Such a reorganization of human relations is what liberation psychoanalysis is about, and it entails reckoning with *cultural difference* without it slipping into *colonial difference*—for instance, Graeber and Wengrow (2021) show, through an extensive archeological archive across a long period of time, that "highly egalitarian organization has been possible on an urban scale" (p. 297). Cultural difference is *a Real difference beyond differences in language, religion, mode of production, customs, and traditions*. It is a paradoxical difference, which is lost in translation, because it is *a difference at the level of libidinal economy*, which has to do with enjoying a certain way of life, beyond questions of morality or even truth—except the subjective truth of unconscious desire, of course, which is singular in any case, hence, our uneasiness in culture. Cultural difference cannot be translated; however, it can be interpreted and (re)constructed, which is to say it cannot be decoded, but can be recoded through a tool such as liberation psychoanalysis. Bridging cultural difference entails an analectical sublation that does not resolve contradictions, but places them side by side as one constellation among many in an expanding pluriverse. This is what Dussel means by transmodernity.

André Patsalides, being of Greek origin, begins his essay with the Greek origin of the signifier 'palimpsest.' He writes that the word comes from 'palimpsestos,' which means "rubbed again" (1992, p. 1). Aside from the sexual associations with the act of rubbing, the repetition of this rubbing is what interests me, as indicated by the signifier 'again.' André did not mention that this signifier of traumatic enjoyment has a Proto-Indo-European root, which comes from *kwel- that becomes 'PIE' and then 'palin,' and eventually 'palim' through Greekification.

The root *kwel-, which can be traced back to Sanskrit among other ancient languages, means circle, and this image or symbol of a wheel (*chakra*) implies repetition. In other words, we are dealing with the drive, hence, the repetitive rubbing. When Hamlet fantasizes about suicide, he is speaking of the death drive, "To die, to sleep./To sleep. perchance to dream. Ay, *there's the rub,*/For in that sleep of death what dreams may come/When we have shuffled off this mortal coil/Must give us pause" (emphasis added). The rub, in Hamlet's soliloquy about being vs. nonbeing, is a reference to the traumatic Real, for the absolute master (death) is beyond symbolization.

Safouan (2002) confirms my thesis when he reframes Hamlet's famous statement to connect the question of being with the trauma of desire in relation to the phallus (-φ): "To be the phallus or not to be" (p. 85). For Safouan, Hamlet's "malediction of being" is a "phallo-narcissistic condition," which is a function of "primary masochism" (p. 85). Life is suffering, but death is unknown and unknowable; consequently, Safouan argues that "the destructive drive, hate, is the reaction of the creature to the negative force of the phallic image as *minus phi*" (p. 85, emphasis in original). What is worse: knowable suffering or the unknowable?

The colonial distinction between being and nonbeing is not merely a political or social reality, for it is internalized on a psychic level, manifesting as a *jouissance* of one's own suffering, a concept we will now explore. Being implies suffering, but nonbeing signifies thinking, that is, unconscious desire. Hence, Hamlet's analogy between dying and dreaming. The ego must die in order for the subject to dream. Hamlet's contemplation on ego-death is a sign of subjective destitution and marks his dissatisfaction (*duḥkha*) with unhappy consciousness as well as his curiosity about unconscious desire, which is uncertain (like death) because it is disguised or distorted by the rub. The rub, as an obstacle, structures our wish-fulfillment: we *do not know* what we want because *we do not wish to know* our desire. This not-knowing, at the heart of our nonbeing, drives our palimpsestic enjoyment.

Writing (like analysis) implies reading, and rewriting. When we write, we rub against what we read. So, we rewrite in order to rub again, but this time against what we just wrote: the Letter. This is the death-driven enjoyment of reading, writing, and rewriting; the enjoyment of what is literary, littoral, or literal, for the Letter kills. We enjoy this cycle, but this enjoyment is, of course, traumatic; it involves the negation of some signifiers, which structure what we write in the form of *traces*.

For me, this *supplementarity* is the dimension of culture not as a Symbolic order, but as a Real instance of the materiality of the signifier: the spirit that gives life.

The question of culture—as the regulation of human relations, which separates us from non-human animals (Freud, 1927)—is important because it has to do with the Symbolic order (of language and Law); therefore, it is a crucial theoretical question in psychoanalysis (cf. Zaretsky, 2004). The radical potential of psychoanalysis has to do, in many ways, with the radical Exteriority of Freud, being a non-European (Jew) in the anti-Semitic milieu of Vienna around the turn of the century, particularly under the mayorship of Karl Lueger, who inspired Adolph Hitler and provided him with a proto-Nazi model of fascist politics. This ideological and material contingency resulted in a bifurcation in the history of psychoanalysis. Freud was alienated between *assimilating into a racist European culture* and *critiquing this culture.*

Freud's (1913a) assimilation of racist ethnology represents *the ego of psychoanalysis*, which the school of ego psychology most concretely epitomizes, particularly with its misreading of *Wo Es war, soll Ich werden* as a strengthening of the analysand's ego through an identification with the analyst. Ego psychology's misreading reveals an assumption that follows the linear developmental logic of racist ethnology: savage id (analysand) → civilized ego (analyst).

Lacan's (2006) translation, or rewriting, corrects this error: "Where *it* was, there must *I* come to be as a *subject*" (p. 734, emphasis added). Becoming a subject is a cyclical process characterized by a constitutive lack, which must be subjectified as one's own. Furthermore, Freud's (1930/1961) critique of our *uneasiness in culture* sheds light on the radical potentiality of *the unconscious*. Kovačević (2007) makes this radical potentiality explicit in relation to *Wo Es war, soll Ich werden* when he writes:

> the subject enters the dimension of truth when it reveals itself as desiring. This leads to the establishment of a standard of truth independent from the standards, norms, and values of the existing social and political order, and hence opens an ethical dimension for refusal and revolt.
>
> (p. xiii)

Liberation psychoanalysis—*qua* the actualization of the radical potential of the unconscious—stems from the hysterical subject's fidelity to an ethics of desire as the foundation for a scientific politics capable of articulating unconscious truths. However, to sublate critique into praxis, hysterization must always be accompanied by analysis, as Nathan Adler (1992) argues:

> It is the task of psychoanalysis as a critical psychology to overcome the banality of secondary process, and to expose the unconscious which has been denied, disavowed, negated, isolated, repressed, and whose traces have to be decoded in manifest speech. Such a psychology reveals the heteroglossic and the polyphonic that the canon excludes, the decenteredness and plurality of the segmented self, as well as the pluralistic otherness of the other.
>
> (p. 13)

Whereas the ego of psychoanalysis may be characterized as European, the unconscious of psychoanalysis is most certainly non-European. The latter statement can be interpreted in at least two ways: either *the non-European unconscious is a negative universal* or *the (non)European unconscious is a complex pluriverse*. I see the validity of both interpretations, but I side more with the second interpretation, that is, of a pluriversal and complex (non)European unconscious.

One of my contributions, as an *analyst-in-(de)formation*, is to intervene through my cultural experience as an Arabic-speaking subject, who grew up in Egypt. This question of (de)formation is a topological distortion effected by the cause of analysis. As Said (1975) argues:

> a text is not whole, but *distorted*. For writing is not coterminous with nature, and therefore it *deforms* its subjects ... more than it forms them. Reading and writing have this in common: they are particular *distortions of general realities*. There is violence in texts, which is answered by the *reconstructions* of the examining critic.
>
> (p. 59, emphasis added)

As an examining critic, my reconstruction of analysis is a function of the toplogical distortions that stem from the fact that I speak and write from the position of a North African or Global Southern subject—a lacking subject of the (non)European variety, which entails *critique of the Other* and *self-criticism of the Other of the Other*. As such, I desire to work primarily with non-European analysands because I am skeptical about the assimilationist model of psychoanalysis, which presents itself as value-free when it is inherently Eurocentric, if not racist. Do non-European analysands need saving? Certainly not. They demand a critical space, within Totality or Exteriority, in which they can freely associate. The question is not "can non-European analysands speak?" Rather, "can European analysts listen?" Culture is paradoxically what prevents or allows free speech and ethical listening.

To clarify, by claiming that the unconscious of psychoanalysis is (non)European I am invoking the Exterior dimension of the Other of the Other, which is beyond the European unconscious *qua* the Other of psychoanalysis within Totality. It is my way of deconstructing the arbitrary distinction between Europeanness and non-Europeanness, which stems from not only cultural difference, but also colonial difference.

My intervention is not about an Imaginary identification between Arabic-speaking analysands and analysts, but concerns the specificity of the Arabic unconscious *vis-à-vis* the Symbolic and the Real registers (cf. Bou Ali, 2020). The same can be said about other non-European unconscious formations. However, I am speaking of the Arabic unconscious since I am most familiar with that. After all, Arabic is my mother tongue, despite my mOther being Polish.

André writes about the exilic nature of psychoanalytic subjectivity in relation to one's desire, a feature of modernity. This state of exile, however, is not merely metaphorical for Indigenous, Black, and Global Southern subjects here in the U.S.

Consequently, it is vital that psychoanalysts on Turtle Island consider the alterity of non-European unconscious formations as unique relations to time and place. For example, we must consider how the Real of coloniality—the underside of modernity—compounds the state of exile for non-European subjects. Hence, we must distinguish between *metaphorical exile* and *literal exile* when thinking about subaltern desire and enjoyment, as questions determined by the politico-libidinal economy.

There is no universal subject; there are pluriversal subjects. The myth of a universal subject is an ideology created by a specific cultural subject: the European bourgeois subject (Rozitchner, 2022). This ideology presents non-European proletarian subjects with an alienating illusion of choice: *either you are with us, or you are with the terrorists*—the T word is a contemporary substitute for barbarians, primitives, or savages.

I wrote my first book in the trilogy on this question (Beshara, 2019a), and I have argued for *an antiterrorist ethic beyond the discourse of (counter)terrorism*, which affords us *not-terrorist* and *not-counterterrorist* subjectivities. Should the reader experience a sense of resistance toward these claims, it may be productive to consider the frequency with which the psychoanalytic subject—though ostensibly universal—is functionally reduced to a masculine position within the existing literature. Is that universal or père-versal? A Lacanian may argue: "At least, Lacan spoke of feminine or Other jouissance." He sure did, but he never explicitly addressed how *jouissance* relates to the material history of European colonization, which made the theorization of psychoanalytic (modern) subjectivity possible.

In other words, I am pointing to the Real traumatic enjoyment associated with any particular culture, while thinking specifically of the asymmetrical (historical and material) power/knowledge dynamics between the Global North and the Global South. Patsalides writes, "Psychoanalysis has to clarify and articulate with precision its ongoing relation to religion, art and science" (1992, p. 4). Furthermore, he acknowledges the "local context of cultural specificities" (p. 5). These cultural questions are not separate from historical and material processes. The dialectic between *culture as ideology* and *the material forces of history* informs my thinking about psychoanalysis as a praxis that appears at a certain point in time and place. While psychoanalysis may not be universal, it has the radical potential to become pluriversal. I call this concretization—or this immanent critique of assimilationist psychoanalytic culture—*the worlding of psychoanalysis*, which resonates with what Derrida (1991) terms *geopsychoanalysis* and what Rahmat (2020) calls *planetary psychoanalysis*.

André writes, "The psychoanalytic project does not resemble religion" (p. 4). I do not find that statement satisfactory, and I doubt that psychoanalysis can pass the duck test. My argument is that psychoanalysis can function either as *an ideology* or as *a critique of ideology*. I have already associated the critical, or hysterical, approach with (non)European Otherness. The analectical move is to recognize these two contradictory tendencies within psychoanalysis, for they will certainly appear in our clinics, particularly when working with non-European analysands. I prefer to use the vague term 'non-European' over 'non-white' because I think that 'race' is not only a social construction, but also a racist formation (Gilroy, 2002). Therefore, 'non-European' does not refer to "non-white races," but to social groups that were racialized and/or continue to be negated by the Totality of modernity/coloniality through different forms of oppression and violence. Furthermore, (non)European indicates the interdependence between Europe and its doubly negated Other: ~~the Other of the Other~~.

Adler (1992) is also critical of the "immanent, universal, ontic process" with its "univocal unilinear elaboration" (p. 2). He adds that psychoanalysis "cannot establish absolutes or universals and must be embedded in socio-cultural and historic dimensions" (p. 15). Besides, he recognizes what I have alluded to as the *pluriversal unconscious*, particularly when he writes about "polyphonic others" (p. 8). My use of the loaded signifier 'culture' throughout is not meant to imply a retreat to identity politics; rather, with it, I wish to index the complex social world to which any singular subject is dialectically, or analectically, tethered. Another name for this dialectic, or analectic, is the psychosocial subject, as the fantasmatic link between the psychic (the ego, the unconscious) and the social (the *objet a*, the barred ~~Other~~). However, this singularity of being is not the one "the bourgeois order insists on" (p. 7), as Adler warns.

In sum, a decolonial palimpsest is an attempt at translating or rewriting, which delinks *coloniality as a logic* from the *rhetoric of Euromodernity*. As such, it is a meta-palimpsest (a palimpsest of a palimpsest) that aims to reveal an Other doubly negated by psychoanalysis: ~~the Other of the Other~~. The palimpsest of Euromodernity—to which psychoanalysis as a discourse belongs—is premised on the colonial erasure of non-European cultures and languages, that is, the overwriting of their ways of thinking and being. This colonial erasure is either *literal* through genocide and enslavement along with their ongoing racist legacies or *metaphorical* through the so-called civilizing mission with its deployment of Indian boarding schools and Christian missionaries. The aim of colonial erasure is assimilating difference into the same: Totality.

Given the location of LSP in San Francisco (on the unceded land of the Ramaytush Ohlone), it is central for us to think about the relationship between psychoanalysis and settler colonialism, for if this relationship is not theorized or, at least, spoken of, then we can fairly assume that coloniality—as a psychic remainder—is at work unconsciously not only in our clinics but also in our schools.

According to Bay Area Equity Atlas:

> The Ohlone are the predominant Indigenous group of the Bay Area, including the Chochenyo and the Karkin in East Bay, the Ramaytush in San Francisco, the Yokuts in South Bay and Central Valley, and the Muwekma tribe throughout the region. Other Indigenous groups include the Graton Rancheria community (Coast Miwok and Southern Pomo), Kashaya, Patwin, and Mishewal Wappo in the North Bay, and the Bay Miwok in the East Bay.

Naming these Indigenous tribes is beyond virtue signaling or fetishization since they are not abstract signifiers that denote some premodern history of no relevance today. These concrete signifiers are *transmodern signifiers par excellence*. For example, I am located in northern New Mexico on primarily Tewa land, and many of my students are Indigenous subjects, who are members of one or more of the eight Northern Pueblos of New Mexico: Taos, Picuris, Santa Clara, Ohkay Owingeh, San Ildefonso, Nambé, Pojoaque, and Tesuque—not to mention Navajo Nation (Diné). I am a guest on this land, neither native nor settler (Mamdani, 2022). Therefore, I am translating or rewriting my experience as an Egyptian immigrant, who is in solidarity with oppressed (ancestors and descendents) on Turtle Island. This is my positionality, or where I am coming from, and how it informs my politics of affiliation.

Psychoanalysis is irrelevant if it is merely a theoretical palimpsest that overwrites non-European ways of knowing. Psychoanalysis, however, can become radical when we are able to freely associate about what it is overwriting and erasing, so that we can organize around these questions in an effort to (re)construct more ethical clinics and institutions. Shedding light on the colonial logics of psychoanalysis stretches the theory and makes it worldly in its application. In other words, what is the political unconscious of psychoanalysis in the U.S. (Jameson, 1981), a settler-colonial society founded upon the genocide of Indigenous peoples and the enslavement of African peoples?

Racial capitalism is, first and foremost, a function of "primitive accumulation"—as an accumulation of not only capital but also waste (Kadri, 2023). Primitive accumulation explains the colonial structure of over-exploition through chattel slavery, which made European patriarchs extremely wealthy after the 15th century. Without primitive accumulation there would have been no industrial revolution in the 18th century. These oppressive and violent colonial conditions, among others, eventually led to the possibility of psychoanalysis existing as a modern praxis in the late 19th century. In other words, psychoanalysis is neither outside time and place nor beyond material and historical forces. As such, desire and enjoyment have everything to do with culture! This is not a call for canceling psychoanalysis, far from it. This is a call for uncanceling that which has already been canceled by centuries of colonial palimpsests: *the non in (non)European*. This uncancelation is the decoloniality of power, knowledge, and being.

Chapter 4

Lacan and Said

Edward Said had a passion for psychoanalysis, as Jacqueline Rose (2017) argues. This passion was twofold: (1) Said (1999) was in analysis for most of his adult life, as he confesses in his memoir *Out of Place*, and (2) he engaged with psychoanalytic theory since the late 60s to the extent of being of the main scholar who introduced psychoanalytic criticism to U. S. academia. In *Freud and Said* (2021a), I wrote about his theoretical engagement with Freud, particularly in three of his books: *Beginnings* (1975), *Orientalism* (1978), and *Freud and the Non-European* (2003). In this chapter, I wish to highlight some connections between Lacan and Said while thinking further about the centrality of psychoanalysis for Said's decolonial project *vis-à-vis* Orientalism in general and Israeli settler-colonialism in particular.

Said introduced Lacan as part of "French theory." To acknowledge Said's role, Timothy Brennan (2021) dubs him "the cicerone of French theory" (p. 168). Brennan adds, "His analysis was, to most ears, astoundingly novel and well ahead of its time. For it is easy to forget that most of these figures [e.g., Lacan] in French theory were still untranslated at the time" (p. 168). Said read French theorists in French and quoted them using his own translations. Said would later become disillusioned with "French theory," particularly the work of Michel Foucault, but he never gave up on Freud and psychoanalysis.

Curiously, Said found Lacan's psychoanalytic theory of language—with its emphasis on speech acts—more convincing than Noam Chomsky's cognitive theory of universal grammar. In 1971, with the publication of "Linguistics and the Archeology of the Mind," Said sided with Lacan over his close friend and comrade Chomsky, who was "utterly astonished that Ed could even begin to take *this stuff* seriously" (as cited in Brennan, 2021, p. 141, emphasis added). Said remained politically on Chomsky's side, but theoretically, he found "this stuff" or Lacan's theory of "language as pure creative expression" and "as the mirror of the unconscious and the structure of social and libidinal desire" more appealing.

In 1972, Said published a positive review of Paul Goodman's *Speaking and Language* titled "A Good Man Against Theories," which upset Chomsky because the book was critical of his linguistic theory. According to Brennan, Said recommended that Chomsky read Roland Barthes and Émile Benveniste, which Chomsky refused

DOI: 10.4324/9781003768104-4

to do. The latter regarded Goodman's approach to be "irreverent non-specialism" (p. 141)

Brennan (2021) explores the importance of psychoanalysis for Said in *Places of Mind*. For example, he writes, "Psychoanalysis stands as another neglected facet of Said's intellectual makeup" (p. 267). Brennan then quotes Said's childhood friend, Andre Sharon, who claimed psychoanalysis "is the key to Said" (p. 267). Brennan also confirms that Said was in personal analysis for more than 50 years: "Said began intense analysis as an undergraduate at Princeton and remained in therapy until the end of his life" (p. 268). One of my motivations for writing *Freud and Said* was to bridge the theoretical gap between psychoanalysis and postcolonialism–an artificial gap characterized by suspicion, hostility, or often ignorance. Brennan continues:

> [Said] threw himself into the psychoanalytic literature in the early 1970s, keeping close at hand a comprehensive bibliography prepared at the University of Buffalo's Center for the Psychological Study of the Arts ... He was, we know, busy at work in October 1968 preparing a piece (never published) on the connection between linguistics, psychology, and psychiatry for *The Hudson Review* that placed Lacan's 1953 Rome lectures on, among other things, speech and language in psychoanalysis and Chomsky's theories face-to-face.
>
> (pp. 268–269)

Said bent psychoanalysis to his will, and he stretched the theory in the direction of poetry and away from psychologization (in the spirit of Martín Baró)—as such, we can characterize his effort as a critical psychological intervention. According to Brennan, Said read not only Freud and Lacan, but also André Green and Christopher Bollas. As I show in *Freud and Said*, he was particularly impressed with Freud, not as a human scientist but as a modern writer. For Said, "the first psychologists were poets" (as cited in Brennan, 2021, p. 271).

Said was interested in developing an "Arab theory of mind" but never did. Brennan writes, "With 'self' on the agenda, psychoanalysis was on full display in the 'Withholding' essay, which Said described as 'a critical psychohistory of contemporary Arab reality'" (p. 144). Said wrote the Arabic essay "Withholding, Avoidance, and Recognition" (1972), which was published in the literary journal *Mawaqif* (Beirut); it addressed Arab intellectuals in the aftermath of the *al-Naksah* (setback) of 1967—an event that politicized Said's consciousness and the consciousness of all Arabs at the time, including the Syrian Marxist Sadiq Jalal al-Azm, who wrote *Self-Criticism after the Defeat* (2011), and was one of Said's staunchest critics along with Aijaz Ahmad.

As such, the seeds for Said's 1978 magnum opus *Orientalism* can be traced back to his earliest response to *al-Naksah* with his first political essay, "The Arab Portrayed" (1968). "The Arab Portrayed" began Said's unfinished project of an "Arab theory of mind." In 1972, Said wrote, "The Arabs since Avicenna [Ibn Sina] and Ibn Khaldun (who borrowed from Aristotle) have never produced a theory of mind" (as cited in Brennan, p. 269). Said intended to produce this theory through his passion for psychoanalysis and Arabic literature, particularly the writings of Naguib Mahfouz, whom Said praised for the "psychological depth of his representations of character and for capturing the 'special mode of Arabic psychological experience'" (p. 269).

In "Linguistics and The Archeology of Mind," Said (1971) writes, "Within the Freudian project, psychoanalysis is not only a technique of interpretation, but also an archeological exploration of the patient's subjectivity" (p. 105). He then adds, "It is to these oppositions [such as 'the opposition between the apparent stability of discursive language … and the discontinuities of the essential human functions'] that on the one hand the psychological linguistics of Noam Chomsky and, on the other, the linguistic psychoanalysis of Jacques Lacan address themselves" (p. 108). Whereas Chomsky's model is an "archeological quest," or a search for origins, Lacan's model acknowledges "the absence of a continuous sequence of dimensions, the absence of a road with signs" (p. 107). While Chomsky "hopes for an achieved discovery," Lacan realizes "that the object of the quest, the *arché* or Origin" is either "unreachable" or "indescribable" (p. 107, emphasis in original). This theoretical distinction explains Said's later preference for beginnings over origins in his overlooked masterpiece, *Beginnings: Intention and Method* (1975).

Said writes about Lacan in a flowery manner. He recognizes him as "the center in France of Freudian thought," particularly because of his "celebrated return to Freud" (p. 124), and describes him as "a first-rate clinician" (p. 125). Still, Said confesses, "A simple characterization of Lacan's theories is impossible" (p. 124). He continues, "Reading Lacan is quite unlike reading anyone else. His *style* bears no resemblance whatever to Freud's" (p. 124, emphasis added). This question of style is central to Said's project because it concerns *subjective (de)formation*, or how the subject is formed *and* deformed by language (cf. Said, 2006), which I referred to in the previous chapter in terms of *topological distortions*. Lacan's late style, in particular, is known for being the least accessible as a result of his turn to the Real, which is accomplished through an adventurous—and at times, nonsensical—exploration of set theory, topology, knots, and algebraic mathemes.

Said writes that Lacan's "manner is aphoristic and declaratory, and what he seems to be trying to create is a disturbing psychodrama" (p. 125). Lacan was known to be bombastic during his Seminars, exuding an expressionistic performance style informed by surreal aesthetics and traceable to his early affiliations with Salvador Dalí and André Breton. For Brennan, French theory is "speculative aestheticism" (2021, p. 1411). Nevertheless, even though Said finds Lacan's style profoundly challenging, mirroring the opacity of the unconscious itself, he admires his "constant striving for density, poetic insight, and anti-literal expression" (p. 125).

While Said was sympathetic toward French theory and unimpressed by the cognitive revolution, heralded by Chomsky, he also wanted to position himself in a third place, uniquely his own, which would eventually lead him to establishing "postcolonial studies" with the publication of *Orientalism* in 1978, the first book in a trilogy that also includes *The Question of Palestine* (1979) and *Covering Islam* (1981).

Orientalism was interestingly followed by a sidequel, *Culture and Imperialism* (1993), which addressed the methodological deficiencies of Foucault's archeological/genealogical method of discourse analysis.

In *Culture and Imperialism*, Said develops an original decolonial methodology—a contrapuntal reading strategy—and moves beyond a mere discursive analysis of Orientalism by highlighting numerous examples that function as counter-discourses/counter-practices (or praxes) of cultural resistance in subaltern literature and beyond. Said's disillusionment with "French theory" comes to its zenith in 2000 with the publication of "My Encounter with Sartre" in *London Review of Books*. While the story dates back to 1979, a year after the publication of *Orientalism*, the timing of the publication is significant: The Second Intifada. Said's reevaluation, twenty-one years later, amounts to an indictment of French theory's idealism, or its disconnection from material practice:

> When I arrived, I found a short, mysterious letter from Sartre and Beauvoir waiting for me at the hotel I had booked in the Latin Quarter. 'For security reasons,' the message ran, 'the meetings will be held at the home of Michel Foucault.' I was duly provided with an address, and at ten the next morning I arrived at Foucault's apartment to find a number of people – but not Sartre – already milling around. No one was ever to explain the mysterious 'security reasons' that had forced a change in venue, though as a result a conspiratorial air hung over our proceedings. Beauvoir was already there in her famous turban, lecturing anyone who would listen about her forthcoming trip to Tehran with Kate Millett, where they were planning to demonstrate against the chador; the whole idea struck me as patronising and silly, and although I was eager to hear what Beauvoir had to say, I also realised that she was quite vain and quite beyond arguing with at that moment. Besides, she left an hour or so later (just before Sartre's arrival) and was never seen again.

Said (2000) continues:

> Foucault very quickly made it clear to me that he had nothing to contribute to the seminar and would be leaving directly for his daily bout of research at the Bibliothèque Nationale. I was pleased to see my book *Beginnings* on his bookshelves, which were brimming with a neatly arranged mass of materials, including papers and journals. Although we chatted together amiably it wasn't until much later (in fact almost a decade after his death in 1984) that I got some idea why he had been so unwilling to say anything to me about Middle Eastern politics. In their biographies, both Didier Eribon and James Miller reveal that in 1967 he had been teaching in Tunisia and had left the country in some haste, shortly after the June War. Foucault had said at the time that the reason he left had been his horror at the 'anti-semitic' anti-Israel riots of the time, common in every Arab city after the great Arab defeat. A Tunisian colleague of his in

> the University of Tunis philosophy department told me a different story in the early 1990s: Foucault, she said, had been deported because of his homosexual activities with young students. I still have no idea which version is correct. At the time of the Paris seminar, he told me he had just returned from a sojourn in Iran as a special envoy of *Corriere della sera*. 'Very exciting, very strange, crazy,' I recall him saying about those early days of the Islamic Revolution. I think (perhaps mistakenly) I heard him say that in Tehran he had disguised himself in a wig, although a short while after his articles appeared, he rapidly distanced himself from all things Iranian. Finally, in the late 1980s, I was told by Gilles Deleuze that he and Foucault, once the closest of friends, had fallen out over the question of Palestine, Foucault expressing support for Israel, Deleuze for the Palestinians.

Said was disillusioned with French theory because it was not a praxis that could be applied to material problems, such as the Israeli–Palestinian 'conflict.' Toward the end of his life, Said returned to Freud, but this time the return was not mediated through Lacan or French theory. Said (2003) saw himself in Freud, a racialized subject living in the west: a (non)European.

For Said, Freud embodied a radical third position beyond Lacan and Chomsky, which opens up the possibility for revolutionary praxis. For Freud (1939), Moses was an Egyptian (i.e., non-Jewish). For Said, Freud was Jewish (i.e., non-European). The psychoanalytic lesson here is that *non-identity politics* is the necessary foundation for solidarity between Jews and Palestinians as (*non*)Europeans. Instead of identifying as Jewish or Arab, the lesson that Said draws from Freud is that we must identify with the negative, the *non*: the unconscious.

Chapter 5

The Importance of Freudo–Lacanian Psychoanalysis to Liberation Praxis

In this chapter, I argue for the importance of Freudo–Lacanian psychoanalysis to liberation praxis by briefly unpacking the following concepts: language, the unconscious, the Gaze, and singularity. But, before I do that, I would like to begin by defining *liberation praxis*. *Praxis*, a key signifier for both Marx and Freire, is the merging of theory and practice or reflection and action. In this sense, psychoanalysis, as a science of the unconscious, is a praxis: a theory of psychical structures (neurosis, perversion, and psychosis), as functions of different forms of negation (repression, disavowal, and foreclosure), which is applied in the clinic and beyond. In essence, psychoanalysis entails working through numerous forms of negation.

The praxis of psychoanalysis is *dyadic*, between analyst and analysand, and *dialectical* in the tradition of Socrates, Hegel, Marx, and Freire. The dialectic between analyst and analysand echoes the one between the subject and the Other—any representative of the Symbolic order for the subject. This Symbolic Other is distinguished from Imaginary others (other egos) because it is an abstract authority figure, whose representative function transcends any concrete subject or being. The Symbolic order is the register of language and Law in which we are born and which, subsequently, forms us as subjects to it. The praxis of psychoanalysis has a radical potential because its dialecticism is not merely dialogical but, more significantly, psychosocial. The analectical moment (i.e., transmodernity/decoloniality) is a further sublation of the Totality of modernity from the perspective of Exteriority.

What of liberation? The meaning of the dialectic, as a liberatory tool, has changed over time, for it is a method of working out contradictions in order to arrive at truth (and, by extension, justice): for Socrates, the method was through dialogue between two individuals; for Hegel, it was through the sublation of two opposing ideas; for Marx, it was the historical struggle between two classes (the bourgeoisie and the proletariat); and for Freire, it was the codependent relationship between the oppressor and the oppressed, which can manifest, on a micro scale in the classroom, as the teacher–student dialectic, or, on a macro scale, as the interdependent relationship between the colonizer and the colonized.

The analyst and the analysand are certainly two individuals or subjects, but they can also represent two ideas or positions (*a* and $), come from different classes, and reenact oppressive dynamics that exist in our larger social context. At the heart of

DOI: 10.4324/9781003768104-5

psychoanalytic praxis is a Real antagonism between the individual and the collective, which must be dialecticized: we are who we are as a function of our place in the collective, yet our singular being is a symptomatic form of existence that also leads to our sense of uneasiness in the culture (*das unbehagen in der kultur*).

In other words, we yearn to become liberated from oppressive individuals, ideas, and groups. But this unconscious desire is inherently psychosocial or extimate; therefore, liberation praxis is *the collective liberation of all speaking beings* at the very least, but I would go further, following both the bodhisattva ideal and kincentric ecology, and ambitiously call for *the collective liberation of all sentient beings*. Potawatomi botanist Robin Wall Kimmerer (2013) grounds the bodhisattva ideal in a concrete utopian framework of kinship that is materially embedded in the very Indigenous language of Bodwéwadmimwen itself:

> In Potawatomi 101, rocks are animate, as are mountains and water and fire and places. Beings that are imbued with spirit, our sacred medicines, our songs, drums, and even stories, are all animate. The list of the inanimate seems to be smaller, filled with objects that are made by people. Of an inanimate being, like a table, we say, "*What* is it?" And we answer *Dopwen yewe*. Table it is. But of apple, we must say, "*Who* is that being?" And reply *Mshimin yawe*. Apple that being is.
>
> *Yawe*—the animate *to be*. I am, you are, s/he is. To speak of those possessed with life and spirit we must say *yawe*. By what linguistic confluence do Yahweh of the Old Testament and *yawe* of the New World both fall from the mouths of the reverent? Isn't this just what it means, to be, to have the breath of life within, to be the offspring of Creation? The language reminds us, in every sentence, of our kinship with all of the animate world.
>
> (p. 56, emphasis in original)

This shift from 'what' to 'who' represents a Symbolic order that negates the mechanistic othering of the natural world (Merchant, 1980)—which reduces it to a series of Imaginary objects (commodities) for the ego's consumption and fetishization—instead affirming the Real Otherness of nature, where the breath of *yawe* functions as the *objet a*, the elusive spark of life and spirit that forever eludes total human mastery. The facticity of our *interbeing* (Hạnh, 1998) provides us with more clarity, as we think and act through the ongoing environmental breakdown, which is a function of a modern/colonial binary opposition: 'man' vs. nature.

Carolyn Merchant (1980) argues that the Scientific Revolution effected a total transformation of the western worldview, shifting from an *organic model*—which viewed nature as a living, nurturing mother—to a *mechanistic model* that reconceptualized the Earth as a dead, inert machine. This "death of nature" stripped the environment of its inherent spirit and agency, removing the moral constraints that had previously limited its exploitation. By reducing the natural world to predictable, mathematical matter, Enlightenment thinkers, like Francis Bacon and René Descartes, justified a relationship of mastery and domination, where 'man' stands apart from and superior to a de-animated world. Significantly, Merchant reveals that this shift was not just a scientific advancement, but a cultural and patriarchal project that redefined nature as a mere commodity to be managed and consumed.

The 'man' vs. nature binary opposition, however, is not dialectical; it is a false dilemma that follows an alienating either/or rhetoric, which is sustained by a self-over-Other logic. A dialectical approach, like analectical materialism, situates the human subject in the materiality of their environment without reducing them to a biological essence, such as 'race.' *Man* is code for so-called European humanity, while *nature* subsumes non-European sub-humanity, that is, material resources or things to be extracted, commodified, over-exploited, and/or exterminated.

The 'barbarian' lives outside of Totality, while the 'primitive' exists in pre-modernity. The over-exploitable 'savage' becomes civilized through their assimilation into the here and now of Totality—as such, *assimilation is the double negation of non-European difference*. The *man vs. nature* binary opposition is the instrumental reason of modernization/colonization, but it gets twisted under fascism to become *man vs. culture*, wherein the fascist subject is conceived as an organic part of nature while culture becomes an index for non-European, or non-Aryan, *things* (e.g., Jews, Roma, Slavs, etc.) that endanger the fantasy of a perfect union. In other words, under fascism, nature becomes a *substitute* for civilization, while culture *displaces* savagery. While Merchant's liberal 'man' sees nature as a dead machine to be used and abused, the fascist 'man' sees nature as a blood-and-soil essence that justifies his terroristic violence. In both cases, the Real Otherness of the living world is ignored in favor of an ideological fantasy of Imaginary (w)holeness through total instrumental mastery or mythic organic unity.

However, the human subject cannot be reduced to a cultural essence, which is the narcissistic tendency of any form of nationalism and the core of all authoritarian (fascist/totalitarian) projects. The human subject is *the Real gap between biology and culture*. Biological and cultural racists reduce the Other to an essence in an effort to suture this Real gap that characterizes all speaking beings.

Rather than Being-in-the-world, we are *interbeing-with-the-environment*, which does not suggest that interbeing and environment are ontologically identical. Instead, it is a realization of our intricate, interconnected relationship with all forms of life—one based on a model of kinship, not just identity. This distinction is crucial. History has shown how a philosophical concept like 'Being' can be used to justify exclusion and harm. Heidegger's idea of 'world' came to mean *the Nazi world*, which excluded the 'Being' of the non-Aryan Other (Di Cesare, 2017). Therefore, my use of the signifier 'environment' indexes a far more expansive *world*, for it refers to the biosphere as a global life system—a Real Otherness, an animate materiality that actively participates beyond the idealism of the modern world system, but whose demands for regeneration, integrity, reciprocity, and autonomy are denied within the ideological matrix of Totality. This is an important distinction because, in the narrow and delusional world of racial capitalism, the environment is often ideologically reduced to 'nature' as a *thing* to be tamed, a savage site of infinite material resources to be extracted, commodified, and over-exploited—if not exterminated.

Language

Lacan (1966/2006) famously wrote, "the unconscious is the Other's discourse" (p. 10, emphasis in original). Psychoanalysis, known facetiously as the talking cure, is radical in its emphasis on language, the site for unknotting complexes in the psyche. The talking cure aims not to make us normal, or even normative, within the Law, but to help us find a singular way of speaking that is not just a carbon copy of the Other's discourse. This insight stems from the reality that we are born into a pre-existing Symbolic order—a concept Lacan adapted from Lévi-Strauss—whereby the structures of society function like the rules of grammar. Within this system, we are split. Drawing on Benveniste's distinction between the enunciating subject and the subject of the statement, the "I" who speaks is never identical to the biological being represented by this linguistic marker or shifter.

Upon entering language—a process mediated by our primary caregivers—we become barred subjects ($), caught in the tension between our biological needs and the cultural demands of the Symbolic order. Our entry into language is simultaneously an entry into the Law, wherein, as subjects, we are forced to trade our animal immediacy for a place within a pre-existing system of social mediation and linguistic exchange. Having internalized this strange and complicated system called language, we begin to articulate our desire through it, albeit through the distorted topology of the symptom.

For Lacan, the subject is a product of the signifier rather than its master. The barred subject ($) represents the internal division created when the Saussurean *bar*—the line separating the signifier (*S*) from the signified (*s*)—*cuts* through the individual, alienating them within a *gap* between instinctual needs and cultural demands. The process of subjectification, according to Lacanian psychoanalysis, is more sophisticated than Althusser's Marxist theory of ideological interpellation, for ideology is a discursive-fantasy, which does not take into account the materiality of the Real—a traumatic materiality that is not only economic but also libidinal.

Consequently, the cut that results from the alienating or castrating effects of the sign is the very birthplace of desire. Simultaneously, the linguistic bar implies a gap, which is filled by the signifier as "what represents the subject to another signifier" (Lacan, 1966/2006, p. 964). Because our needs can never be fully represented by the signifiers we use to express them, a *surplus* remains. This psychic remainder is desire, which is forced to circulate endlessly through the metonymic chain of signifiers, forever seeking a satisfaction that language itself has rendered impossible. Liberation psychoanalysis must work through the coloniality of desire, that is, the unconscious desire for coloniality.

While desire follows a somewhat linear, metonymic chain of signification—constantly sliding from one signifier to the next—the drive is nonlinear, and its inertia gets disrupted by a distortion in the Symbolic fabric of spacetime: the gravitational pull of the *objet a*. The drive is thus caught in the orbit of this object-cause of desire, circling a central lack—the hole in our tubular Symbolic order. This repetition of the drive represents the materiality of the signifier in its most insistent form. Here, the Letter does not communicate or convey meaning; it anchors the subject in a singular, repetitive circuit of *jouissance*.

This is how the Letter kills: it imposes a signifying fixity upon the body, transforming libido into a site of the death drive. In this distorted topology, the subject fantasizes about a dark, twisted satisfaction in the symptom—a repetitive script that simultaneously voices their desire and bars them from realizing their fantasy of organic unity. What we want, as subjects of the signifier, is unconscious and comes to us from outside.

As a "virus from outer space," language carries an external morality that precedes us; we do not just learn to speak, we are spoken—or, rather, infected—by a system of repression and oppression. Subjectivity, then, is the complex of signifiers that informs *what we desire* and *how we enjoy our symptoms*. Liberation praxis involves moving from being a *parlêtre* (a being spoken by the Other) to a driven subject who can traverse the fantasy. If language is a virus, then praxis is a mutation, effected by the cause of liberation.

Because the unconscious is the Other's discourse and is "structured like a language" (Lacan, 1966/2006, p. 737), it is inherently psychosocial and not personal or individual. We desire through the Other, we desire the Other, we desire to be desired by the Other, and we desire what the Other desires. Desire is a linguistic phenomenon that has to do with the movement of signifiers (e.g., metaphoric condensation and metonymic displacement). This psychoanalytic emphasis on language is not a denial of the body; on the contrary, language is inscribed on our very bodies, it is materially embodied, which is why we experience symptoms that do not have a biological cause, yet are bodily symptoms. This is what Lacan refers to as *the materiality of the signifier*. The Letter kills because it is the inscription of the symptom, which is another way of speaking about how the death drive structures our singular form of enjoyment beyond the pleasure principle.

It is precisely within this materiality of the signifier that the possibility for liberation praxis resides. By traversing the fantasy of organic unity and confronting the lack in the Other, the subject can move from being a passive victim of the drive's inertia (the subject-as-demand) to an active agent (the subject-as-drive). Liberation, then, is not an escape from language, but a reconfiguration of the Letter—transforming the symptom into a *sinthome*, a singular tool for navigating the Symbolic order without being crushed by its weight.

The Unconscious

The unconscious decenters the ego and sheds light on the primacy of the psychosocial over the psychic. If the unconscious is psychosocial, then it is also the site where the Law is most fragile. Consciousness-raising is important, but it will not succeed without *unconsciousness-raising*, which is a political intervention at the level of the Other's discourse. According to Malherbe (2023):

> Unconsciousness-raising initiatives strive to recognize how unconscious desire obstructs and/or advances the political goals of the collective, thereby allowing subjects to change their relationship to their desires, or indeed use these desires to foster solidarity and bolster their commitment to a collectively constituted emancipatory project.
>
> (p. 460)

In other words, to be antiracist one has to also speak of an *antiracist unconscious*, which implies transforming *the culture of racism* and replacing it with an *antiracist culture*. To put it differently, *the subject cannot be antiracist as long as the Other is racist*. We may look at the racist Other in a judgmental way, but that will not alter the fact that we are locked into the habit of racializing others, whom we (mis)perceive to be different from us. 'Race' is indeed a social construction, a function of the racist Other's Gaze. Every subject living inside a racist culture internalizes racism regardless of their 'race.' However, not everyone is racialized in the same way.

The *colonial unconscious* is the logic sustaining the rhetoric of the modern subject. For Dussel (1995), "The 'I-conquistador' [or 'I-conqueror'] forms the protohistory of Cartesian *ego cogito* and constitutes its own subjectivity as will-to-power" (p. 43, emphasis in original). Grosfoguel (2013) develops Dussel's argument further and writes:

> What links the 'I conquer, therefore I am' (*ego conquiro*) with the idolatric, God-like 'I think, therefore I am' (*ego cogito*) is the epistemic racism/sexism produced from the 'I exterminate, therefore I am' (*ego extermino*). It is the logic of genocide/epistemicide together that mediates the 'I conquer' with the epistemic racism/sexism of the 'I think' as the new foundation of knowledge in the modern/colonial world. The *ego extermino* is the socio-historical structural condition that makes possible the link of the *ego conquiro* with the ego cogito.
>
> (p. 77, emphasis in original)

For Žižek (1998), the Cartesian subject is the "monster" that remains when we subtract from the subject the wealth of self-experience that constitutes subjectivity (p. 7). In other words, the Cartesian, or modern, subject of psychoanalysis is a dehumanized/dehumanizing subject that has not come to terms with the traumatic Real of coloniality: the double negation of the being and thinking of non-Europeans.

Given the Cartesian cogito's, or the modern subject's, foundation in coloniality, it is essential that we try and conceive of *a pluriversal subject* from the perspective of transmodernity. Dussel's (2002) notion of transmodernity, as the sublation of modernity and its alterity, affords us such a possibility. The colonial difference between Totality and Exteriority has resulted in a further division of subjectivity: *double-unconsciousness*.

My theorization of double-unconsciousness is grounded in W. E. B. Du Bois's (1903/2007) account of "double-consciousness," which results from the "two-ness" of non-European subjects. Non-European subjectivity is doubly divided, particularly in the context of Totality. For Du Bois, 'race' is a veil, which screens racialized subjectivity. Coloniality is a further abyssal layer beyond modern alienation, as explicated by Descartes (being vs. thinking) and Freud (ego vs. unconscious). 'Race' is a screen onto which racist fantasies are projected, and which also functions opaquely to block the consciousness of the Euromodern subject from perceiving the Exteriority of non-European ways of being and knowing.

For Du Bois, two-ness is not only a curse, but also a gift of "second-sight," which allows the non-European subject–specifically, the African American subject–to perceive both themselves in their Exteriority and how they are (mis)perceived, or racialized, within Totality. Liberation praxis treats the unconscious as a map of the enemy's territory within us—this is a function of internalization. By unknotting the complexes, we reclaim the libido that was previously used to maintain a destructive symptom and redirect it toward collective action or creative production in the form of a creative *sinthome*.

The cultivation of an antiracist unconscious is not merely a cognitive shift but a topological one. If the double-unconsciousness of the racialized subject provides a second-sight, it also provides the raw material for a *pluriversal subject*. Liberation praxis here involves more than recognizing how the Other racializes us; it requires using the second-sight of Exteriority to map the *ego extermino* that haunts the modern psyche. By redirecting the libido away from the racist Other's demands and toward a pluriversal praxis of liberation, the subject undergoes a *transmodern becoming*. In this state, the subject no longer seeks to be seen, recognized, or validated by an oppressive/violent Totality, but instead acts from the singular authority of their own *sinthome*, effectively raising the political unconscious of the collective toward a kinship model that transcends the Totality of the modern/colonial world system.

The Gaze

Unfortunately, many confuse the look with the Gaze. The confusion can be traced back to early psychoanalytic film theory, which is known as Screen Theory. In her 1975 essay, "Visual Pleasure and Narrative Cinema", Laura Mulvey wrote about film spectatorship *qua* the "male gaze." While this phrase is popular today and sounds feminist, it is actually non-psychoanalytic and maybe even antifeminist, since it equates spectatorship with maleness.

In her 1989 essay, "The Orthopsychic Subject: Film Theory and the Reception of Lacan," Joan Copjec not only cleared the confusion between the look and the Gaze in psychoanalytic film theory, she also inaugurated Lacanian Film Theory by anchoring it in the register of the Real—that which can neither be imaginarized nor symbolized. The confusion between the look and the Gaze is a function of Screen Theory being more Foucaultian than Lacanian, wherein the Gaze is conceptualized in terms of panopticism, as exemplified by the all-seeing eye of the guard in the Jeremy Bentham's Panopticon. The *panoptic look* is shot through with misrecognition (*méconnaissance*), for it is essentially an Imaginary look of mastery that has to do with a power/knowledge fantasy, rather than unconscious desire *per se*.

The *anamorphic Gaze*, on the other hand, is on the side of the screen (not the spectator), or on the side of the prisoners (not the guard). In other words, the Gaze is always on the side of the object (not the subject), for it is the form of the *objet a* in the scopic drive. To put it differently, the Gaze is that which we cannot see but which causes our desire through its absence. This absence is not necessarily a lack in the image, but is often a distortion in the visual field, a stain, or an opacity, which requires effort from the spectator (subject) in order to be experienced.

Lacan's (1977/2004) most famous example of the Gaze is a 1533 painting by Hans Holbein called *The Ambassadors*. In the painting, Holbein used a technique called *anamorphosis*, wherein a distorted human skull at the bottom center of the painting can only be seen from a specific angle. The skull, which symbolizes the absolute master (death), stains the painting by reminding viewers that the vain merchants, who are showing off their wealth, are mortal beings, as are the spectators.

Because anamorphosis drives the viewer to move in order to see the distorted object, this example demonstrates that the viewer is not a passive recipient of the painting but an active participant, a subject, whose unconscious desire is caused by the painting's Gaze. The same principle is at work in cinema, but given the wide range of dynamic film techniques, there are more opportunities for film spectators to experience the Gaze. Todd McGowan has written extensively on the filmic Gaze, most importantly in *The Real Gaze: Film Theory After Lacan*.

The example that I would like to use is Albrecht Dürer's (1525) *Draughtsman Drawing a Recumbent Woman* (see Figure 5.1). The draughtsman on the right exemplifies the subject's look, as informed by the structure of male fantasy; however, the recumbent woman on the left represents the *objet a*'s anamorphic Gaze. In other words, she is not only objectified by the male fantasy, but also subjectifies

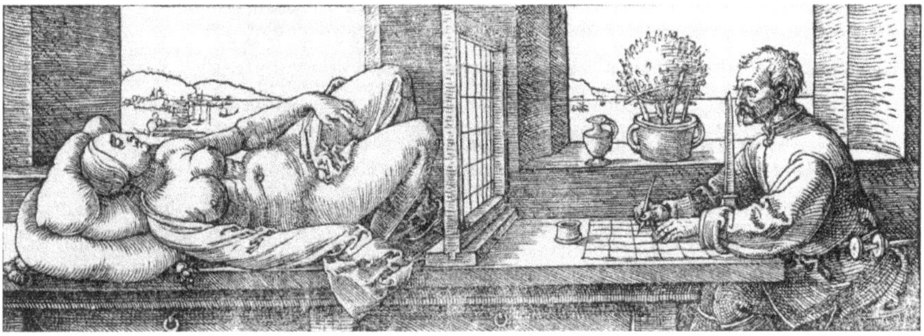

Figure 5.1 Draughtsman Drawing a Recumbent Woman (Dürer, 1525)

the draughtsman by causing his desire—like an analyst *vis-à-vis* an analysand in the clinic.

The Real Gaze is a more nuanced approach than that of the "male gaze," which actually negates female, and feminine, subjectivity. The look-Gaze dialectic may be applied beyond sexual difference to colonial difference, for instance, wherein we can speak of *a colonial patriarchal look* vs. *a decolonial feminist Gaze*. Liberation requires subjective destitution—the moment when the subject realizes that the Other (e.g., patriarch) does not exist or is itself lacking. When *the pluriversal subject-as-drive* stops mistaking *the look of the other* for the Real Gaze, they are finally free—beyond the fundamental fantasy of good and evil—to enjoy their existence. This decolonization of the Real Gaze, through anamorphically subjectifying the cause of one's desire, is empowering, to say the least.

Singularity

There is a transversal link between the singular and the universal. It is this link, which illustrates the continued relevance of psychoanalysis, as a science of the unconscious. However, given the specific context of the development of psychoanalysis in Austria in the late 19th and early 20th centuries, we must also speak of *pluriversality* in order to acknowledge the cultural difference between the Global North (the west) and the Global South (the rest). This cultural difference is Real—that is, politico-libidinal—as a function of the hegemonic dominance of the racial capitalist order of Totality (modernity/coloniality) since 1492.

In other words, there is universality to psychoanalytic concepts *vis-à-vis* modern subjectivity, but this universality must be put into question, if we are interested to account for transmodern subjectivity from the decolonial perspective of Exteriority. As such, we must think about not only the singularity of being, but also *the singularity of becoming*. The being-nonbeing dialectic is structured by the material history of colonial difference; however, analectical materialism moves us in the direction of *transmodern becoming*.

Identity politics is premised on the primacy of particularity, which is rooted in cultural essentialism. The question of cultural difference is one of linguistic and historical materiality *vis-à-vis* modernity/coloniality. For example, while I was born and raised in a particular culture (Egypt), I am a singular subject who can only represent himself, however imperfectly. My historical link to my particular culture is both linguistic and material, but that does not mean that my politics is premised on my identification with being Egyptian. On the contrary, I am much more interested in identifying with a non-identity politics of affiliative solidarity that links singular transmodern subjects with a pluriversal praxis of liberation, and this is what I mean by *transmodern becoming*. As such, the task of liberation psychoanalysis is decolonizing both *the Other through ideology critique* and *the Other of the Other through self-criticism*. The aim of our task is to traverse colonial and antimodern fantasies, which ideologically sustain the apparatus of racial capitalism in both Totality and Exteriority.

True liberation praxis, therefore, does not aim at restoring a lost wholeness or returning to a pre-linguistic nature, both of which are Imaginary traps. Instead, it seeks to identify the subject's singularity of being. This singularity resides in the *sinthome*—the specific, irreducible way in which a subject knots together the Real, the Symbolic, and the Imaginary to survive the lethal power of the Letter. While the universal Law of the Other demands conformity and produces suffering, the *sinthome* is a creative compromise with the drive's unceasing inertia. Liberation lies in identifying with one's symptom—transforming the repetitive, dark satisfaction of the drive into a singular form of enjoyment that no longer seeks validation from the Other. In this shift from symptom to *sinthome*, the subject is no longer a victim of a viral language, but a singular mutant of their own enjoyment.

Chapter 6

A Liberation Psychoanalytic Account of Racism

Lacanian Psychoanalysis as a Theoretical Resource for Critical Psychologists

Lacanian psychoanalysis has been a theoretical resource for critical psychologists at least since the 1970s in the English-speaking academic world. Lacanian psychoanalysis particularly found a place for itself in the journal *Ideology & Consciousness*, which years later metamorphosed into an important edited volume titled *Changing the Subject: Psychology, Social Regulation and Subjectivity* (Henriques, Hollway, Urwin, Venn, & Walkerdine, 1984/1998).

Ian Parker (1999) writes that *Changing the Subject* "was a powerful inspiration for *those* who wanted to rebuild something of the 1970s radical psychology movement in the 1980s" (p. 5, emphasis added). In a sense, Parker was partly referring to himself when he wrote "those;" his reference was more generally representative of the Discourse Unit, which he co-founded with Erica Burman in 1990. I say this because his record (Parker, 2001, 2003a, 2005, 2010a,b, 2011, 2014a,b) dwarfs similar contributions from his colleagues in terms of quantity—Parker happens to be the most cited critical psychologist and Lacanian, according to Google Scholar, with more than 25 thousand citations. However, in terms of quality, there is significant scholarship on Lacanian critical psychology from Parker's comrades (e.g., Malone, 2000; Pavón-Cuéllar, 2010). As a Marxist psychoanalyst, Parker has written extensive critiques of capitalism and psychology, but the work of critiquing racism and colonialism is being carried out by a new generation of Lacanian critical psychologists. Hence, Lacanian critical psychology is broader than any one master; it is the praxis of many scholars, activists, and practitioners.

Parker has indisputably been the most productive critical psychologist writing on Lacanian psychoanalysis, which will be my main focus in this section as a way of introducing this chapter. Parker's productivity, as a Lacanian leftist, is punctuated by a radical ethico-political commitment to comradeship beyond the bourgeois academic sphere. This is the theme underlying his recent collaboration with Pavón-Cuéllar, for instance, *Psychoanalysis and Revolution: Critical Psychology for Liberation Movements* (Parker & Pavón-Cuéllar, 2021).

DOI: 10.4324/9781003768104-6

In addition to *Ideology & Consciousness*, it is also worth mentioning another journal of import, namely *PsychCritique: The International Journal of Critical Psychology*. Parker (1999) writes that this journal "started from the premise that psychoanalysis was the basis for an adequate critique of psychology" (p. 4). The reasoning for this is clear in Henriques et al.'s (1984/1998) section on theorizing subjectivity, wherein they argue that Lacanian psychoanalysis essentially provides us with a psychosocial account of subjectivity beyond the "individual–society dualism" (p. 203) because of its emphasis on language since "the workings of language provide a key to unconscious mental processes" (p. 213). Nevertheless, the authors are quick to list "some problems with Lacan's account" (pp. 216–218). Similarly, Parker, who is a practicing Lacanian psychoanalyst, does not use Lacanian theory as a critical psychological panacea, which is why the Discourse Unit relies on four theoretical resources, wherein each one keeps the other three in check:

> Marxism attempts to place feminism only within a socialist feminist framework, finds in Foucault much abstract talk about power which ignores class privilege in capitalist society, and sees psychoanalysis as the reflection of and prison of individualised misery. Feminism in turn is concerned at the way Marxism conceals the oppression of women in its narrative of the history of classes, the way foucauldians sabotage the idea of gender solidarity and consciousness, and the way psychoanalysis keeps smuggling in normative accounts of sexual desire. Foucauldians meanwhile are indignant at Marxism's continued adherence to totalising grand theory, at feminism's identification of power only with male designs, and at the psychoanalytic spiral of oppressive and self-blaming confession. Psychoanalysis then responds by characterising Marxism as the infantile search for ideal conflict-free worlds, feminism as pathological denial of sexual difference, and foucauldian work as a warrant for perversity.
>
> (Parker, 2003b, p. 9)

I want to end this section with a significant innovation from Parker, which sits at the intersection between critical psychology and Lacanian psychoanalysis, namely: Lacanian Discourse Analysis (LDA). LDA is a radical qualitative research method in critical psychology, which applies Lacanian theory, as a discursive analytic tool, to any and all textual material, such as transcripts of interviews, speeches, etc. LDA owes a great deal of debt to Jacques Lacan's Seminar XVII, *The Other Side of Psychoanalysis*, which primarily deals with his theory of four discourses (i.e., Master, University, Hysteric, and Analyst). There are undoubtedly important contributions—for an overview see Beshara (2019a, pp. 1–31)—between the publication of that Seminar (Lacan, 1991/2007) and Parker's writings on LDA, such as Mark Bracher's (1993) *Lacan, Discourse, and Social Change: A Psychoanalytic Cultural Criticism*.

In addition to the articles dealing with the method, which are about a dozen or so, there are primarily three books that fully explore LDA: *From the Conscious*

Interior to an Exterior Unconscious: Lacan, Discourse Analysis and Social Psychology (Pavón-Cuéllar, 2010); *Lacan, Discourse, Event: New Psychoanalytic Approaches to Textual Indeterminacy* (Parker & Pavón-Cuéllar, 2013); and *Decolonial Psychoanalysis: Towards Critical Islamophobia Studies* (Beshara, 2019a).

In this section, I have established Lacanian psychoanalysis as a major theoretical resource for critical psychologists, particularly as represented by the writings of Parker and his colleagues—a diverse group to which I belong. Furthermore, the reader is encouraged to explore the open-access peer-reviewed journal published by the Discourse Unit (*The Annual Review of Critical Psychology*), particularly volume 7 on "Lacan and Critical Psychology" (2009), and the two book series edited by Parker for Routledge: *The Lines of the Symbolic in Psychoanalysis* and *Concepts for Critical Psychology*.

What is critical psychology? For some, critical psychology is a sub-field within psychology, which critiques the discipline in order to save it from itself. For others (such as Parker et al.), critical psychology enacts a transdisciplinary deconstruction of the discipline of psychology from without. This *without* is psychoanalysis, the other side of mastery. In essence, psychology is a university discourse, which is subservient to the apparatus of racial capitalism, manifesting ideologically as the master's discourse of liberalism or conservatism. As such, for Lacanian leftists, psychoanalysis must be an antiracist (humanist) and anticapitalist (socialist) discourse.

In the next section, I evaluate some of the key Lacanian psychoanalytic accounts of racism (i.e., Lacan, Miller, Žižek, Seshadri-Crooks, and George) while bracketing some important interventions in the process (e.g., Khan, 2018; Lane, 1998; Mitchell, 2012) due to the limitations of space. Unquestionably, racism is not only a research topic that is poorly studied in mainstream (Euro-American) psychology, which Wetherell (2012) qualifies as "the prejudice problematic;" it is also, and more significantly, a psychosocial problem that necessitates an antiracist praxis from critical psychologists. In other words, we, as Lacanian leftists, must act upon our reflections if we are to eliminate racism from our societies.

Lacanian Psychoanalytic Accounts of Racism

In this section, I will be reviewing some of the major Lacanian psychoanalytic accounts of racism beginning with Lacan's brief remark on the topic. However, it is important to bear in mind the contentious place of 'race' and racism in psychoanalysis, so that the reader does not get the wrong idea that Freudo–Lacanian psychoanalysis is somehow inherently progressive as a critical psychological tool: "anthropological theories are to be found throughout Freud's work, giving rise to a covert racist subtext within the discourse of psychoanalysis" (Brickman, 2018, p. 3). The clearest example of this covert racist subtext is Freud's use of the psycho-anthropological concept of *primitivity*, which Brickman (2018) argues "is not simply a disinterested term signifying the earliest and often repressed stage of individual psychic development" but also a signifier that "functioned for Freud both as a psychological category and an anthropological one" (p. 4). Brickman (2018) adds:

> For the nineteenth-century anthropology from which Freud borrowed, the *primitive* referred to the earliest and most rudimentary stages of a universally conceived human evolution. In this anthropological sense, it referred to "savages" who were considered, by virtue of their differences from European cultural norms and their darker skins, to be less evolutionarily advanced than their European cousins. But for Freud *primitivity* also referred to the earliest psychosexual stages of development of the white, European child. The overlap of these two meanings meant that the concept of *primitivity* would move throughout Freud's work with metonymic force, allowing for the possibility of a continuous slippage between psychological and anthropological registers. *Primitivity* is thus the key to the racial economy of psychoanalysis, the watchword of a psychologizing discourse behind which is concealed an ideology of race.
>
> (p. 4, emphasis in original)

To be clear, I follow Alana Lentin (2020) in her formulation of "race as a technology for the management of human difference, the main goal of which is the production, reproduction, and maintenance of white supremacy on both a local and a planetary scale" (p. 31). Consequently, I understand racism as "a global hierarchy of human superiority and inferiority, politically, culturally and economically produced and reproduced for centuries by the institutions of the 'capitalist/patriarchal western-centric/Christian-centric modern/colonial world-system'" (Grosfoguel, Oso, & Christou, 2015, p. 636).

Television

The following excerpt is from a text titled *Television*, which was published in English for the first time in 1987 based on a 1973 program for French TV featuring Lacan lecturing and being interviewed by Jacques-Alain Miller (his son-in-law and the current leader of the Lacanian right):

> *From another direction, what gives you the confidence to prophesy the rise of racism? And why the devil do you have to speak of it?*
>
> Because it doesn't strike me as funny and yet, it's true. Without our *jouissance* going off the track, only the Other is able to mark its position, but only insofar as we are separated from this Other. Whence certain fantasies—unheard of before the melting pot. Leaving this Other to his own mode of *jouissance*, that would only be possible by not imposing our own on him, by not thinking of him as underdeveloped. Given, too, the precariousness of our own mode, which from now on takes its bearings from the ideal of an overcoming [*plus-de-jouir*], which is, in fact, no longer expressed in any other way, how can one hope that the empty forms of humanhysterianism [*humanitairerie*] disguising our extortions can

> continue to last? Even if God, thus newly strengthened, should end up existing, this bodes nothing better than a return of his baneful past.
>
> (Lacan, 1987, pp. 36–37, emphasis in original)

Even though Lacan never fully addressed the topic of racism beyond this brief exchange in *Television* and another passing reference in one of his most obscure texts known as *L'étourdit* (1973/2009), there are a number of theoretical insights that are worth unpacking from the above-quoted statement. First, Lacan links racism with *jouissance*—that is, enjoyment beyond the pleasure principle, which is sometimes rendered paradoxically as *painful-pleasure*. This linkage is foundational for later theoretical elaborations from Jacques-Alain Miller to Sheldon George.

For Lacan, racial difference (and consequently, racism) is premised on a difference in modes of *jouissance*, which is a non-essentialist account that goes even further than social constructionist theorizations of 'race.' In other words, the European racist subject looks down on the racialized non-European Other because of how they enjoy differently. However, the racist fantasy is inherently ambiguous, for it typically consists of two contradictory but superimposed fantasies: phobic and philic ones. For example, the racist dual-fantasy can manifest as overzealous admiration (e.g., "I love your hair, can I touch it?") mixed with subtle disgust (e.g., "how do you wash it?"). For this reason, in my research on Islamophobia, I radically ground antiracism in a third position beyond liberal-conservative modes of racist *jouissance*: learned ignorance (Beshara, 2019a). In this sense, *learned ignorance* provides antiracists with a way of traversing racist fantasies.

Second, Lacan frames racism not in terms of a civilizational clash, but in terms of *a clash of fantasies*. In fact, the most antiracist aspect here is Lacan's rejection of developmental logic—"not thinking of him as underdeveloped"—both as an economic discourse (i.e., the developed v. developing world) and a psychological discourse (e.g., Freud's stages of psycho-sexual development). Ultimately, as illustrated above, the rhetoric of psycho-economic development is rooted in a racist (anthropo)logic regarding non-European *primitivity*.

Third, when Lacan is talking about "the ideal of an overcoming" which drives "the empty forms of humanhysterianism," he is specifically diagnosing liberal racism—that is, the conceited position of most neoliberal subjects in the Global North today: "I am not racist, but…"—*vis-à-vis* humanitarianism-as-false-generosity (Freire, 1970, p. 54), or what has been aptly characterized as "humanitarian imperialism" (Bricmont, 2005) in the context of the endless "war on terror" (WOT).

The overcoming, or more specifically *plus-de-jouir*, which Lacan refers to is an ambiguous neologism that signifies both a lack and an excess of enjoyment. The ideal of overcoming at the heart of liberal racism, or even antiracism, explains why these strategies will always fail, for they are premised solely on conscious (mis) recognition, or a politics of *méconnaissance*, when they should be engaged in a radical effort of delinking from the racist unconscious, that is, the racist discourses of the modern/colonial Other. While not writing from a psychoanalytic angle, Kwame Ture and Charles Hamilton (1967) were aware of these two dimensions of racism (i.e., conscious–unconscious racism) when they distinguished between *overt–covert racism* and *individual–institutional racism.*

Finally, Lacan's prophecy about the rise of racism as a function of "the melting pot" ideology is salient because while some might imagine, for instance, one of the effects of globalization and mass immigration since the end of the Second World War being a reduction in the liberal subject's fantasies about Others; the lack of separation (i.e., the so-called melting pot, which is a monocultural metaphor) has the exact opposite effect: a clash of fantasies, which manifests in terms of nationalism, racism, fundamentalism, etc.

Lacan argues against subjects from a hegemonic culture imposing their own *jouissance* (e.g., 'freedom' and 'democracy' as empty signifiers) onto subaltern Others. To reiterate, the key is *separation,* for without it there is no difference. Here Lacan is clearly arguing for cultural pluralism, or a pluralism of modes of *jouissance*, which can neither be fantasmatically nor discursively sutured. Subsequently, cultural pluralism is another name for the traumatic Real beyond the ideological reality of the Symbolic-Imaginary order. The only way we can live with this traumatic Real is, I argue, through *the praxis of learned ignorance.* The *learned* aspect speaks to our conscious but radical antiracist effort of delinking from the racist unconscious. And the *ignorance* aspect points to our unconscious acceptance of Real (sexual–cultural–colonial) difference, that is, the incomprehensible mode of Other *jouissance.*

Extimité

Jacques-Alain Miller, Lacan's son-in-law and the editor of his Seminars among other things, developed Lacan's earlier account by emphasizing his psychosocial concept of extimacy (*extimité*), which signifies that the exterior (unconscious) is present in the (conscious) interior:

> In racism, for example, it is precisely a question of the relation to an Other as such, conceived in its difference. And it does not seem to me that any of the generous and universal discourses on the theme of "we are all fellow-beings" have had any effectiveness concerning this question. Why? Because racism calls into play a hatred which goes precisely toward what grounds the Other's alterity, in other words its jouissance. If no decision, no will, no amount of reasoning is sufficient to wipe out racism, it is indeed because it is founded on the point of extimacy of the Other. It is not simply a matter of an imaginary aggressivity which, itself, is directed at fellow-beings. Racism is founded on what one imagines about the Other's jouissance; it is hatred of the particular way, of the Other's own way of experiencing jouissance. We may well think that racism exists because our Islamic [sic] neighbour is too noisy when he has parties; nevertheless it is a fact that what is really at stake is that he takes his jouissance in a way different from ours. Thus the Other's proximity exacerbates racism: as soon as there is closeness, there is a confrontation of incompatible modes of

> jouissance. For it is simple to love one's neighbour when he is distant, but it is a different matter in proximity. Racist stories are always about the way in which the Other obtains a "*plus-de-jouir*": either he does not work or he does not work enough, or he is useless or a little too useful, but whatever the case may be, he is always endowed with a part of jouissance that he does not deserve. Thus true intolerance is the intolerance of the Other's jouissance. Of course, we canot [sic] deny that races do exist, but they exist in so far as they are, in Lacan's words, races of discourse, i.e., traditions of subjective positions.
>
> (Miller, 1988, pp. 125–126, emphasis in original)

It is not a coincidence that Miller, a French citizen, cites "our Islamic neighbour" in the context of his discussion of racism—it is also worth noting his error in using the adjective 'Islamic' to refer to Muslims. France happens to be one of the most Islamophobic countries in the Global North (Wolfreys, 2018), which attempts to impose its specific (read: ideological) mode of *jouissance* (i.e., secularism or *laïcité*) onto its Muslim subjects in particular, many of whom being the descendants of colonized subjects. France occupied Algeria, for example, for 132 years from 1830 to 1962. Decolonization was successful due in large part to the sustained anti-colonial efforts between 1954 and 1962 of the *Front de Libération Nationale* (FLN), which included revolutionary psychiatrist Frantz Fanon among its ranks.

Wolfreys (2018) characterizes French Islamophobia using the phrase "respectable racism," which is another way of describing the new or cultural racism of liberals as opposed to the old religious and scientific racisms of conservatives. Wolfreys (2018) writes with a psychoanalytic sensibility:

> The new racism is genteel and respectable, providing users with a sophisticated upgrade on the old while operating in a similar way. Metonymy, for example, the use of objects [e.g., the *ḥijāb*] to symbolise or embody race without having to spell out their meaning, is simply applied to a different set of things.
>
> (p. 41)

States legitimize Islamophobia, or render this form of racism respectable, particularly through the WOT discourse, which is sustained ideologically by fantasies about Islam being a 'primitive' religion or culture that is incompatible with, and therefore will endlessly clash with, modern/colonial civilization and its values. One does not need to deny the present reality of Islamic terrorism in order to clearly see the historical effects of the *longue durée* of colonial terrorism, from the colonization of the Americas beginning in 1492 to the scramble for Africa in the 19th century—not mentioning the rise of fascism in the 20th century, two world wars, and the so-called cold war.

While the 1.8 billion diverse groups of Muslims in the world are not a 'race,' they are certainly racialized metonymically (or with metonymic force), particularly in the Global North, in the context of the WOT discourse, which dates back to Ronald Reagan's first presidential term in the early 1980s. Therefore, while the (counter)terrorism discourse is fairly recent, the Islamophobia/Islamophilia fantasy predates the discourse by close to five centuries (Beshara, 2019a).

In sum, the extimacy of the Islamic, or non-European, Other—its own way of experiencing *jouissance*—is that which the European racist subject hates. Miller (1988) writes, "the Other's proximity exacerbates racism" (p. 125), which we can read historically in terms of the Judeo-Islamic Other's proximity in al-Andalus for close to 800 years—a fact that is repressed in the Euromodern unconscious. 1492 indexes both the collapse of al-Andalus—as a polycultural Caliphate—and the beginning of the colonization of the Americas. Anti-Semitic and Islamophobic fantasies are old, for they date back to the 11th century or since the Crusades, and they are foundational for later racist fantasies because they were projected onto, for example, the Indigenous peoples of the Americas (Beshara, 2019a, pp. 32–64).

Islamophobia is a reaction formation to the presence of Muslims in the Global North, who are positioned as outsiders (or immigrants) when they really signify the return of the repressed. For instance, in the case of the U.S., Muslims have been present on Turtle Island since at least the 16th century, with a case in point being the presence of Mustafa Azemmouri (1500–1539)—an enslaved Moroccan explorer—in what is now known as the State of New Mexico. But, more significantly, the transatlantic slave trade (16th–19th c.) brought to the Americas a large number of enslaved African Muslims: "between 2.25 and 3 million Muslims" according to Diouf's (1998, p. 48) estimate.

The Judeo-Islamic Other has been the exterior unconscious of the Euromodern subject (present in its conscious interior) since at least the 8th century. This extimacy, this proximity, is what makes Judeo-Islam and Jews/Muslims—as representatives for non-Europeans in general in the Euromodern unconscious—so disturbing to Euro-Christian racist subjects. At the heart of this violent (us v. them) dualism and oppressive hierarchy (civilized v. savage) is an attachment to a discourse or tradition of subjective positions—that is, an essentialist myth about racial origin (e.g., Europe is Christian, Greece is the cradle of Western civilization, etc.), hence, the ongoing clash of fantasies. A cosmopolitan sensibility towards world history, and particularly one grounded in learned ignorance, can provide us with the possibility of traversing racist fantasies: "Because I do not (and may never) understand the Other's mode of enjoyment, I accept that my specific mode of enjoyment is neither better nor worse, but different."

However, the real challenge is undoing racism at the cultural (or ideological) level, that is, exploding racist discursive-fantasies embedded deeply within the Symbolic-Imaginary order. Furthermore, the consequence of traversing racist fantasies may be moral relativism, which is a whole other can of worms. Suffice to say that this chapter is driven by *an ecocentric ethic* that I say more about later. I wish to end with the aporia that Miller has become of late a vocal representative of the Lacanian right. For example, he frequently indexes Islamophobic, anti-Arab, and anti-trans tropes in some of his recent writings and social media posts.

The Sublime Object of Ideology

Slavoj Žižek's (1989) first book in English, *The Sublime Object of Ideology*, was a very influential intervention in contemporary continental philosophy, which introduced the English-speaking world to the Lubljana school of psychoanalysis known for its unique synthesis of the ideas of Hegel, Marx, and Lacan. Žižek (1989) analyzes anti-Semitism, which for him is "the purest … form of racism" (p. 128), through the Lacanian concept of '*Che vuoi?*' (What do you want?). Žižek (1989) writes:

> in the anti-Semitic perspective, the Jew is precisely a person about whom it is never clear 'what he really wants' – that is, his actions are always suspected of being guided by some hidden motives …The case of anti-Semitism also illustrates perfectly why Lacan put, at the end of the curve designating the question *'Che vuoi?'* the formula of fantasy ($ ◊ *a*): fantasy is an *answer* to this *'Che vuoi?'*; it is an attempt to fill out the gap of the question with an answer … The crucial point that must be made here on a theoretical level is that fantasy functions as a construction, as an imaginary scenario filling out the void, the opening of the *desire of the Other*: by giving us a definite answer to the question 'What does the Other want?', it enables us to evade the unbearable deadlock in which the Other wants something from us, but we are at the same time incapable of translating this desire of the Other into a positive interpellation, into a mandate with which to identify.
>
> (p. 128, emphasis in original)

In other words, for Žižek, racism is a function of the European racist subject not knowing what the non-European Other wants, whose obscure desire, and therefore enjoyment, is a cause of anxiety. Once more, the radical antiracist lesson here is that one must be able to sit with this anxiety: "the unbearable deadlock" of not knowing the Other's desire. Racist fantasies are comforting to the anxious racist subject, for they suture the void of desire with "an imaginary scenario … a definite answer." Learned ignorance, on the other hand, is uncomfortable and even "unbearable" since it entails living with the anxiety of open questions. Learned ignorance is how we can translate the desire of the Other "into a positive interpellation, into a mandate with which to identify."

Žižek's analysis of anti-Semitism in *The Sublime Object of Ideology* and in some of his other works, such as *The Plague of Fantasies* (Žižek, 1997), represents the first sophisticated Lacanian psychoanalytic account of racism. Elsewhere in the book, Žižek (1989) formalizes Lacan's and Miller's crude theorizations of racism through his conception of "the *subject presumed to enjoy*" (p. 212, emphasis in original)—a variation on the *subject-supposed-to-know*. The racist subject, for Žižek (1989), is an obsessional neurotic, who fantasizes about saving "the Other from his [sic] *jouissance*, even at the price of destroying him or her" (p. 212, emphasis in original), which again explains the humanitarian imperialist impulse. The non-European Other, for the racist subject, "is always presumed to have access to some specific enjoyment, and that is what really bothers us" (p. 212).

In *Decolonial Psychoanalysis* (Beshara, 2019a), I draw a clear link between anti-Semitism and Islamophobia, particularly through the ideological figure of the *Muselmann*, which is the signifier that Nazis used for Jews in concentration camps because of how they would collapse on their knees from starvation and exhaustion. The Nazis used this signifier because they fantasmatically associated Jews, in those sadistic conditions, with *sujūd* (prostration) in Muslim prayer (*salah*). While I draw on Žižek's excellent analysis in my work, I also lament him for his under-theorization of Islamophobia given its affiliation with anti-Semitism since the Reconquista.

Desiring Whiteness

Kalpana Seshadri-Crooks's (2000) *Desiring Whiteness: A Lacanian Analysis of Race* is the first book-length treatment of 'race' and racism from a Lacanian perspective and it is an erudite study that builds upon the previous works I reviewed thus far through an engagement with what she calls "the system of 'desiring Whiteness'" (p. 9). For Seshadri-Crooks (2000), the foundational problem is 'race' itself rather than racism *per se*, particularly because of how the discourses of 'race' along with fantasmatic racializations sustain the ideology of whiteness, which informs how we desire and enjoy. She writes, "racial anxiety, the unconscious anxiety that is entailed by the sight of racial difference, has its cause not in ideology, but in the structure of race itself, and in the functioning of its master signifier, 'Whiteness'" (Seshadri-Crooks, 2000, p. 32). Whiteness, for Seshadri-Crooks (2000), is "the inaugural signifier of race" that "implicates us all equally in a logic of difference" (p. 3). She adds:

> By Whiteness, I refer to a master signifier (without a signified) that establishes a structure of relations, a signifying chain that through a process of inclusions and exclusions constitutes a pattern for organizing human difference. This chain provides subjects with certain symbolic positions such as "black," "white," "Asian," etc., in relation to the master signifier. "Race," in other words, is a system of categorization that once it has been organized shapes human difference in certain seemingly predetermined ways. We will therefore have to see how this symbolic structuration is related to visibility.
>
> (Seshadri-Crooks, 2000, pp. 3–4)

In the hollow structure of 'race' (even as a social constructionist discourse), racializations—or (mis)perceiving Others through the lens of 'race'—function as the fantasmatic quilting points (*points de capiton*), which suture the ideology of whiteness and, hence, give it its Symbolic-Imaginary coherence. In other words, racialization (and racial visibility) is always from the perspective of ideological invisibility (or whiteness), which leads Seshadri-Crooks (2000) to distinguish between the invisible white subject of the Imaginary and the hypervisible racialized subject of the Gaze:

> The difference between the visible body as an ego function, and the visible body as a function of Whiteness or racialization, can be understood as the difference between seeing and being seen. The subject of the imaginary is constituted as *seeing* by the signifier, whereas the subject of race is constituted as *seen*, the subject of the gaze, through a certain logic of the signifier.
>
> (p. 38, emphasis in original)

Seshadri-Crooks (2000) concludes her analysis with a radical antiracist thesis that traversing the fantasy of ideological whiteness can be accomplished through "symbolic passing," which she defines as

> one's relation to the signifier that is redefined. One neither submits nor resists its marking; rather, one assumes it and thereby makes it one's own. The (anxious) object of racial visibility has been traversed. It is "subjectified" to the point that it can no longer sustain the subject in the circuit of desiring Whiteness. One *passes* for what one *is*—a being in the world. The Other is simply snowed.
>
> (p. 131, emphasis in original)

Seshadri-Crooks's (2000) strategy of *Symbolic passing* aligns with Lacan's (2009) argument in *L'étourdit* that 'race' is "constituted according to the mode in which symbolic places are transmitted by the order of a discourse" (p. 15). In order words, the strategy of Symbolic passing problematizes and disturbs Imaginary, or anthropological, accounts of 'race,' which continue to be central to scientific and cultural forms of racisms.

Trauma and Race

Sheldon George's (2016) *Trauma and Race: A Lacanian Study of African American Racial Identity* explains 'race' and racism, particularly *vis-à-vis* the African American experience, as iterations of "a transhistorical *jouissance*" knotted around the "traumatic past of slavery" (p. 13). George (2016) writes:

> This past of slavery has produced both race and racism as modes of *jouissance*, as methods of accessing being. *Jouissance*, I would suggest, is embedded in the very signifiers of race themselves, which enable remanifestation of structures of enjoyment that bind subjects equally to concepts of race and to practices of racism.
>
> (p. 13, emphasis in original)

Like Seshadri-Crooks before him, George is problematizing the notion of 'race' itself, particularly because of how it has historically been cathected with a traumatic charge, since its *jouissance* can be traced back to the period of slavery. In other words, the signifiers of 'race' are haunted or cursed to the extent that there is no way of undoing racism without simultaneously undoing 'race,' for it is "a Symbolic remnant ... a link ... to the traumatic Real of slavery's *jouissance*" (George, 2016, p. 36, emphasis in original). The problem precisely is how to undo 'race' without falling back into facile post-racial discursive-fantasies of colorblindness. George (2016) continues:

> slavery and racism seek to bring about precisely a traumatic confrontation with lack and an unveiling of the subject's status as signifier. I call this confrontation the trauma of slavery, an assault directed not simply at the slave him- or herself but, more critically, at the very fantasies that sustain subjectivity ... I suggest that because the slave and his African American descendants continually confront obstacles in their efforts to manipulate the discourses that define them, these racialized subjects often struggle more than is usual to maintain their safe distance from the traumatic *jouissance* of lack. My argument is that slavery and racism become traumatic because they seek to inhibit the subjectifying function of fantasy, aiming to confront African Americans with the very lack that is necessarily masked in the Lacanian subject.
>
> (p. 21, emphasis in original)

In other words, the lack that racialized subjects, especially African Americans, experience is much more unbearable—than the lack experienced by the Lacanian (read: Euromodern) subject—because of the trauma of slavery. This logic can be extended to Indigenous subjects, too, through a conception of *the trauma of genocide*. In sum, while all racialized subjects experience lack in a significantly more traumatic way, our politico-libidinal analyses must be nuanced to reflect historical and material differences *vis-à-vis* modernity/coloniality, that is, our varied subjective experiences of intergenerational trauma (e.g., genocide, slavery, forced displacement, etc.).

A Liberation Psychoanalytic Account of Racism

In the previous section, I have reviewed some of the major Lacanian conceptualizations of racism. In this final section, I will propose a liberation psychoanalytic account of racism as an analectical materialist praxis (cf. Pavón-Cuéllar, 2017; Reich, 1934/2012; Tomšič, 2015). I have written about decolonial psychoanalysis (Beshara, 2019a) as a way of decolonizing psychoanalysis from the perspective of the damned, and I have also theorized contrapuntal psychoanalysis (Beshara, 2021a) as a liberation praxis, which takes into consideration both (post)colonial and decolonial psychoanalyses.

Liberation Psychoanalysis as an Analectical Materialist Praxis

Liberation psychoanalysis as an analectical material praxis names a positive process, which goes beyond ideology critique and, therefore, attempts to delink itself from modernity/coloniality. It is clearly inspired by Freire's (1970) *Pedagogy of the Oppressed* and Martín-Baró's (1996) *Writings for a Liberation Psychology*. Gaztambide's (2019) *A People's History of Psychoanalysis: From Freud to Liberation Psychology* is a one-of-a-kind study, which traces the theoretical and practical linkages between psychoanalysis and liberation psychology. Gaztambide (2019) shows that the seeds for social justice are there in the early history of psychoanalysis, particularly in the works of Freud, Ferenczi, Fenichel, Reich, and Fromm. This is the revolutionary legacy of "radical psychoanalysis" (Parker, 2022), or the Freudo-Lacanian left.

However, with the institutionalization and globalization of psychoanalysis by the International Psychoanalytic Association in tandem with a later neoliberal tendency to psychologize, or reduce psychosocial distress to the level of the psyche *qua* brain, behavior, and/or cognition, psychoanalysis today is at best a liberal project (if not a conservative one) that has adapted to its ordinary unhappiness within the global racial capitalist apparatus. Liberation psychoanalysis, on the other hand, reactivates the radical potential of psychoanalysis as a social justice oriented praxis of not only changing the subject, but also, and more importantly, changing the Other—that obscure representative of the Symbolic order. For instance, free association is not only a technique in psychoanalysis, but also an anarcho-communist praxis.

Liberation psychoanalysis reactivates the radical potential of psychoanalysis, especially from the decolonial perspective of the damned (i.e., the poor, the racialized, the oppressed, etc.), who can become transmodern subjects. My point is not to repeat Gaztambide's (2019) excellent historicization here, but to theorize racism (and oppression more generally) through the lens of what I am calling liberation psychoanalysis, which builds upon the findings reviewed in the second section of this essay, but grounds them analectically in the materiality of history.

The signifier 'psychosocial' names an analectical reality, that is, the antagonistic relationship between the subject and the Other. This relationship is ideological in at least two ways: discursively and fantasmatically. Lacan (1966/2006) famously wrote, "*the unconscious is the Other's discourse*" (p. 10, emphasis in original), which means that unconscious racism is a function of the racist Other, hence, why radical antiracism must be analectical (i.e., not only an individual effort). Elsewhere, Lacan (1966/2006) writes, "unconscious desire is the Other's desire" (p. 528), hence, his formula for fantasy ($ ◊ *a*)—the key link between the subject and the Other. Fantasy is ambiguous because desire is polysemous: the subject desires the Other, through the Other, and/or what the Other desires. Lacan's formula reads: the barred subject's unconscious desire for the *objet a* (the object-cause of desire). How then do we traverse racist ideologies (discursive-fantasies)?

The racialized (or oppressed) subject is doubly barred because of the traumatic legacies discussed above (genocide, slavery, forced displacement, etc.). Furthermore, they are also the *objets a* of racism, that is, they take the form of phobogenic/philogenic object-causes of anxious desire in racist fantasies. In writing about dialectical materialism, Leon Trotsky (1939) made a very relevant point,

"Consciousness grew out of the unconscious," which is premised on Karl Marx's (1859/1978) argument, "It is not the consciousness of men [and women] that determines their being, but, on the contrary, their social being that determines their consciousness" (p. 4). In other words, from a dialectical materialist perspective: social being → the unconscious → consciousness.

The primacy of our social being—*qua* speaking being (*parlêtre*)—emphasizes the material (politico-libidinal and economic) conditions that give rise to both the unconscious and consciousness. Therefore, our ideology critique of racist discursive-fantasies must be grounded in a material analysis of the means and relations of production that position us as a specific social being within a racial capitalist apparatus: an alienated, over-exploited, and racialized (lumpen)proletariat. This form of material alienation, from our own labor and from our comrades or co-workers, precedes ideological alienation, which is of great interest to psychoanalysts. Racial capitalism, which is what liberation psychoanalysis as an analectical materialist praxis aims to dismantle, refers to "a racially hierarchical political economy constituting war and militarism, imperialist accumulation, expropriation by domination, and labor superexploitation" (Burden-Stelly, 2020). Its dialectical opposite is "antiracist socialism" (Burden-Stelly, 2020).

Furthermore, we can speak of not only the juridico-linguistic bar dividing the subject of the Law/signifier, but also the politico-libidinal and economic bar dividing the subject of racial capitalism. The subject, according to liberation psychoanalysis, is split between a bourgeois ego and a proletarian unconscious. In other words, we must pay attention to both juridico-linguistic (or ideological) oppression and politico-libidinal and economic (or material) violence, that is, the extraction of surplus-*jouissance* and the extraction of surplus-value. Racist *jouissance*, then, is only possible because of the existence of a racial capitalist apparatus driven by oppression and violence.

Additionally, it is worth noting Lacan's (1966/2006) discussion of "the materiality of the signifier" (p. 16) or how a given S_1 (master-signifier) subjugates us under it as an alienated subject ($). A clear example is how the rhetoric of modernity is founded upon a colonial logic. In other words, the discourse of modernity necessitates not only colonial fantasies—i.e., the desire of colonizers for everything—but also the Real of coloniality, as a material structure premised on the over-exploitation of colonized objects (nonbeings/nonthinking things). We can formally locate the Real of coloniality (its materiality) in both the bar splitting the modern/colonial subject ($), and dividing the world into zones of being and nonbeing, as well as the phobogenic/philogenic *objets a* of racism—that is, the racialized (lumpen) proletariat.

Decolonizing Dialectics | Metonymic Decolonization | Grounding Psychoanalysis

Before ending this section with a historical materialist timeline of racism, I would like to state a few caveats regarding decolonizing dialectics, metonymic decolonization, and grounding psychoanalysis. In a recent essay for Aeon, Avram Alpert (2020) provocatively exposes "the racist history of the dialectic going back to Rousseau." Alpert's point, however, is not for us to cancel dialectics, but for those who have historically been the objects of dialectics (i.e., the colonized) to decolonize these modern notions and methods the way Césaire, Fanon, and other transmodern/decolonial subjects did. George Ciccariello-Maher (2017) makes a similar argument when he writes, "I approach the task of decolonizing dialectics by excavating a largely subterranean current of thought, what I call a *counterdiscourse*, that I argue constitutes a radicalization of the dialectical tradition while also opening outward toward its decolonization" (p. 6, emphasis in original). Ciccariello-Maher (2017) decolonizes dialectics chiefly through the works of Fanon and Dussel, the latter being "sharply critical of dialectics," embracing instead "what he calls an *analectics* rooted in the embrace of the Other as exteriority" (p. 8, emphasis in original).

My use of the term 'decolonization' brings to mind Tuck and Yang's (2012) critical essay, *Decolonization is not a metaphor*, wherein they argue against the metaphorization of decolonizing discourses in an effort to remind readers of the literal meaning of *decolonization as a praxis of unsettling*: "decolonization specifically requires the repatriation of Indigenous land and life" (p. 21). An example of decolonization as a praxis of unsettling is the decolonization of Asia and Africa between 1945 and 1960. While I certainly agree with Tuck and Yang's (2012) call for "the demetaphorization of decolonization" (p. 10), I want to make a counterargument for *metonymic decolonization.*

For a recent critique of Tuck and Yang's (2012) influential essay from the perspective of Black studies, the reader is encouraged to survey Garba and Sorentino's (2020) case for "the slave metaphor" being "central to the logics of slavery, not an after-effect" (p. 11). Their rebuttal rests on the seemingly counterintuitive thesis that "*slavery is (nothing but) metaphor*" (p. 3, emphasis in original), which for them is premised on the argument that "anti-Blackness is animated by the gratuitous substitution that marks metaphoricity" (p. 3). In other words, slavery as metaphoric condensation is a symptom of the traumatic Real of coloniality.

Whereas *metaphoric decolonization* is based on an Imaginary fantasy of oneness (e.g., the masses identifying with a charismatic decolonial politician), *metonymic decolonization* is based on a Symbolic alignment of desire (e.g., we want landback, reparations for slavery, prison abolition, etc.), which is analectical, for it is premised on difference (the 'we' is made up of Indigenous, Black, and Global Southern subjects in solidarity with Euromodern comrades).

Metonymic decolonization, as a metonymy of desire, can be a source of collective *jouissance* (or comradeship). Metonymic decolonization is founded upon "true solidarity with the oppressed," which "means fighting at their side to transform the objective reality which has made them these 'beings for another'" (Freire, 1970, p. 49)—that is, phobogenic/philogenic *objets a* in racist fantasies. Freire (1970) emphasized that the oppressed must occupy the subject-position of revolutionaries leading the way toward a humanizing liberation for all. How else can we (the oppressed) subjectify our metonymic desire for decolonization?

To say that psychoanalysis is *worldly* is to ground it historically and materially, which means that it is an "event" that is "part of the social world, human life, and of course the historical moments in which [it is] located and interpreted" (Said, 1983, p. 4). Furthermore, psychoanalysis is "materially bound to [its] time" (Said, 1983, p. 25), for it is neither ahistorical nor immaterial. For example, psychoanalysis, as a modern science of the unconscious, began in late 19th century Vienna with its founder (Freud) being an atheist Jew working in an anti-Semitic Christian milieu, which literally became colonized by Nazis in 1938.

The radical worldliness of psychoanalysis, which has been deemphasized over more than a century through institutionalization and psychologization, contains within itself the seeds for its (and our) decolonial liberation: free association. Furthermore, I encourage grounding liberation psychoanalysis in radical Indigenous, Black, and Global Southern theories and practices.

A Historical Materialist Reading of Racism

Civilization

I will end the chapter with a swift historical materialist reading of racism as a "social relation of oppression" (Camfield, 2016) as opposed to "racism-as-ideology" (p. 40). Paradoxically, slavery was a product of civilization as a function of social stratification during the first agricultural revolution (c. 10,000 BCE). As Derrick Jensen (2004) shows, "Slaves built the levees, canals, and granaries vital to the agricultural revolution. They built the pyramids of Egypt and the great hydraulic systems of China … Indeed, without slave labor there would have been neither Bronze nor Iron Ages" (pp. 141–142). He adds,

> until modern times, no sane person ever uncoerced became a mine worker … Only prisoners, captives, and slaves—three branches from the same tree—ever entered the underworld, and even then did so only under the lash, or at the point of a sword.
>
> (p. 142)

"Slavery's use," Jensen (2004) continues, "was so central to the foundation of civilization that it dictated the design of early cities" (p. 143). He then concludes, "To undo slavery—if this argument holds—would be to undo the civilization we—at least those of us who might be considered slaveholders—all enjoy" (p. 145).

One hundred and twenty five years earlier, Friedrich Engels (1877/1939) made a similar argument in *Anti-Dühring*:

> It was slavery that first made possible the division of labour between agriculture and industry on a considerable scale, and along with this, the flower of the ancient world, Hellenism. Without slavery, no Greek state, no Greek art and science; without slavery, no Roman Empire … no modern Europe.
>
> (p. 206)

From the perspective of 'civilization,' we can then understand who are the ones framed as 'barbarians' or 'primitives' and why (Mignolo, 2007). 'Barbarians' were/are those racialized beings living in the periphery, that is, Exterior to the core of Euromodernity; in other words, non-Europeans or Orientals (Said, 1978), particularly Muslims and Arabs. 'Primitives' were/are those racialized beings lagging behind the scientific advances of Euromodernity; in other words, Amerindian, African, and Asian tribes. The first term designates *spatial colonial difference*; the second one signifies *temporal colonial difference*.

Slavery

According to Niall McKeown (2011), a "third of the population of classical Athens [were] slaves" (p. 20). Three preconditions gave rise to chattel slavery in ancient Greece and Rome: "(1) Large, privately controlled farms ... (2) The development of market exchange ... (3) Crucially, a lack of internal source of labour" (p. 21). Further, McKeown (2011) argues, that "rather than democracy helping to create slavery, slavery helped the development of democracy by allowing farmers time to engage in politics" (p. 21). Slavery certainly existed in the pre-modern world, particularly in Greece, Rome, and Africa.

However, the Atlantic slave trade (15th–19th c.)—the largest forced migration in modern history with over 9.5 million Africans enslaved and worked to death on plantations in the Americas (Rawley & Behrendt, 1981/2005, p. 4)—represents a massive acceleration of the institution of chattel slavery, which was instrumental for establishing the hegemony of the modern/colonial world-system. Rawley and Behrendt (1981/2005) note, "It is not a paradox that the start of the Atlantic slave trade coincides with the dawn of modern Europe. The trade was closely interwoven with the major changes that are associated with the making of the modern era" (p. 8). Modernity/coloniality signifies that modernity was/is founded upon coloniality.

Rawley and Behrendt (1981/2005) add, "The [Atlantic slave] trade formed a part of Europe's transition to capitalism, the nation-state, and imperialism" (p. 360). They conclude, "The [Atlantic slave] trade illustrates various stages in the history of capitalism, moving from mercantilism and state-conferred monopoly to free trade and individual enterprise to concentration, and from royal to bourgeois direction" (p. 364). Racial capitalism, as a concept, seeks to capture all these different historical iterations of capitalism given their material basis in slavery.

Following from this traumatic legacy of slavery, it makes sense from a historical materialist perspective to read racism today through the lens of Marx's (1867/1978) theory of commodity-fetishism in *Capital, Volume One*. While the racialized subject is no longer a commodity in a literal sense, for he or she is not a chattel slave, they still retain the "mystical character of commodities" (p. 320). Racialized subjects exhibit an "enigmatical character" and appear as "a mysterious thing" in the eyes of the racist commodity-fetishist. Racialized subjects are thingified, or positioned as fantasmatic phobogenic/philogenic *objets a*, as a function of how they are anxiously fetishized both ideologically and materially within the oppressive and violent apparatus of racial capitalism.

Racism

Religious Racism. Historically, there have been three main types of racism, which often overlap. Presented chronologically, these three types are: religious racism, scientific racism, and cultural racism. Fredrickson (2002/2015) writes, "In the twelfth and thirteenth centuries the attitudes of European Christians toward Jews became more hostile in ways that laid a foundation for the racism that later developed" (p. 19). Fredrickson (2002/2015) adds:

> the racism or protoracism of the late Middle Ages extended well beyond the Jews. As the core of Catholic Europe expanded, conquering and colonizing the periphery of the continent, attitudes of superiority to indigenous populations anticipated the feelings of dominance and entitlement that would characterize the later expansion of Europeans into Asia, Africa, and the Americas. If the demonization of the Jews established some basis for the racial antisemitism of the modern era, the prejudice and discrimination directed at the Irish on one side of Europe and certain Slavic peoples on the other foreshadowed the dichotomy between civilization and savagery that would characterize imperial expansion beyond the European continent.
>
> (p. 23)

Scientific Racism. To recap the historical materialist argument thus far: civilization → slavery → religious racism (Figure 6.1). This means that slavery existed before racism, and racism existed before the modern concept of 'race'—whose etymology is the Spanish word *raza*, which is based on the Arabic term رأس or *ra's* (literally, headland, as in place of origin). As Fredrickson (2002/2015) shows, "The modern concept of races as basic human types classified by physical characteristics (primarily skin color) was not invented until the eighteenth century" (pp. 52–53). Further, "The notion that there was a single pan-European or 'white' race was slow to develop and did not crystallize until the eighteenth century" (p. 53). Therefore, the invention of scientific racism and whiteness coincided with the modern conception of 'race': "The scientific thought of the Enlightenment was a precondition for the growth of a modern racism based on physical typology" (p. 56).

As I mentioned before, these types of racism are not mutually exclusive; in fact, they often overlap. For example, some may think that today we live in a post-racial society or that one can be colorblind because slavery and segregation are no longer legal; however, sexual trafficking and forced child labor, for instance, are contemporary forms of slavery. While it is true that we see more racialized folks represented in politics and culture, we continue to use the modern concept of 'race,' most obviously in the U.S. Census, which includes five racial categories (i.e., white, Black, American Indian, Asian, and Native Hawaiian) even though

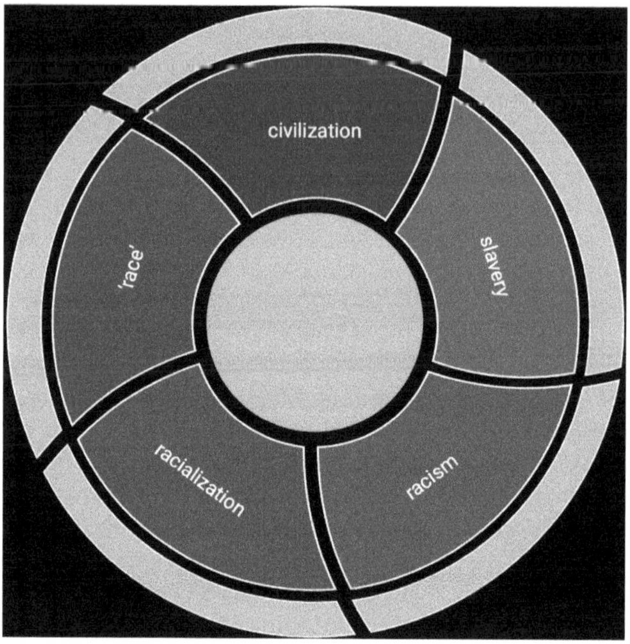

Figure 6.1 The 'race'-racism paradox

'race' is a social construction that has no material basis. So, why does 'race' continue to be ideologically salient? The next type of racism may provide the answer.

Cultural Racism. Cultural racism, the most popular type of racism today, is not premised on phenotype or skin color alone, but employs stereotyping, prejudice, and/or discrimination on the basis of any cultural marker of difference (e.g., clothing, language, religion, accent, food, facial hair, etc.) that signifies Otherness from the perspective of hegemonic subjects, who are often, but not necessarily, of European descent.

In many ways, cultural racism is quite insidious because while it may appear benign, it is the culmination of the two types of racism that preceded it. For instance, racists today, typically from a Euromodern nationalist perspective, will argue that some cultures (or religions) are inferior to others. This covert practice of cultural racism—or "racism without races" (Balibar & Wallerstein, 1988/1991)—indexes the signifiers 'savage,' 'barbarian,' and 'primitive' *vis-à-vis* subaltern cultures without mentioning any 'races' and so reverts back to a civilizational discourse, which is the beginning of the problem anyway.

Racialization

Racializing—or (mis)perceiving the Other through the lens of 'race'—is inherently problematic because of how racism historically preceded the concept of 'race.' In other words, the concept of 'race' is tainted and may never be salvageable. However, colorblindess—or pretending that we do not (mis)perceive 'race' or racialize—is equally (if not more) problematic. This is the paradox facing radical antiracists. We know from mainstream psychological studies of perception that misperception is baked into the process of perceiving itself, as is clear from how the brain automatically changes what we see, particularly in the face of optical illusions (e.g., the Moon illusion).

In other words, it is impossible to override misperception, even if we consciously understand the logic of why we are misperceiving. Similarly, Lacan (1966/2006) addressed Imaginary misrecognition (*méconnaissance*), which is something that the ego cannot avoid and which typically leads to narcissism and aggressivity *vis-à-vis* Imaginary others, that is, other egos; therefore, the point of learned ignorance is knowing that we will always (mis)perceive difference when faced with the Other without reverting to categorizing this difference in a hierarchical way. This anti-hierarchical stance is simultaneously an anti-civilizational stance. Like Wahba (2022), I believe in the worldcentric idea of *one civilization with many cultures*, and I am against the ethnocentric thesis of a "clash of civilizations" (Huntington, 1993).

Antiracist Ecosocialism

In sum, liberation psychoanalysis, as an analectical materialist praxis, is a contribution to the destruction of racial capitalism and the construction of antiracist ecosocialism. Whereas whiteness is a racialist ideology, Indigeneity, Blackness, and other transmodern/decolonial ways of being are an *antiracist praxis* against "environmental racism" (Anthony, 1995)—and in alignment with social ecology (Kadalie, 2019). Therefore, radical non-European ways of being and knowing are driven by an *ecocentric ethic of liberation*, which necessitates *an ecopsychoanalysis of the ecological unconscious* (Roszak, 1992).

Unlike whiteness, which is an ideological fantasy that sutures class struggle among those of European descent in settler-colonial societies, terms associated with the racialized (lumpen)proletariat signify human difference along a horizontal axis of power (i.e., non-hierarchically) without occluding class struggle—since whitening is a bourgeois aspiration. As Cedric Robinson (1984) puts it succinctly: "We will be Black [or Indigenous or Global Southern] not because we are not white, but *because of our history and the achievements of our struggle*" (p. 27, emphasis added).

Chapter 7

The Psychoanalysis of Racism and the Racism of Psychoanalysis

Psychoanalysis, like subjectivity, is divided. On the one hand, it is a praxis whose orientation revolves around listening to, and deciphering, the unconscious. As such, it is a powerful tool for both *theorizing unconscious racism* and *practicing antiracism*. On the other hand, psychoanalysis is a discipline that arose within *a particular material history*; psychoanalytic clinics and institutions also operate under *specific ideological conditions*.

Therefore, it is vital to think of the oppressive dimensions of psychoanalysis, as a function of its being a European modern/colonial project invented around the time of new imperialism. However, I will argue for the worlding of psychoanalysis through both *an immanent critique* and *a decolonial reading*. The first approach critiques psychoanalysis from within its own logic in an effort to emphasize its radical potential. The second approach critiques psychoanalysis from without through the Exterior lens of the non-European Other *qua* A^2. Ultimately, the analectical move is to be able to both appreciate what psychoanalysis has to offer us today in terms of praxis while also critiquing the false universality of ethnocentric psychoanalytic notions.

There is a bifurcation in psychoanalytic theory that parallels Freud's division as a subject. I characterize this bifurcation in terms of two strands inherent within psychoanalysis: *a liberal-conservative strand* and *a radical one*. I qualify the liberal-conservative strand as *colonial secularism* and the radical strand as *decolonial secularization*.

Psychoanalysis as colonial secularism either furthers, or adapts itself to, the ongoing machinations of racial capitalism. According to Ruth Wilson Gilmore (2020), "capitalism requires inequality and racism enshrines it." Racial capitalism does not denote a type of capitalism, rather it names the very fact that *capitalism was always racial*. Similarly, Charisse Burden-Stelly argues that the analytical framework of racial capitalism "helps us see that race and class–or racialized oppression and capitalist exploitation–are mutually constitutive" (as cited in Kelley & Burden-Stelly, 2021). On the conservative end of the spectrum, psychoanalysis is used as a colonial tool to enact the civilizing mission of modernity/coloniality in the way that it furthers the logics of racial capitalism through imperialism. On the liberal end of the spectrum, psychoanalysis is a silent bystander on questions of oppression and violence, thereby adapting to modernity/coloniality through humanitarianism.

DOI: 10.4324/9781003768104-7

What do I mean by colonial secularism? In order to answer that question, I must first define *secularism*. According to Talal Asad (2003), secularism is both a "political doctrine [which] arose in modern Euro-America" (p. 1) and "an enactment by which a *political medium* (representation of citizenship) redefines and transcends particular and differentiating practices of the self that are articulated through class, gender, and religion" (p. 5, emphasis in original).

"The difficulty with secularism as a doctrine of war and peace in the world," Asad continues, "is not that it is European (and therefore alien to the non-West) but that it is closely connected with the rise of a system of capitalist nation-states" (p. 7). In other words, the problem with secularism is that *it is not truly secular* since it is a modern Euro-American political doctrine housed within the apparatus of racial capitalism, which is ideologically promoted as a universal panacea, particularly to non-European subjects. While I am for secularization as an autochthonous process, I am against secularism as a Euromodern ideology (see Wahba, 2022), which is secretly Christian.

Similarly, Alberto Toscano (2009) critiques secularism as a "normative political notion" (p. 105), which displaces the so-called Judeo-Christian (European) heritage. Toscano shows that the psychoanalytic institution can problematically function as the "midwife of secularism" when it "takes the parameters of acculturation (and of pathology, anomaly and dislocation) provided by Western Christendom and its secular inheritance as somehow normative" (p. 112). He warns of "the dangers of secularizing the psychoanalytic subject, and of turning psychoanalysis into a secular clinic" (p. 112). Psychoanalysis fails when it is an ideological clinic dedicated to converting non-European subjects (particularly Muslims) to secularism (e.g., Benslama, 2009).

In sum, the aim of Toscano's critique is to distinguish between secularism's "normative narrative" and "the methodological atheism of psychoanalysis" (p. 114). By *methodological atheism*, he means "a praxical, materialist and naturalist inquiry into transindividual behaviour and psychic structure which … is not generative of further political fantasies, illusions of autonomy, or cultural superiority" (p. 117). To put it differently, the methodological atheism of psychoanalysis is a form of *decolonial secularization*, which affords psychoanalytic subjects a pluriverse of ontologies and epistemologies that are not possible within the false universality (Totality) of secularism since it is, in essence, a provincial ideology that furthers the civilizing mission of global racial capitalism.

Psychoanalysis, as decolonial secularization, is a radical liberation praxis, which implies that it is actively both anticapitalist (socialist) and antiracist (humanist). Stephen Frosh (2020) writes, "psychoanalysis needs and can never escape its Jewish provocations; and in these can be found some of the energy with which it is possible for psychoanalysis to contribute to the ongoing struggle for a decolonized world." His notion of "psychoanalysis as decolonial Judaism" is not equivalent to the Nazi characterization of psychoanalysis as a "Jewish science"; rather, it is an echo of the argument that "the contributions of Freud are to be understood largely as a contemporary version of, and contribution to, the history of Jewish mysticism" (Bakan, 1958/1975, p. 25).

According to David Bakan, "Freud, consciously or unconsciously, secularized Jewish mysticism; and psychoanalysis can intelligently be viewed as such a secularization" (p. 25). This insight sheds light on Freud's subjective division between *assimilated European* and *racialized Jew*. Edward Said (2003) calls the unconscious dimension of Freud's subjectivity "non-European" since it functioned as the repressed for Freud, which explains his racist projections onto so-called 'primitives' (cf. LaMothe, 2023). Let us simply recall the subtitle of Freud's (1913a) *Totem and Taboo*: "Resemblances Between the Psychic Lives of Savages and Neurotics." That subtitle, which can be seen on the cover of the 1918 English translation by A. A. Brill, was later removed—censored, repressed—from the cover of the translation by James Strachey, who edited the *Standard Edition of the Complete Psychological Works*.

As Bakan shows, Freud's secularization of Jewish mysticism was a practical response to the heightened anti-Semitism of his time, particularly in 1882; Freud's self-censorship—his negation of his alterity—was a survival strategy in the face of the collective racist enjoyment commanded by the superegoic anti-Semitic Other (Gilman, 1993). I also read Freud's negation of Jewish mysticism as a defense mechanism to both *fortify his European ego* and *disown his Jewish unconscious*.

Freud (1939) faced his Jewish unconscious head-on in his last book, *Moses and Monotheism*, and it is for this reason that Said, who enjoys idiosyncratic late style, returns to this text, at the end of his life, to highlight Freud's radicalism, such as his emphasis on non-identity politics as a praxis of affiliative solidarity. To say that Moses, the founder of Judaism, is Egyptian means that *politics is the grounding of identity* and not the other way around (Mignolo, 2007).

To put it in Lacanian terms, non-identity politics eschews Imaginary identifications–the essence of any form of nationalism—in favor of *a politics of difference centered on desiring and enjoying the commons*. In other words, comrades are in solidarity not because they are the same but because *they desire and enjoy commoning*. The praxis of liberation entails a political movement away from all kinds of oppression and toward egalitarian forms of power. Freud's free clinics exemplified the radical political potential of psychoanalysis as decolonial secularization (cf. Danto, 2005), for there is no social justice without psychic justice and vice versa.

This is the radical potential of psychoanalysis as decolonial secularization, which is inherent in the praxis, alongside the more reactionary strand of colonial secularism. We must ask ourselves: Is my use of psychoanalysis furthering, or undoing, the logics of racial capitalism? Decolonial secularization, as a method, delinks *psychoanalytic modernity* from *psychoanalytic coloniality*. The key is keeping the former, but expanding it through non-European worlding, and excising the latter, which is *the psychic remainder of colonialism*.

If we choose to commit to radical psychoanalysis, then our task entails fidelity to decolonial secularization as a transmodern methodology; transmodernity combines the best of modernity and its alterity, particularly when it comes to questions of truth and justice, such as how social oppression is linked to psychic repression, as

I illustrated earlier in relation to Freud's alienation. The answer to assimilation is *integration*. I say more later about the colonial logic, which functions as the unconscious of psychoanalysis, but, for now, let us turn to the psychoanalysis of racism.

The Psychoanalysis of Racism

Psychoanalysis is a powerful tool for both *theorizing unconscious racism* and *practicing antiracism*. In this section, I will share some of my thoughts on the psychoanalysis of racism (cf. Eng & Han, 2018; Cheng, 2001; Dalal, 2006; Keval, 2016; Khan, 2018; George, 2016; George & Hook, 2021; Lane, 1998; Seshadri-Crooks, 2000); however, I will not perform an exhaustive survey of the Lacanian literature on racism—as in Chapter 6—since I wish to raise specific points for the reader instead. Also, I want to highly recommend the excellent book *Internal Racism*, which is written by Fakhry Davids (2011). In *Internal Racism*, Davids does not merely apply psychoanalysis to racism; rather, he analytically works through the internal racism, which surfaces in the clinic, in order to theorize this phenomenon of internalization that affects us all (cf. Richards, 2023). Echoing some of Davids's arguments, I have written elsewhere:

> Consciousness-raising is important, but it will not succeed without *unconsciousness-raising*, which is a political intervention at the level of the Other's discourse. In other words, to be antiracist one has to also speak of an *antiracist unconscious*, which implies transforming the culture of racism and replacing it with an *antiracist culture*. To put it differently, the subject cannot be antiracist as long as the Other is racist. The paradoxical question of racism is: how do we acknowledge human, and cultural, differences beyond racial categories without being color-blind? In other words, we must collectively come to terms with both the denial of racism (which is also a denial of colonialism) and the overpresence of racial discourses as an effect of religious, scientific, and cultural racisms. We do not yet have a post-racial language and we may not have one anytime soon since undoing modernity/coloniality may take hundreds of years, but we can at least try to prefigure a transmodern/decolonial world-system through our liberation praxis.
>
> (Beshara, 2020, emphasis in original)

We all internalize the racist unconscious as the discourse of the racist Other because we all live in a racist culture. We have not transcended racism because we are still attached to racial categories, which inform our racializations or (mis)perceptions of racial difference. It is not a question of subscribing to post-racial color-blindness, but of how to enact *radical humanism*, as an antiracist praxis beyond the concept of 'race.' I have opted in this book, for example, for the concept of the (non)European, as a way of speaking around the Real of cultural difference without trying to translate it too much. I am particularly interested in the *non*, the productive negativity that is in an analectical relationship with the European. While it is often positioned in a zone of nonbeing due to colonial difference, this *non* also contains the seeds for the zone of becoming—the transmodern ground for collective liberation.

Theorizing unconscious racism

If we accept Lacan's (1966/2006) axiom that *the unconscious is the discourse of the Other*, then we can theorize *unconscious racism as the discourse of the racist Other*. In other words, unconscious racism is a psychosocial phenomenon that is located in the fantasmatic link between the modern subject and the colonial Other. Therefore, antiracism cannot be reduced exclusively to the psychic level of the subject. To put it differently, racism exists not because racist individuals exist, but because racism enshrines the inequality required by racial capitalism as a system. The phrase 'racial capitalism' signifies the historical and ongoing structural (material and ideological) interdependence between racism and capitalism.

The ideology of racism comprises two parts: (1) racist discourses and (2) racist fantasies. The materiality of racism is a function of enacting the racist ideology on two levels: (1) the individual level and (2) the institutional level. But what is 'race'? According to Lentin (2020), 'race' is "a technology for the management of human difference, the main goal of which is the production, reproduction, and maintenance of white supremacy on both a local and a planetary scale" (p. 24). She adds,

> race is about the delineation not only of whites from non-whites, but of the essence of Europeanness from that of non-Europeanness. Therefore, race is above all else a project of colonial distinction and a system of legitimation to justify oppressive and discriminatory practices.
>
> (p. 27)

As such, the technology of 'race' is, *ipso facto*, racist.

The antiracist challenge, then, is accounting for human (or cultural) difference without falling into the hierarchical trap of managing difference through *méconnaissance*, which Davids (2011) qualifies as a paranoid (us v. them) construction (p. 37). For Davids, this paranoid construction is part of 'normal' (neurotic) psychosexual development, and his name for this defensive system is: "*internal racist organization*" (p. 31, emphasis in original). The function of the internal racist organization is to reduce the anxiety that results from human difference, particularly along the racial axis.

The racial axis is Aníbal Quijano's (2000) term for how the idea of 'race' was used by the Spanish conquistadors in the 15th century as part of their modern/colonial model of power. In other words, the idea of 'race' made possible the definition of the modern subject (the universal subject of psychoanalysis), as a racializing subject in contradistinction from the colonized/racialized object, who was positioned as not only Exterior but also inferior on the basis of arbitrary markers of human difference and consequently managed by a supposedly superior imperial subject.

What rendered these arbitrary categorizations a technology of "colonial domination" was their definition by the European colonizers followed by their deployment of said categories "as instruments of basic social classification" (p. 534). These dynamics constitute the unconscious of psychoanalysis, or what Davids characterizes as "the psychoanalytic silence on race" (p. 144). I have explained this silence earlier in terms of Freud's repression of Jewish mysticism in the anti-Semitic context of late 19th century Vienna—a practical strategy of survival.

But Freud's other defense, which supports the thesis of internal racism, is the displacement of his Jewish unconscious onto non-European 'primitives,' thereby splitting his non-Europeanness and projecting it elsewhere, Exterior to his psyche, so he can feel less anxious. Therefore, working with racism entails working with the anxiety around human difference, which is exacerbated by the apparatus of racial capitalism. Racial capitalism thrives on power asymmetry, hence, why it manages human difference through the technology of 'race' and the surplus-*jouissance* of racism.

As Miller (1988) puts it, "Racism is founded on what one imagines about the Other's jouissance; it is hatred of the particular way, of the Other's own way of experiencing jouissance" (p. 125). In other words, we are commanded to unconsciously enjoy racism and there is no way of ending this mythic libidinal economy without abolishing the political economy of racial capitalism. If abolishing racial capitalism is not possible in the foreseeable future, then how can we turn our clinics and institutions into antiracist (humanist) and anticapitalist (socialist) spaces?

Practicing antiracism

Consequently, practicing antiracism must involve two strategies: (1) a critique of the racist ideology and (2) an antiracist/anticapitalist praxis. The critique of the racist ideology entails theoretical critiques of both racist discourses and racist fantasies. In other words, the task here is to show how racism works ideologically in an effort to dismantle both its discursive rhetoric and fantasmatic logic, and in this realm, psychoanalysis has a lot to offer.

For example, racist discourses tend to manifest in at least one of three forms: (1) the master's discourse, (2) the university discourse, and (3) the capitalist discourse (cf. Lacan, 1991). The first form is the most dominant one, wherein racism is embedded ideologically so as to appear commonsensical on all levels of society; this is typically the ideological position of the State. Therefore, we can call this form: institutional or State racism.

The second form supports the first one and we can label it: scientific racism. It can be overt in its indexing of pseudoscientific 19th century ideas from eugenics on human difference, or it may be covert in its reliance on more contemporary concepts from psychology or psychoanalysis that supposedly explain human difference through a focus on intelligence or development.

The third form capitalizes on racism, particularly as a type of surplus-enjoyment. This third form, in many ways, is the most ambivalent one because it involves contradictory passions, that is, not only phobic but also philic dimensions. The phobic dimension is the dimension of hate when it comes to racism, but the philic dimension is that of love. The philic dimension may come across as a celebration of multiculturalism, for example, but it typically sutures cultural difference through two-dimensional stereotypical and paranoid representations, such as the "good Muslim" vs. the "bad Muslim" (Mamdani, 2005). The phobic dimension tends to manifest in terms of prejudice or discrimination, that is, in terms of hateful affects or acts, respectively. Cultural racism, or racism without races, is ideologically supported by both institutional racism and scientific racism.

In sum, within the apparatus of racial capitalism, racism is structured through three nodes: institutional racism, scientific racism, and cultural racism. Therefore, in addition to critiquing the ideology of racism in its many forms, we must also engage in an antiracist/anticapitalist praxis (e.g., liberation psychoanalysis), which is how we disrupt the surplus-enjoyment generated by racism. Antiracist/anticapitalist praxis is the name for our solidarity or free association, as psychoanalytic theorists and practitioners committed to radical humanism and libertarian socialism. Liberation psychoanalysis entails comradeship among those who wish to live in a truthful and just world beyond racial capitalism. So, in a sense, this praxis involves prefiguring the desire and enjoyment for this world-to-come in our relationships today with our colleagues, analysands, etc.

Liberation psychoanalysis is the question of accounting for human, or cultural, difference while bracketing the ideological coordinates of racial capitalism, which hierarchize us on the basis of translating the untranslatable into the same. For this reason, learned ignorance (as opposed to crass ignorance) is a central feature of antiracist/anticapitalist praxis. Lacan characterized learned ignorance as a passion, which is linked to unconscious know-how (as cited in Soler, 2016, p. 86). I define learned ignorance as *a critical epistemological attitude of knowing what we do not know.* This paradoxical but practical know-how is opposed to thinking that we know when our paranoiac knowledge, in many cases, is but an internalization of modern/colonial epistemology. Modern/colonial epistemology is a racist epistemology of crass ignorance, for the most part, as far as non-European ways of knowing are concerned. This is what Said (1978) showed *vis-à-vis* Orientalism, for example. As such, I regard learned ignorance to be a central feature of liberation psychoanalysis.

The Racism of Psychoanalysis

Psychoanalysis is a discipline that arose within a particular material history; psychoanalytic clinics and institutions also operate under specific ideological conditions. Therefore, it is vital to think of the oppressive dimensions of psychoanalysis (cf. Stoute & Slevin, 2022), as a function of its being a modern/colonial project invented around the time of new imperialism.

The material history of psychoanalysis as a discipline

Psychoanalysis did not materialize out of thin air in the late 19th century, the discipline's beginning coincides with the birth of psychology as a scientific discipline separate from philosophy and theology. The psyche, in both psychoanalysis and psychology, used to be understood, from the Ancient Greeks onwards, as the soul, the breath of life, spirit, or even *al-nafs* in Arabic. The definition of psyche changed in the late 19th century to mean mind (or cognition). Since the 20th century, psyche has come to also be conceptualized as behavior and brain. This naturalization of psyche is a function of psychologization (cf. Martín-Baró, 1996)—a symptom of psychology's physics envy. In other words, psychology's *raison d'être* stems from its identification with the natural sciences, hence, its quest for objectivity through experimentation.

However, Freud was part of a human scientific movement dedicated to the empirical study of psyche from a subjective viewpoint. Therefore, Freud was building on a humanistic tradition with origins in philosophy. He learned about this tradition first and foremost from Franz Brentano, who also taught Edmund Husserl (the founder of phenomenology). Brentano, of course, wrote *Psychology from an Empirical Standpoint*, which was published in 1874 or 21 years before Freud and Breuer's (1895) *Studies in Hysteria*. More can be said certainly about the intellectual genealogy that influenced Freud and led to the beginning of psychoanalysis (from Schelling to Nietzsche); however, my point here is to historicize and theorize the modern unconscious *vis-à-vis* colonialism and coloniality.

Colonialism is the material colonization of peoples and their resources (land, water, oil, etc.). Coloniality is *the psychic remainder* of this system, which is not only a historical event, but also an ongoing structure that manifests as either *settler-colonialism* or *franchise colonialism* (Wolfe, 2001). For example, whereas the U.S. is a settler colonial society, the territory of Puerto Rico is a franchise colony. Significant variations on these two forms include neo-colonialism (Nkrumah, 1965), which is more economic than political, and internal colonialism (Blauner, 1969), which is an autoimmunitary form of endo-colonization (Virilio, 2006).

Settler colonialism typically morphs into internal colonialism, wherein Indigenous and Black natives experience being subjects more than citizens. Similarly, franchise colonialism transforms into neo-colonialism over time, which is the case with Egypt, for example. It used to be a franchise colony of the British Empire, and now it is a neo-colony of the U.S., as the second largest recipient of foreign military financing after Israel.

My effort, as I shall argue later, is not merely to critique psychoanalysis, but, more importantly, to world it and stretch it through an emphasis on Exteriority. This intervention is a further development of some of my ideas in *Decolonial Psychoanalysis* as well as *Freud and Said*. My question now is: What is on the Other side of the Cogito? This is a question about the beginning of the modern unconscious. Christopher Columbus did not 'discover' the

Americas in 1492. By the same token, Breuer and Freud did not 'discover' the unconscious in 1895.

Freud is credited to have said, "The poets and philosophers before me discovered the unconscious. What I discovered was the scientific method by which the unconscious can be studied" (as cited in Lehrman, 1940). In other words, Freud is the first to theorize the modern unconscious. Some attribute the invention of the unconscious to Schelling (Ffytche, 2011; McGrath, 2012) or Nietzsche (Katsafanas, 2016; Lehrer, 1994), but Descartes undoubtedly provided the philosophical foundation for the modern unconscious (Žižek, 1998).

I want to pause for a moment on this image of Freud the conquistador, an intriguing identification with Columbus, which links his 'discovery' of the unconscious to the latter's 'discovery' of the New World. In a letter to Wilhelm Fliess on February 1, 1900 (Freud & Fliess, 1985), Freud wrote: "I am by temperament nothing but a *conquistador*–an adventurer, if you want it translated–with all the curiosity, daring, and tenacity characteristic of a man of this sort" (as cited in Masson, 1985, p. 398, emphasis added). There is also, of course, Freud's use of archeology as a metaphor for what analysts do during (re)construction as opposed to interpretation. Freud is a psychic adventurer, but what is he digging for? What is the psychic equivalent of gold? Is it feces perhaps?

The following lengthy passage from Khanna's (2003) magnum opus demonstrates that the ideological 'discovery' of material (in Columbus's case) and psychic (in Freud's case) "dark continents" is a question of not only exploitation and alienation, but also accumulation and fungibility:

> Psychoanalysis is a colonial discipline. A colonial intellectual formation disciplines a way of being as much as it establishes a form of analysis based in the age of colonialism and constitutive of concepts of the primitive against which the civilizing mission could establish itself. It brought into the world an idea of being that was dependent on colonial political and ontological relations, and through its disciplinary practices, formalized and perpetuated an idea of uncivilized, primitive, concealed, and timeless colonized peoples. As a discipline, it formalized strategies to normalize a form of civilized being constituted through colonial political dynamics. In the space between the earth and the colonizing world of late-nineteenth and early-twentieth-century Europe, a national-colonial self was brought into existence, or perhaps more accurately, into unconcealment. And it situated itself, with fascination, in opposition to its repressed, concealed, and mysterious "dark continents": colonial Africa, women, and the primitive.
>
> (p. 6)

Along similar lines, Justin Clemens (2013) explores the relationship between psychoanalysis and slavery, or the importance of Symbolic slavery in Lacanian psychoanalysis, in particular, as informed by Aristotle's distinction between natural slavery and political slavery as well as Hegel's master–slave dialectic. Clemens writes that the problem of slavery or "the biopolitical problem of the genesis of irreparable inequality [is] at the centre of the psychoanalytic project" (p. 64). Clemens adds:

> the slave – the subject of the signifier – *is not really correlated with the master at all.* This may seem like a preposterous remark. Yet what is important here is that the 'mastery' of which Lacan most often speaks is correlated with the ego, that is, with the imaginary. As Lacan says, 'we analysts deal with slaves who think they are masters'. Mastery is thus an imaginary function; slavery is a symbolic one. The subject is a subject insofar as it subsists in a state of servitude, servitude to the signifier.
>
> (p. 75, emphasis in original)

However, I must ask: What of the Real of slavery? Is *that* the repressed unconscious of psychoanalysis itself? A source of its racist *jouissance* perhaps? We, of course, know about the analyst's desire, which Bruce Fink (1997) describes as "purified desire" or a "desire that focuses on analysis and only on analysis" (p. 6). He also calls it "the motor force of analysis" (p. 7). Nevertheless, is the psychoanalytic clinic an acontextual space? Or is it a psychosocial space that is linked with what is going on materially and ideologically in the world? Is the practice of psychoanalysis ahistorical? Or is it a function of a specific form of reason?

I ask these political questions in order to think about not only the analyst's desire, but also the *jouissance* of analysis, which is rarely theorized. The metaphorization of slavery, or psychoanalysis *qua* Symbolic slavery, seems to me like a defense against the traumatic Real of slavery, which is not properly historicized in relation to psychoanalysis. The following passage from Saidiya Hartman (1997) sheds light on my claim about the unaccounted for shift from the analyst's desire to the *jouissance* of analysis:

> The relation between *pleasure* and the possession of slave property, in both the figurative and literal senses, can be explained in part by the *fungibility of the slave*—that is, the joy made possible by virtue of the replaceability and interchangeability endemic to the commodity—and by the extensive capacities of property—that is, the augmentation of the master subject through his embodiment in external objects and persons. Put differently, the fungibility of the commodity makes the captive body an abstract and empty vessel vulnerable to the *projection* of others' feelings, ideas, desires, and values; and, as property, the dispossessed body of the enslaved is the surrogate for the master's body since it guarantees his *disembodied universality* and acts as the sign of his power and dominion. Thus, while the beaten and mutilated body presumably establishes the brute materiality of existence, the materiality of suffering regularly eludes (re)cognition by virtue of the body's being replaced by other signs of value, as well as other bodies. Thus the *desire* to don, occupy, or possess blackness or the black body as a sentimental resource and/or locus of *excess enjoyment* is both founded upon and enabled by the material relations of chattel slavery.
>
> (p. 21, emphasis added)

So, how did psychoanalysis get here, to this place of *excess enjoyment*? I argue that it is a function of the modern unconscious being the Other side of the Cogito. As Žižek (1998) puts it, "the subject of psychoanalysis is none other than the Cartesian *cogito*" (p. 4, emphasis in original). In other words, the modern subject of psychoanalysis, who is divided between being and thinking, is the inverse of the Cartesian formulation: *Cogito ergo sum*. I say the inverse because the modern subject is divided between their false being (articulated in the illusion of ego mastery) and their unconscious thinking.

Mladen Dolar (as cited in Žižek, 1998a) claims there are three Cogitos following Lacan's register theory: (1) The Imaginary Cogito "as the support of an illusory self-transparency that the mirror phase could effectively dismantle"; (2) the Symbolic Cogito "as the best way to conceive the subject of the signifier ... and its relation to the unconscious"; and (3) the Real Cogito, or the acephalic subject of drives as the "symptomatic nodal point ... that pushes subjectivity first 'beyond' the imaginary 'I,' then 'beyond' the symbolic subject" (pp. 36–37).

I think of the three Cogitos in terms of the three substitutional metaphors of alienation, separation, and traversal of fantasy, which indicate the progression of the analytic subject's unconscious thinking from meaning to sense and beyond. In alienation, the *subject as demand* is dominated by the (non)meaning of the master signifier, which comes from the Other. In separation, the *subject as desire* is lured by the unconscious (non)sense of fantasy *vis-à-vis* the *objet a*. In the traversing of fantasy, the *subject as drive* subjectifies the cause of their existence by reconfiguring their enjoyment in relation to their symptom.

Having said that, the subject of psychoanalysis is not a universal subject. Dolar (as cited in Žižek, 1998) asks: "*is there an unconscious outside of cogito?*" (p. 14, emphasis in original). He answers in the negative following Lacan. I answer in the affirmative: *the transmodern unconscious*. The subject of psychoanalysis, he adds, is "the subject of modern science" (p. 15). Dolar continues: "For being empty, it can be universal, and it can indeed be seen as the form of subjectivity implied by science, a *merely formal subjectivity*" (p. 15, emphasis added). I wish to problematize this *merely formal subjectivity* while confirming Dolar's assertion that "[the] Freudian unconscious is the unconscious of cogito" (p. 15). Finally, Dolar (1998) asks "how does the subject of the unconscious, as cogito, relate to *jouissance*?" (p. 15, emphasis in original).

I would like to historicize this question in the context of European colonialism. Unlike Dolar and—as you shall see in a moment—Žižek, I believe that the alienation and nonbeing of the colonized subject is not a psychical metaphor, but a Real historical materiality. In fact, one could argue that *the Cogito's literal assault on the being and thinking of non-Europeans* is one of the essential features of colonialism.

In writing about modern subjectivity, Žižek (1998a) does not hide what is obvious to him: the excremental subject of modernity is a Christian, European man. He writes:

> modern subjectivity is not announced in the Renaissance humanist celebration of man as the "crown of creation", that is, in the tradition of Erasmus and others (to which Luther cannot but appear as a "barbarian"), but rather in Luther's

> famous statement that man is the excrement who fell out of the God's anus. Modern subjectivity has nothing to do with the notion of man as the highest creature in the "great chain of being," as the final point of the evolution of the universe: modern subjectivity emerges when the subject perceives himself as "out of joint," as *excluded* from the "order of the things," from the positive order of entities. For that reason, the ontic equivalent of the modern subject is inherently *excremental*: there is no subjectivity proper without the notion that, at a different level, from another perspective, I am a mere piece of shit.
>
> (p. 4, emphasis in original)

For Žižek (1999), the excremental core of Cartesian modern subjectivity has an "excremental objectal counterpart" (p. 157), which is labor-power. However, Žižek (1999) argues that "being reduced to an excremental remainder" has revolutionary potential, especially for proletarian subjects, because it is a form of "radical 'subjective destitution'" (p. 161). Žižek (1999) reads what he calls "excremental identification" following the Lacanian logic of *identification with the symptom* (p. 228), which signifies assuming one's unique way of enjoying while renouncing the search for completeness in the Other. As such, it is a creative enjoyment of the symptom, whose function, as the *sinthome* in particular, anchors the subject and knots their Real, Symbolic, and Imaginary registers together.

Nevertheless, while I value the subject-as-drive, I would argue that the transmodern subject should be less driven by feces and more driven by the Gaze and/or the Voice. Therefore, I am skeptical about the revolutionary potential of regressive drives since their modes of enjoyment correspond to early childhood. Like Antoine de Sainte-Exupéry, I am committed to being in touch with one's inner child; however, there is an important distinction between being childish and childlike. Embracing the latter entails post-phallic forms of enjoyment, such as latent, genital, scopic, and invocatory enjoyments, to mention a few.

The ideological conditions governing psychoanalytic clinics and institutions

What historians call new imperialism, or the period in European colonialism between 1875 and 1914, is another ideological context for the founding of psychoanalysis as a discipline. What is being disciplined? The unconscious as a signifier of Otherness, or non-Europeanness. We are currently living in the era of humanitarian imperialism, which is a variation on the civilizing mission. However, to understand the development of European colonialism, we must return to what Grosfoguel (2013, p. 17) labels the four genocides and epistemicides in the long 16th century, for that traumatic history can shed light on the unconscious of psychoanalysis.

First, the genocide/epistemicide against Muslims and Jews in the conquest of al-Andalus in the name of "purity of blood." Second, the genocide/epistemicide against Indigenous peoples, first in the Americas and then in Asia. Third, the genocide/epistemicide against African peoples with the captive trade and their enslavement in the Americas. Fourth, the genocide/epistemicide against women who were accused of being witches and then burned alive.

These four genocides/epistemicides were essentially against non-European peoples who were perceived as premodern or uncivilized 'savages.' The genocides were essentially against 'non-beings' from the totalitarian perspective of Totality and the epistemicides were against their 'non-thinking,' which was considered irrational by the Euromodern Cogito. Therefore, non-Europeans were positioned as outside the "merely formal" or excremental subjectivity of modern science. However, I am trying to argue that they are Exterior or extimate, there is a perverse affirmation in their negation.

What is of concern to us today is that

> [i]n the analytical experience there is an oppressed person, the psychoanalyzed, whose need for communication is exploited and who (in the same way as the witches could, under torture, only repeat the language that the inquisitors wanted to hear) has no other choice ... than to attempt to say what she is supposed to say.
>
> (Wittig, 1992, p. 24)

In short, psychoanalysis, by design, excludes non-European subjects by negating their so-called 'savage' being and 'primitive' or 'barbaric' knowing. But why?

The colonial unconscious is the logic sustaining the rhetoric of the modern unconscious. Therefore, to unravel the unconscious of psychoanalysis, we must conduct a genealogy of the Cogito. Dussel, and Grosfoguel after him, show that the *ego cogito* of the 17th century was structured upon the *ego conquiro* of the 15th century. Dussel (1995) writes, "The 'I-conquistador' [or ego conquiro] forms the protohistory of Cartesian *ego cogito* and constitutes its own subjectivity as will-to-power" (p. 43, emphasis in original). Grosfoguel (2013) also posits an *ego extermino* in the 16th century:

> What links the 'I conquer, therefore I am' (*ego conquiro*) with the idolatric, God-like 'I think, therefore I am' (*ego cogito*) is the epistemic racism/sexism produced from the 'I exterminate, therefore I am' (*ego extermino*). It is the logic of genocide/epistemicide together that mediates the 'I conquer' with the epistemic racism/sexism of the 'I think' as the new foundation of knowledge in the modern/colonial world. The *ego extermino* is the socio-historical structural condition that makes possible the link of the *ego conquiro* with the *ego cogito*.
>
> (p. 77, emphasis in original)

For Žižek (1998a), the Cartesian subject—from the 17th century to this day—is the "monster" who "remains when we subtract from the subject the wealth of self-experience that constitutes subjectivity" (p. 7). The Cartesian (or modern) subject of psychoanalysis is a dehumanized/dehumanizing subject, a monster, who has not come to terms with the Real of coloniality. This negated monstrosity is projected onto the colonized, the enslaved, the over-exploited, and the sexually oppressed; this projection, which blames the victims—and denies the being and thinking of non-Europeans—demarcates the line between the zones of being and nonbeing.

Liberation, then, necessitates a different type of subjectivity, one that can account equally for the humanity of both Europeans and non-Europeans. I call it transmodern (contrapuntal, pluriversal, decolonial) subjectivity and Freud exemplified it even when he did not always embody it in his writings. Transmodern subjectivity accounts for both modernity and its alterity, and it does so from the Exterior perspective of decoloniality—which is the name for any methodology that delinks coloniality from modernity. Modernity is the baby worth saving, coloniality is the bathwater to be thrown away.

Dussel (2002, p. 235) provides us with a powerful model for how to enact this delinking through what he calls *the new transmodern system*, which is Exterior to the Totality of the modern/colonial world system and yet integrates this Totality in a way that supersedes the efforts of postmodern and critical modern approaches. For him, an innovative transmodernity is constructed from the synthesis of three elements: (1) the innovative interpellation before modernity, (2) the subsumption of modernity's positivity, and (3) the affirmation of the Other in its Exteriority. Dussel's model is a critique of approaches that either name the limit of modernity but stop there or that aim to assimilate the Other into the Totality of the same.

The Worlding of Psychoanalysis

In this final section, I wish to argue for the worlding of psychoanalysis through both *an immanent critique* and *a decolonial reading*. The first approach critiques psychoanalysis from within its own logic in an effort to emphasize its radical potential. The second approach critiques psychoanalysis from without through the Exterior lens of the non-European Other *qua* A^2. Ultimately, the analectical move is to be able to both appreciate what psychoanalysis has to offer in terms of praxis while also critiquing the false universality of ethnocentric psychoanalytic notions.

By using the term 'worlding,' I am for one indexing Said's (1983) notion of *worldliness*, which signifies that texts—including this one—are "part of the social world, human life, and of course the historical moments in which they are located and interpreted" (p. 4). In other words, psychoanalytic texts are always situated. However, with 'worlding' I am also invoking Fanon's (1961/2004) practice of *stretching theory*, which I see as a move from ethnocentrism to worldcentrism—with the caveat that I believe, following Freire, in the leadership of the oppressed (i.e., the proletariat, the racialized, and the sexualized), which entails working through sub-oppression. This chapter has been one attempt of stretching psychoanalysis beyond its comfort zone in Totality in order to shed light on the zone of nonbeing—the unspeakable Real of coloniality—which points the way to *the zone of becoming*. The zone of nonbeing is a traumatic zone, and who is more qualified to confront it than liberation psychoanalysts?

An immanent critique of psychoanalysis

An immanent critique of psychoanalysis means critiquing the praxis from within its own logic; as such, it involves critical reflexivity on the part of the psychoanalytic practitioner and/or theorist. I also think of immanent critique as *a critique grounded in love*. I would not spend so much time and effort critiquing something I do not care about. As I write elsewhere in this book:

> The radical potential of psychoanalysis is grounded in two basic principles: ethical listening and free association. Ethical listening means listening to the unconscious of the speaker, which requires a certain level of compassion or empathy and is not a question of over-interpretation (i.e., wild analysis); in other words, ethical listening entails practical ethics much more than theoretical knowledge. The analyst's lack of ethical listening correlates to reports from analysands of abuse in the clinic. This abuse is a result of the link between theoretical knowledge and mastery … Further, institutions in general tend to function aggressively like an ego while forgetting about their unconscious, that is, what they institutionally repress. Therefore, psychoanalytic institutions that encourage silencing or censorship are paradoxically non-psychoanalytic, for they essentially embody the complete opposite of the principle of free association, which should only be limited by the confidentiality binding the analyst to the analysand.

A decolonial reading of psychoanalysis

Double-unconsciousness and two-ness

A decolonial reading of psychoanalysis is an engagement with the praxis from without, particularly through the Exterior lens of decoloniality. As such, I would like to end the chapter by highlighting the work of a few non-European theorists on a further division of psychoanalytic subjectivity: *double-unconsciousness* or *two-ness*. For example, Safouan (2007) writes about how the Arab subject, as in the Arabic-speaking subject, is a diglossic subject, as a function of the gap between Classical Arabic and spoken Arabic dialects. This schism between a high formal language and a low vernacular one has both material and ideological effects. Safouan argues that diglossia creates a situation, where the formal language of the Symbolic order (Classical Arabic) is completely detached from the vernacular language of lived experience and desire. As such, he calls for *vernacularization of the lifeworld*, or the use of spoken, everyday language in education and public life.

The Arab subject's unconscious is formed in the vernacular. However, the language of authority, science, and education is a different, learned language. This forces a further split in the Arab subject: the subject that speaks the vernacular and the subject that must learn and use the formal language. This creates a state of *linguistic narcissism*, where individuals who master the formal language form a separate, elite class of scribes and experts, further alienating the general population. Since the language of desire is the vernacular, and the language of authority is a separate system, there is no linguistic space to articulate one's unconscious desires within the socio-political sphere. This lack of a bridge between the two linguistic registers leads to a disavowal of desire.

The formal language becomes a tool for an impersonal and bureaucratic barrage of statements, while the enunciating subject remains in the negated realm of the vernacular. A core principle of psychoanalysis is that the subject must be able to speak their truth freely to an Other. Safouan argues that without a unified vernacular language, a society cannot form a truly democratic subject. Political participation becomes difficult because people feel powerless and unable to articulate their thoughts in the language of authority. This linguistic gulf between the people and the elites contributes to authoritarianism and a lack of genuine public discourse, as the unconscious truths of the collective remain unspeakable. This explains the problem of an Arab nationalism based on linguistic or cultural sameness, as opposed to politico-economic cooperation. Therefore, I would argue for an Arab internationalism, as a unity in difference, grounded in a material project of liberation and not merely a regression to an ideological fantasy of oneness.

For Safouan, the diglossic subject, particularly in the Arab world, engages in a form of societal disavowal. The subject knows that their lived experience is in the vernacular, and that their desires and truths are linked to this spoken language. However, they disavow the reality that this language of the self is not the language of social power, authority, and knowledge. This dynamic of disavowal has several key psychoanalytic consequences.

According to Lacan, the subject enters the Symbolic order by accepting the Name-of-the-Father. For the diglossic subject, this process is fractured. The Name-of-the-Father is presented in a foreign, formal language, while the mOther's desire and the subject's early identity are formed in the vernacular. This leads to a Symbolic split rather than a unified entry into the social order. The diglossic subject is forced to split themselves further. One part knows the truth of the vernacular's primacy for subjectification. The other part accepts the authority and superiority of the formal language. These two parts do not integrate, but, rather, coexist in a state of disavowal. Since the language of the unconscious desire is systematically excluded from the public sphere, it cannot be articulated in the formal language of political and social life. This linguistic aporia contributes to political stasis and an inability to challenge authority, as the fundamental desires of the populace are not given a voice in the dominant Symbolic register.

The liberatory potential within psychoanalysis stems from the fact that Freud theorized the science of the unconscious from an ambivalent position: being a racialized subject while thinking he can assimilate into the anti-Semitic environment of late 19th and early 20th century Vienna. In the end, Freud was proven wrong and had to flee from Nazi-occupied Austria to England. Therefore, we should think about Freud's theorization of divided subjectivity with two-ness or double-alienation in mind, "Where it was, I must come into being" (as cited in Lacan, 1966/2006, p. 435). The original in German is *Wo Es war, soll Ich werden*, which Lacan (1966/2006) translates as: "I am thinking where I am not, therefore I am where I am not thinking" (p. 430).

Interbeing

In addition to Du Bois (1903/2007), other non-European theorists have written about the double negation (or two-ness) affecting non-European subjects in various ways. For example, Thích Nhất Hạnh (1998) challenges Descartes by arguing from a Zen perspective, "I think, therefore I am not." Right Thinking in Buddhism is the realization that there is no ego or that the ego (i.e., mastery) is an illusion, which is to affirm the unconscious as the psychosocial link between the subject and the Other. The purpose of meditation, in Buddhist practice, is to stop thinking and experience nonbeing, which is framed beyond a western nihilistic reading as a form of *becoming* through a realization of our *interbeing*.

Other-thought

Similarly, Abdelkébir Khatibi (1983/2019) has developed what he calls "other-thought," and Mignolo (2000) credits Khatibi when he writes about "other thinking." Khatibi's concept of "other-thought" (in French, *la pensée-autre*) is a key element of his intellectual framework. It refers to a form of decolonial thinking that seeks to transcend binary oppositions, particularly those rooted in colonialism, such as self/Other, east/west, or even colonizer/colonized. Khatibi uses other-thought to advocate for a plural, non-hierarchical way of thinking that resists dominant narratives and embraces hybridity, multiplicity, and difference. For Khatibi (1983/2019), other-thought is "planetary" and "plural" (p. 21), that is, pluriversal. It is also dialogical:

> What is *necessary* (the duty of an other-thought) is to broaden our freedom to think, to introduce in all dialogue several strategic levers—for example, to eliminate from discourse the absolutes of theology and theocentricism, which shackle the time, space, and edifice of Maghrebi societies. But this is not enough. The dialogue with all thought of difference is monumental. It aims to unsettle all that stupefies us in repetition and reproduction. An other-thought is always a plot, a conspiracy, a perpetual revolt, and a relentless risk. And we are so defenseless in the face of the power of the world. Such is our "history," which will have struck the body.
>
> (p. 19, emphasis in original)

Other-thought is not only dialogical but also dialectical and analectical. Like transmodernity, other-thought aims to sublate modernity and its alterity, thereby traversing the colonial fantasy of power through a subjectification of historical reason as cause:

> *An other-thought, analyzing itself in the words and laws that ground and bear it, works to penetrate the question of nonpower on the one hand and, on the other, to try to go beyond this opposition (power, nonpower) toward a research that would erase itself at the margins of metaphysics. This is what this dialogue aims for in its specific context.*
>
> (p. 25, emphasis in original)

As I have been arguing throughout this book, decoloniality is not antimodernity, premodernity, or nonmodernity. Decoloniality is alter-modernity, the historical reason of non-Europeans. As such, it is opposed to both instrumental reason and irrationalism. This thesis is affirmed by Khatibi when he writes:

> To be decolonized would be the other name of this other-thought, and decolonization would be the silent completion of Western metaphysics. And this is where begins this third speech, this unbinding of Western reason, in its sciences and techniques. How can this researcher bear in himself the Third World—which is a plural question—within a thought that must accept the overturn of all values and hierarchies? Insurgency is an exigency of life and of survival. Once again, there is no choice. Endless debate—let us make a leap.
>
> (p. 28)

Other-thought is post-Marxist *à la* non-aligned libertarian socialism:

> That is why this other-thought that we uphold is neither Marxist in the strict sense nor anti-Marxist in the right-wing sense of the word, but stands at the limits of its possibilities. For we seek to decenter in us Western knowledge, to decenter ourselves with respect to this center, this origin that the West gives itself. This should be done by operating already in the field of a plural and planetary thought, difference that struggles against its own reduction and domestication.
>
> (p. 30)

Other-thought is also deeply tied to Khatibi's linguistic and philosophical reflections on bilingualism and cultural identity, as he explored in his works like *La mémoire tatouée* [The Tattooed Memory] (2016) and *Amour bilingue* [*Love in Two Languages*] (1990). In short, other-thought represents an alternative, decolonial mode of thinking that encourages openness to the multiple, the hybrid, and the non-totalitarian. For Khatibi:

> an other-thought, such as we envisage it, is a *thought in tongues*, a globalizing translation of the codes, systems, and constellations of signs that circulate in the world and above (in a nontheological sense). Each society or group of societies is a relaying of this globalization. A strategy that does not actively work to transform these relays is, perhaps, condemned to eat itself and turn on itself—entropically.
>
> (p. 35, emphasis in original)

Other-thought is part of Khatibi's broader project of *double critique*, where he critiques both the west's dominance in knowledge production and the essentialist responses from postcolonial contexts. The task of double critique arises from the experience of non-European subjects with double-unconsciousness; the point is to not only critique the ideology of Totality (i.e., racial capitalism), but also to engage in self-criticism *vis-à-vis* Exteriority. In other words, the goal is to reject both coloniality and antimodernity. Rather than simply inverting the power relations, Khatibi's other-thought tries to move beyond authoritarian forms of power, creating spaces for intercultural dialogue and new forms of pluriversal subjectivity that are fluid and complex.

> The double critique consists in opposing to the Western episteme its unthought-of outside, while radicalizing the margin, not only in a *thought in Arabic*, but also in an other-thought that speaks *in tongues*, listening to every word–from wherever it comes ... This other-thought, this "as-yet unnameable," is perhaps a promise, the sign of a happening in a world to be transformed. Doubtless, an endless task. However, in thought (let us call it thus), there are no miracles, only ruptures.
>
> (p. 38, emphasis in original)

Caliban's reason

The historical reason of non-Europeans—the alter-modernity of Exteriority is what Paget Henry (2000) calls "Caliban's reason." Caliban is a half-human, half-monster character from Shakespeare's *The Tempest*, enslaved by the wizard Prospero. As such, the play deals with the Hegelian master–slave dialectic. While Prospero (the master) represents power, Caliban (the slave) represents knowledge, particularly practical know-how (*savoir-faire*). Henry reveals the Real of slavery under racial capitalism, which is sutured by the Symbolic slavery of modern/colonial fields such as psychoanalysis:

> Faust, the capitalist developer, was here metamorphosed into Prospero, while his racialized worker was transformed into Caliban. This "Calibanization" of Africans could not but devour their rationality and hence their capacity for philosophical thinking. As a biological being, Caliban is not a philosopher. He or she does not think and in particular does not think rationally. In the European tradition, rationality was a white trait that, by their exclusionary racial logic, blacks could not possess. Hence the inability to see the African now reinvented as Caliban, in the role of sage, philosopher, or thinker. In short, this new racialized identity was also the death of Caliban's reason.
>
> (Henry, 2000, p. 12)

Like Dussel, Grosfoguel, and Hạnh, Henry also problematizes the Cartesian principle of *cogito, ergo sum*, which is foundational for the hyper-individualism of neoliberal subjectivity. Henry accomplishes his critique through the other-thought of C.L.R. James:

> In James, the corresponding formulation could be "I undertake or participate in a historical project, therefore I am." This socially constructed nature of the

> Jamesian self will find some significant echoes in traditional African thought. In this tradition, the thinking or speaking subject was not conceived on the solitary Cartesian model. On the contrary, as Mbiti suggests, it is more a case of "I am, because we are, and since we are, therefore I am."
>
> (pp. 59–69)

Henry also indexes the historical reason of Sylvia Wynter (2003) to expose the coloniality of Cogito when he writes:

> Vulnerability via the necessary misrepresentation of liminal categories is the dynamic principle of epistemic change for Wynter. Because of these categories, discourse production is accompanied by the creating of a shadow that will eventually lead to the downfall of the discourse. Wynter's new vertical drama of cogito consciousness is to make explicit this process of shadow creation through the analysis of the liminal categories of *epistemes*. By making discursive shadow production explicit, Wynter hopes to introduce a qualitatively new type of *episteme*, one that would give us greater control over the misrepresentations that have undermined horizontal projects of emancipation.
>
> (p. 129, emphasis in original)

The vertical drama of ego, or Cogito, consciousness, for Wynter, revolves around the following question: "whether or not as human beings we will be able to increase significantly our consciousness of and control over the auto-poetic processes that ground our discursive practices" (Henry, 2000, p. 141). *Autopoiesis* is a decolonial challenge to what Dussel (2002) refers to as "*the inclusion of the other into the same (the old system)*" (p. 235, emphasis in original). In other words, transmodernity is autopoiesis, for it affirms the Other in its Exteriority and subsumes modernity's positivity. Henry qualifies Africana philosophy as an instantiation of this transmodern autopoiesis (p. 155).

The Other of the Other

In conclusion, the historical division between Totality and Exteriority has resulted in colonial difference: the hierarchical power/knowledge asymmetry between two Others (see Figure 7.1). As such, we must resurrect and redefine a notion abandoned by Lacan: the Other of the Other. For Lorenzo Chiesa (2007), the Other of the Other is the transcendent Law, the universal Name-of-the-Father, or the signifier of signifiers. Lacan ends up abandoning this notion of the Other of the Other in an effort to argue that there is no metalanguage beyond the desire of the mOther. However, this is dishonest because the Other of the Other was foundational for modern science—and, by extension, psychoanalytic subjectivity:

> modern science relies on an anomalous Judeo-Christian tradition which is no longer preoccupied with what goes on in the celestial domain but, rather,

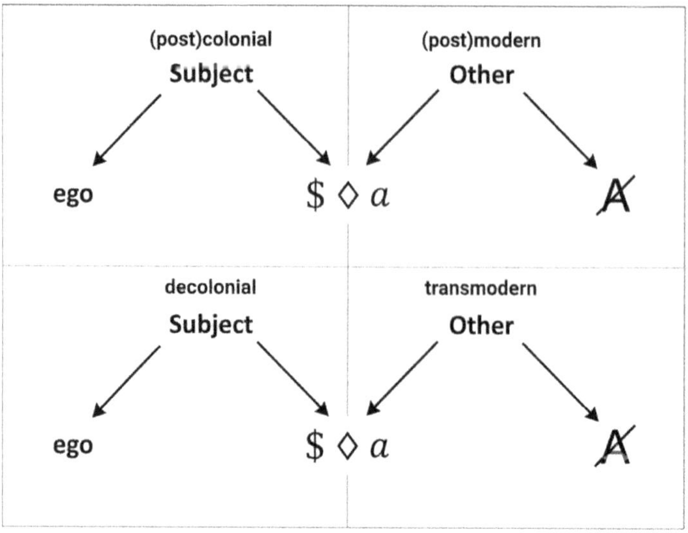

Figure 7.1 The two Others

> secures the Other to a nondeceptive a priori which is itself *symbolic*. This is nothing but Descartes's nondeceiving God. "The notion that the real [everyday reality] is unable to play tricks on us," which is so "essential to the constitution of the world of [modern] science"—and still influences "the mentality of people like us"—ultimately depends on "Descartes' meditation about God as incapable of deceiving us." In other words, for modern science, the Other of the Other is symbolic: this presupposes "an act of faith." Modern science relies on a "unique principle at the foundation, not only of the universe [objects as perceived in everyday reality], but of the law."
>
> (p. 113, emphasis in original)

Chiesa argues that the Totality of modernity was founded historically, while the supposed premodernity of Exteriority was founded retroactively on the basis of a Symbolic Other of the Other:

> Lacan believes that all symbolic systems necessitate a "non-deceptive element," a basic Law that functions as the universal Other of the Other in a given epoch of history, yet he also deems modernity to be special insofar as it founds itself on a symbolic Other of the Other. Having said this, one should not overlook the fact that the precise functioning of premodern symbolic systems is irremediably lost to us—and this independently of whether we still have faith in the Judeo–Christian God. Despite his own endeavor to sketch the foundation of Aristotelian science "from the inside," Lacan believes that we inevitably end up retroactively reinterpreting the Aristotelian (and pre-Aristotelian) universe as being based on

> a *symbolic* Other of the Other: this is the only way in which we can formulate any truth (as fiction) about it.
>
> (p. 113, emphasis in original)

The negation of Otherness describes alienation under modernity. However, we need an account of double-negation (or two-ness) in order to explain the material effects of coloniality—that psychic remainder of colonialism. *Le nom du père* (the No or Name of the Primordial Father) holds the key to this double-negation, particularly since European colonization often engaged materially in the emasculation, or castration, of non-European patriarchs, who were exterminated if not enslaved, raped, and over-exploited: "The basic Law of the prohibition of incest is what one discovers at the root of any historically determined Other of the Other" (Chiesa, 2007, p. 114).

The pluriversal Other of the Other (i.e., the Name-of-the-Father) is Lacan's mythical equivalent to Freud's Oedipus complex—see also Fu Wai (2021) on the Name-of-the-Grandfather in the context of Chinese culture. I say pluriversal when Chiesa says universal because I associate the Other of the Other with Exteriority, and I wish to reclaim this negated alter-modernity:

> From a slightly different angle, we could suggest that, for Lacan, the first mythical emergence of the *universal* Other of the Other—the birth of the Symbolic as such—should be regarded as being homologous with what we now know happens at the *individual* level of the child who resolves the Oedipus complex thanks to the Law of the Name-of-the-Father. The first basic Law of/in history, the beginning of history itself, should thus be associated with the conclusion of an explicitly phallic prehistorical period (the universal correlate of the phallic phase) … As I have just suggested, this first basic Law *qua* universal Name-of-the-Father is, by definition, at the same time the Law that prohibits incest and thus retroactively symbolizes (on the universal level) all the protosymbolic activities of the species that preceded this moment—in simply [*sic*] terms, the allegedly phallic culture of menhirs.
>
> (p. 114, emphasis in original)

Lacan abandons the concept of the Other of the Other after *Seminar V*. His problem with his own structuralist account is that the Other of the Other presupposes *a purely external Real*, a metalanguage outside of the Symbolic order (see Figure 7.2). In my view, the Other of the Other signifies an extimate Exteriority, analectically related to Totality, and marked by the Real of coloniality. The Other represents Otherness within Totality, which can only go as far as postmodernity/postcoloniality, but can never capture the decoloniality of other-thought, the historical reason of non-Europeans or their alter-modernity.

Also, modernity/coloniality presupposes a "pure Real" outside of Totality: the so-called noble savage. This explains why "dark continents" are imagined as exotic resources (i.e., non-European lands inhabited by barbarian peoples) that can be

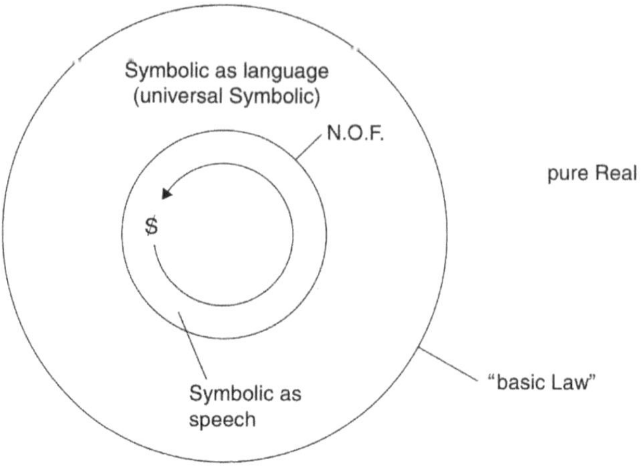

Figure 7.2 The purely external Real

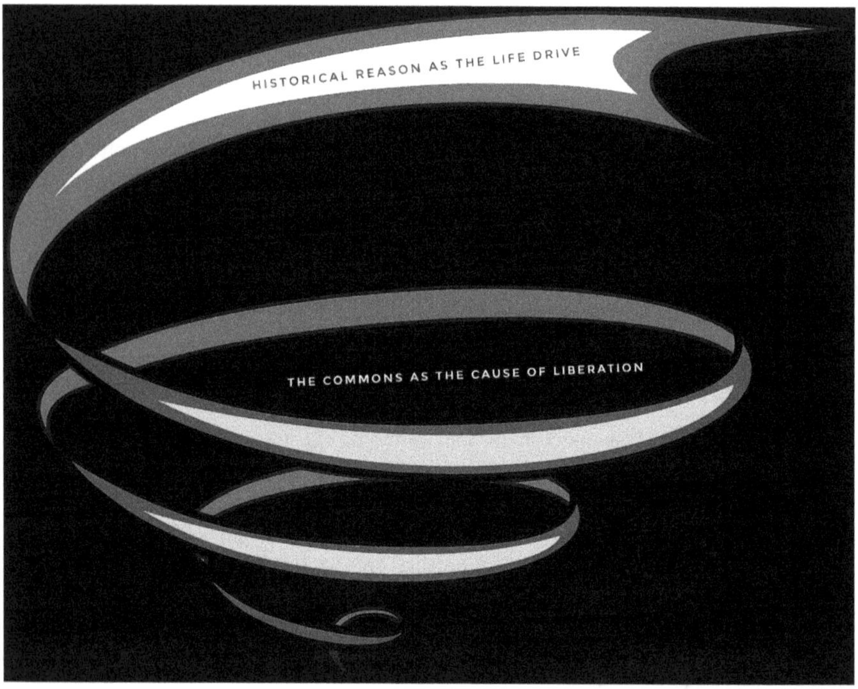

Figure 7.3 The commons as the cause of liberation

extracted, over-exploited, and primitively accumulated. This colonial logic is the surplus-*jouissance* of psychoanalysis, which is not possible without the double-negation of the Other of the Other.

As such, I agree with Lacan that there is no metalanguage, but my argument is that *there is an Other language* signifying an Other system (transmodernity), which is Exterior to modernity and negated by it. This Other system is structured by the logic of *colonial difference*, which precedes, and is foundational for, sexual difference. Masculine *jouissance* and feminine *jouissance* are both forms of mythic *jouissance* in the zone of being predicated on negating the divine *jouissance* of (non)Europeans in the zone(s) of nonbeing/becoming. This difference between mythic and divine *jouissance* is what I term *colonial difference*—the difference between colonial enjoyment and decolonial enjoyment. Transmodernity is the negation of colonial enjoyment and the affirmation of decolonial enjoyment. The latter is the collective enjoyment of the commons, as the cause of liberation, driven by historical reason (see Figure 7.3) via anticapitalism, antiracism, and antisexism, that is, libertarian socialism, radical humanism, and revolutionary feminism.

Chapter 8

The Other Side of Abyssal Psychoanalysis

Let me begin by saying that I read the disturbing reports by seven women accusing Boaventura de Sousa Santos of harassment a few years after I finished writing this text. This, of course, raises the question of whether one can separate the scholar from the scholarship, or whether the personal is political, as second-wave feminists argued. I will most likely refrain from citing de Sousa Santos moving forward; however, I decided to retain my references to his ideas for the purposes of the arguments I develop in this chapter with the caveat that I will always side with the abused, as someone who is committed to ethical listening. Santos denied wrongdoing, which is a classic defense mechanism. While I retain Santos's terminology, my use of his theoretical framework is an act of *subversive appropriation*. By siding with the abused, I am applying a postabyssal ethics to the very production of this text—i.e., using the theory against the theorist.

This chapter is written from the perspective of, and in solidarity with, analysands as an attempt to think critically about psychoanalysis beyond the gatekeepers of power and knowledge—be that in the form of analysts *qua* masters or institutions *qua* universities. This is an intervention at the level of praxis, which undermines psychoanalytic approaches that privilege *theoretical knowledge* over *practical ethics*. Why do we continue to hear about ethical breaches involving abusive analysts as well as institutions that come to their defense to protect their image by silencing the victims? Is it hard to imagine the clinic replicating the oppressive dynamics existing within a given society, particularly in the Global North? Is it impossible to consider the history of colonization vis-à-vis the invention of psychoanalysis in the late 19th century in the context of New Imperialism, especially the Scramble for Africa?

These practical questions concern politics and ethics because the clinic is neither an ahistorical entity nor a neutral space that exists in a vacuum. The clinic is a psychosocial space, wherein *what is psychically repressed is linked to what is socially oppressed*, or, as Lacan (1966/2002) put it succinctly in Seminar XIV, "*the unconscious is politics!*" (p. 122, emphasis in original). While the subject of psychoanalysis may be normative in *theory*, for *he* is often presumed to be 'civilized' (i.e., male, of European descent, and bourgeois), the subject is far from normative in *practice*. Therefore, only through a critical understanding of the field from the

DOI: 10.4324/9781003768104-8

perspective of female, non-European, and proletarian analysands can psychoanalytic scholars and practitioners reconnect with the field's radical potential, but to do so is the work of decolonial critique, which is my task here.

I want to acknowledge that the signifier 'clinic' is a controversial term as shown by numerous anti-psychiatrists (e.g., Laing, 1960; Szasz, 1960). The clinic is historically associated with forced institutionalization and excessive medicalization, so when I invoke the clinic, as a radical humanist, I am thinking of *a safe space where psychoanalysis takes place*, whether that space is actual or virtual. In other words, I am not thinking of an asylum or a psychiatric hospital, and I am certainly indexing neither the pathologizing medical model as a form of social control nor the dehumanizing clinic as a site of coercive power.

The radical potential of psychoanalysis is grounded in two basic principles: *ethical listening* and *free association*. Ethical listening means listening—with "the third ear" (Reik, 1948)—to the unconscious of the speaker, which requires a certain level of openness and is not a question of over-interpretation (wild analysis); in other words, ethical listening entails practical ethics (know-how) much more than theoretical knowledge. The analyst's lack of ethical listening correlates to reports from analysands of abuse in the clinic. This abuse is a result of the link between theoretical knowledge and mastery, which is what Foucault (1980) referred to as power/knowledge and what Lacan (1991/2007) identified in terms of the university and master's discourses—the former being always subservient to the latter. Subsequently, the analyst is not supposed to embody an ontological, or even epistemological, position of mastery, but simply an ethical function within a specific clinical context *vis-à-vis* the analysand, who performs the work of analysis. While the analysand may position the analyst as a *subject-supposed-to-know*, this projection is a fantasmatic trap; it is a transference that must be worked through and dismantled. The *subject-supposed-to-know* is not a position of mastery that the analyst identifies with, as some form of expert on the unconscious.

For example, Lacan founded and dissolved several analytic schools because of the members' transference in relation to him as the analyst *qua* absolute master—a death-driven conundrum. Furthermore, institutions in general tend to function aggressively from the place of their ego while forgetting about their unconscious, that is, what they institutionally repress. Therefore, psychoanalytic institutions that encourage silencing or censorship are paradoxically non-psychoanalytic, for they essentially embody the complete opposite of the principle of free association, which should only be limited by the confidentiality binding the analyst to the analysand.

My attempt here is to theorize the historical conditions, which give rise to the ethical breaches we continue to witness today within the clinic and analytic institutions. Psychoanalysis is not outside these historical conditions; therefore, anyone who is interested in the praxis of psychoanalysis has a responsibility *to sustain fidelity to the field's radical potential, particularly from the perspective of oppressed analysts–analysands*. My dialogue with oppressed analysands is the ethical and political background driving my concerns in this chapter, which is also dedicated to them.

I draw on the work of Boaventura de Sousa Santos, particularly his notions of "abyssal thinking" and "postabyssal thinking" (Santos, 2007), in an effort to distinguish between *abyssal psychoanalysis* and *postabyssal psychoanalysis*. Santos's (2014) overall project is to critique dominant (Euromodern) epistemologies from the Exterior perspective of the Global South, which is not an argument for the superiority of "epistemologies of the South," but, rather, an argument for embracing "ecologies of knowledges." While his focus is on epistemologies in general, I am interested in *psychoanalytic epistemology* in particular because I find it—with its emphasis on the unconscious—to offer both *a damning critique of psychology* and *a theorization of complex subjectivity*.

In my own work (Beshara, 2019a, 2021a), I qualify psychoanalysis—regardless of type—as (post)colonial because, in its different iterations from Freud and beyond, it is primarily a critique of Totality from within, whether it indexes critical modern or postmodern discourses in order to perform this immanent critique. In other words, (post)colonial, or abyssal, psychoanalysis exemplifies a Euromodern rhetoric, which is sustained by a colonial logic—the unconscious of psychoanalysis.

Many of the important insights of psychoanalysis (e.g., the unconscious, desire, enjoyment, fantasy, the drive, etc.) warrant delinking the field's epistemology from its unconscious colonial logic, for example, regarding the so-called primitivity of non-Europeans (see Brickman, 2018). This is the task of liberation, or postabyssal, psychoanalysis, which entails a transmodern critique, that is, a critique of Totality from Exteriority, in an effort to ground the praxis of psychoanalysis in a decolonial, or worldly, logic.

Delinking also leads to a pluriversal verification of psychoanalytic epistemology, which is different from the colonial tendency to *universalize what is provincial*, for example, in relation to theorizing the subject. To put it differently, the Euromodern subject of abyssal psychoanalysis is not a universal subject. On the other hand, *the transmodern subject of postabyssal psychoanalysis is a pluriversal subject*. The transmodern critique renders psychoanalysis—the revolutionary science of the unconscious—falsifiable by exposing its provincial limits and testing its claims against the colonial Real that was previously produced as nonexistent.

By abyssal thinking, Santos (2014, p. x) is referring to how dominant (Euromodern) epistemology makes non-European human and nonhuman realities invisible or even actively produces them as nonexistent. For this reason, he qualifies dominant epistemology, of which psychoanalysis is one example, as an "*epistemology of blindness*" (emphasis in original, p. x).

Khanna (2003) makes this dimension of epistemological blindness *vis-à-vis* psychoanalysis explicit in *Dark Continents*, wherein she writes, "the concepts of self and being that came into existence in psychoanalysis were dependent on strife or violence, that is, on the politics of colonial relations" (p. 2). Postabyssal thinking (and consequently, postabyssal psychoanalysis), then, involves shedding light on these unconscious colonial logics, which inform modern fields of knowledge, in an attempt to delink modernity from coloniality and, therefore, ground our theorizations of the subject in a cosmopolitan sensibility, which I have referred to before as *contrapuntal psychoanalysis* (Beshara, 2021a). In the words of Santos (2014), postabyssal thinking

> is a nonderivative thinking; it involves a radical break with modern Western ways of thinking and acting. In our time, to think in nonderivative terms means to think from the perspective of the other side of the line, precisely because the other side of the line has been the realm of the unthinkable in Western modernity. (p. 134)

In this chapter, I extend Santos's analysis by conceiving of this unthinkable line in terms of a further bar in addition to the one familiar in Freudo–Lacanian psychoanalysis (i.e., the bar that splits subjectivity into ego and unconscious). I attempt to point to an Other bar, which is *the repressed unconscious of psychoanalysis* itself. I also refer to this Other bar as *the bloody shadow of psychoanalytic epistemology*, and I demonstrate my thesis through a critical analysis of Lacanian discourse theory, particularly the master's discourse (see Figure 8.1).

Signifying this Other bar can help us account for the doubly-split subjectivities of those who were socially excluded since the beginning of psychoanalytic epistemology, that is, non-Europeans—be they Indigenous, Black, or Global Southern. These non-European subjects were historically, and continue to be, divided not only by Euromodern discourses, but also by the materiality of colonization, enslavement, over-exploitation, racism, etc. Repressing that colonial materiality manifests itself as a fantasy that sanitizes modernity from this traumatic Real of violence and oppression, and, of course, frames modernity as civilizational. Traversing this fantasy is the central task of postabyssal psychoanalysis.

What, then, is on the Other side of abyssal psychoanalysis? From an abyssal perspective, one encounters the Other side as "only nonexistence, invisibility, nondialectical absence" (Santos, 2007, p. 46). I am referring here not to modernity as the master's discourse, but to its double or bloody shadow, which ideologically—and fantasmatically—sutures the Real of coloniality. Following Santos (2007), a postabyssal psychoanalysis, then, "consists of the symbolic amplification of signs, clues, and latent tendencies that, however inchoate and fragmented, do point to

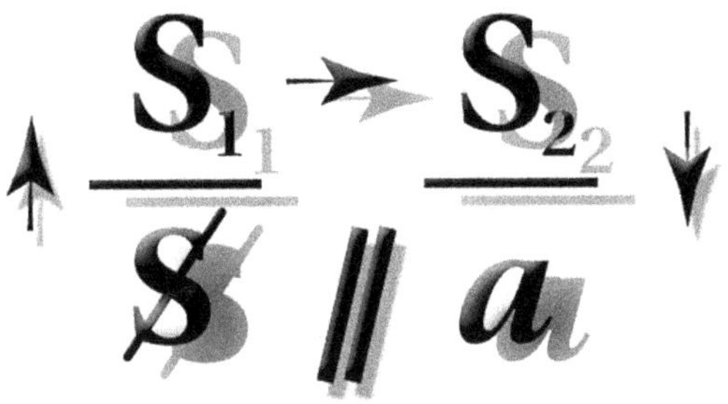

Figure 8.1 The master's discourse and its bloody shadow

new constellations of meaning as regards both the understanding and the transformation of the world" (p. 64).

On the Other side, postabyssal praxis manifests as a decentered clinic. For example, when an analyst engages in ethical listening with a (non)European analysand, they must move beyond interpreting the unconscious solely through the Oedipal triangle (a provincial Euromodern construct). Instead, they adopt ecological thinking, recognizing that the analysand's symptoms may be a legitimate response to the colonial Real—a swerving toward a zone of becoming that requires the analyst to witness historical trauma rather than merely pathologize it. The two characteristics of postabyssal psychoanalysis are: "subaltern cosmopolitanism" (p. 63) and "ecological thinking" (p. 65). Before I unpack these concepts, I shall now turn to a critique of abyssal psychoanalysis.

Psychoanalysis, as a type of modern western (read: abyssal) thinking, is caught up in a "dual modern cartography: a legal [S_1] cartography and an epistemological [S_2] cartography" (Santos, 2007, p. 52). This dual modern cartography, with its two main forms of radical negation (negating what is beyond 'universal,' or European, conceptions of true/false and legal/illegal), results "in a radical absence, the absence of humanity, modern subhumanity" (p. 52). Subhumans are those who are positioned as spectral subjects (objects, commodities, things) below the abyssal line separating Euromodernity from "the colonial zone" (p. 48)—its repressed Other. Subhumans are doubly barred ($\$$) because they represent both "the foundation" of abyssal thinking and the "negation of the foundation" (p. 52). In other words, the colonial zone is repressed in both senses of the word: the political and the psychoanalytic, respectively.

For this reason, we are currently witnessing, particularly since the rise of neoliberalism or global racial capitalism in the 1970s, the return of the repressed *qua* "the return of the colonial and the return of the colonizer" (Santos, 2007, p. 55). The return of the colonial takes one of three forms: "the terrorist … the undocumented migrant worker … and the refugee" (p. 55). In this sense, we can speak both metaphorically and literally of the abyssal bar *qua* cartographic lines, borders, fences, walls, etc., which sustain the appropriation/violence paradigm in the colonial zone.

However, since the colonial zone today is often an "endo-colonial" zone (Virilio, 1983/2008), as is clear from apartheid policing in the Global North, the appropriation/violence paradigm, which used to be restricted to exo-colonial territories, has been seeping for decades into the regulation/emancipation paradigm governing modern social reality, particularly because the abyssal lines today are not as clearly defined as they were in the 15th century. Regardless of their definition, they are still operational, albeit invisible, and as such they inform modern theories and practices grounded in abyssal thinking, such as (post)colonial psychoanalysis.

Furthermore, Santos (2007) characterizes the return of the colonizer in terms of both "new indirect rule," or the privatization of the commons, and "the rise of social fascism" (p. 58). Because the colonial zone is radically negated, the ~~colonial subject~~ is a *homo sacer* living in a "state of exception" (Agamben, 1998), wherein anything goes since he or she is positioned in an extra-legal zone (e.g., Guantánamo). This state of exception is especially evident in terms of the appropriation of, and violence against, Indigenous and/or Black subjects in settler-colonial societies (e.g., U.S.A.), which Virilio (1983/2008) qualifies using the term "endo-colonization" (p. 103). Consequently, the Black Lives Matter movement is a *swerving* from endo-colonial appropriation and violence, which points toward the *zone of becoming*.

Lacan's (1991/2007) formalization, or mathematization, of psychoanalysis, as exemplified by his use of algebraic symbols and diagrams (see Figure 10.1), can be read as a form of "abyssal cartography" (p. 51) since the juridico-epistemological bar, which pushes the modern subject ($) below the master-signifier (S_1), occludes an Other bar: the abyssal bar. The abyssal bar is a function of the cartographic lines that were established as part of the historical imperial process to justify property rights over occupied lands and enslaved peoples.

As illustrated in Figure 8.1, the bloody shadow of the master's discourse is represented by the superimposition of a second bar over the subject. While the first bar represents the standard Lacanian split between ego and unconscious, the second bar signifies the abyssal bar: the literal and material exclusion of (non)Europeans from humanity itself. This doubly-barred subject is not only alienated in language but is structurally produced as subhuman or a thing below the line of civilization.

Santos (2007) writes, "The first modern global line was probably the Treaty of Tordesillas between Portugal and Spain (1494), but the truly abyssal lines emerged in the mid-sixteenth century with the amity lines" (pp. 48–49). In other words, the metaphoric barring (Symbolic-Imaginary castration) of the modern subject is premised on the literal barring (Real castration) of the ~~colonial subject~~, or as Santos (2007) puts it, "the metaphorical cartography of the global lines has outlived the literal cartography of the amity lines that separated the Old from the New World" (p. 53).

As a result, the Symbolic-Imaginary order (e.g., the Euromodern reality of psychoanalysis) is rooted in the "global spiritual order" (p. 49) of Christendom, which rests on repressing the non-European Real. The ~~colonial subjects~~ of the non-European Real, who are Exterior to modern knowledge and Law, include non-Christians *qua* non-Europeans. Having said that, psychoanalysis includes within itself a post-abyssal potential because its founder (Freud) was Jewish and Frosh (2020) even reads psychoanalysis as *decolonial Judaism*.

Nonetheless, because Freud struggled throughout his life to assimilate into anti-Semitic Viennese society, he internalized some of that society's abyssal thinking (e.g., racism), which he clearly struggled with as is obvious in his last book, *Moses and Monotheism* (Freud, 1939)—written in the context of Nazi Germany's annexation of Austria. Said's (2003) final text, *Freud and the Non-European*, highlights how identity, as theorized by Freud, is paradoxical since it is based on non-identity given that the founder of Judaism (Moses) was an Egyptian. Said's reading of Freud's last book allows for a liberatory figuration of *non-identity politics*, or "an *identity based on politics* (and not a *politics based on identity*)" (Mignolo, 2007, p. 492, emphasis in original). Whereas non-identity politics is articulated through both Symbolic alignment of desire and Real *jouissance*, identity politics is nothing but *méconnaissance* since it is premised on Imaginary identifications, which are shot through with narcissism and aggressivity. Non identity politics manifests itself in terms of solidarity and comradeship around common demands; identity politics is caught up in the seductive games of representative democracy, which slide between fascism and totaliarianism.

While psychoanalysis may exhibit abyssal thinking, Lacan's (1966/2006) concept of the Real affords a reading of the colonial zone, or the "zone of nonbeing" (Fanon, 1952/1967), as the colonial Real. The colonial Real is "the realm of incomprehensible beliefs and behaviors which in no way can be considered knowledge, whether true or false" (Santos, 2007, p. 51). The modern Symbolic-Imaginary order radically excludes the colonial Real and produces it as nonexistent. Exterior to Totality. Consequently, Santos (2007) regards the colonial negation of non-European humanity to be the founding negation of modernity, whose function is "sacrificial, in that it is the condition of the affirmation of that other part of [European] humanity which considers itself universal" (p. 52).

Therefore, psychoanalysis, as a (post)modern rhetoric, is logically built upon an abyssal fantasy, which sutures the colonial Real—its bloody shadow. While the hysteric's and analyst's discourses hold within them the radical potential for generating counter-hegemonic discourses *vis-à-vis* the university and master's discourses, respectively; psychoanalysis's repression (and repetition) of the colonial Real—"incomprehensible … subhuman territory" (Santos, 2007, p. 57)—renders the distinctions between the four discourses superfluous and may even lead to the analyst's discourse functioning unconsciously as a master's discourse.

That being the case, psychoanalytic theorists and practitioners must delink the field's modern rhetoric regarding knowledge (S_2) and Law (S_1) from its colonial logic—a delinking, which entails traversing the abyssal fantasy. The colonial Real refers to what is beyond modern western thinking, in particular beyond modern knowledge and Law. The colonial Real is the invisible foundation of the Symbolic-Imaginary order, or the modern world-system, which is the hegemonic global order of racial capitalism since the colonization of the Americas.

I chose to critically analyze the master's discourse, as opposed to the capitalist discourse, because the former is foundational juridico-epistemologically from a historical perspective. As Lacan (1991/2007) shows, the university is always subservient to the master, but even the analyst's and hysteric's discourses, as critical discourses that challenge both mastery and the commodification of knowledge respectively, will eventually circle back to the master's discourse through the generation of new master-signifiers (S_1). Not mentioning how the hysteric's production of critical knowledge (S_2) can eventually become co-opted and commodified by the university in the liberal version of racial capitalism: rainbow capitalism. This is the paradox at the heart of Lacanian discourse theory, which is a challenge for any concrete utopian praxis of liberation.

Furthermore, my theoretical treatment of the master's discourse involves an innovation with my conception of the discourse's bloody shadow, which is the specter of a silenced discourse returning like the ghost of Hamlet's father. In other words, my argument, in short, is that while psychoanalysis has a liberatory potential, which can be designated as postabyssal, the praxis can also slip into a discourse of mastery, or its knowledge of the unconscious can become commodified, as a function of its colonial unconscious, which is the bloody shadow of psychoanalytic epistemology.

The subject of psychoanalysis is the modern subject (the metropolitan and bourgeois European *man* who entered the social contract in order to abandon the state of nature to form civil society). This modern subject ($) was constructed in relation to its negated Other: ~~colonial objects~~ ('savage' peoples or the state of nature where civil society's institutions have no place). Consequently, can psychoanalysis account for ~~colonial subjects~~ ($) beyond their objectification as fantasmatic *objets a*? And is the analyst, as a structural embodiment of the *objet a*, taking the place of a non-European Other in order to functionally cause the desire of the European analysand?

Accounting for (de)~~colonial subjectivity~~ entails moving beyond the abyssal thinking of modernity/coloniality and towards the ecological thinking of liberation psychoanalysis. In other words, the question of cultural, and colonial, difference is at the heart of psychoanalytic epistemology given its "sociology of absences" (Santos, 2014). It is not scientific to universalize what is provincial while repressing what is Other, hence, the necessity for thinking pluriversally about subjectivity and the unconscious.

Liberation psychoanalysis is postabyssal because it is grounded in "subaltern cosmopolitanism," which is a "cultural and political form of counter-hegemonic globalization" and "the name of the emancipatory projects whose claims and criteria of social inclusion reach beyond the horizons of global capitalism" (Santos, 2007, p. 63). One of the features of liberation psychoanalysis is postabyssal thinking, which is "a nonderivative thinking" that "involves a radical break with modern Western ways of thinking and acting" (p. 66).

Postabyssal thinking is *thinking from the perspective of the Other of the Other*, that is, the colonial Real or "the realm of the unthinkable in Western modernity" (p. 66). While Lacan (1966/2006) is correct to argue that "there is no metalanguage that can be spoken" (p. 688), I add that "there are Other languages" (Beshara, 2021a, p. 175). To put it differently, there is something to be said about the cultural specificity of psychoanalytic epistemology given how its knowledge was historically transmitted through particular languages (e.g., German, English, French, etc.).

Postabyssal thinking is "learning from the South through an [Indigenous, African, Latin@, Asian] epistemology of the South … It is an ecology, because it is based on the recognition of the plurality of heterogeneous knowledges" (Santos, 2007, p. 66). Santos adds, "The ecology of knowledges is founded on the idea that knowledge is interknowledge" (p. 66). A great example of postabyssal psychoanalysis in the context of cultural and linguistic specificity is Omnia El Shakry's (2017) *The Arabic Freud: Psychoanalysis and Islam in Modern Egypt*. El Shakry grounds psychoanalysis in the Exteriority of Islamic mysticism (*al-Taṣawwuf*); however, I prefer worlding or stretching psychoanalysis through non-European rationalism; hence, my interest in the philosophy of Ibn Rushd, for example.

Santos (2007) writes about "the hegemonic eye," which "ceases to see and indeed declares as nonexistent the state of nature" (p. 50). This hegemonic eye, which is located in civil society, is also *the hegemonic I of psychoanalysis*—its ego or consciousness (e.g., Descartes's *ego cogito*, wherein thinking = being). Therefore, the state of nature (the colonial Real) is the abyssal unconscious of psychoanalysis, which exposes the repressed "ego conquiro" and "ego extermino" (Grosfoguel, 2013) at the root of the hegemonic I's false being.

Not mentioning that Lacan's (1977/2004, p. 211) account of alienation—nonmeaning as a compromise between the subject's being and the Other's meaning—leaves out the historico-imperial facticity of nonbeing and the potential for transmodern becoming. Colonial *objets a* (who are most often non-European) are those on the Other side of the abyssal line, that is, those living in the colonial zone of nonbeing, which is analectically linked with *the decolonial zone of becoming*.

Fanon (1952/1967) was the first theorist to author a postabyssal psychoanalytic account of the damned from the perspective of, and by someone located in, the zone of nonbeing (the French colonies of Martinique and Algeria). Fanon's analectical account grounded—and, hence, immanently critiqued—psychoanalytic ideology in the Real of colonization in an effort to emphasize the primacy of decolonization, as a permanent revolutionary praxis of collective liberation beyond racial capitalism.

In other words, those of us who are attracted to psychoanalysis must seriously think about the relationship between psychoanalysis, the modern state, and racial capitalism, as functions of the historical imperial process (cf. Hook, 2025). Since that relationship can never be neutral and will always be political, why must psychoanalytic theorists and practitioners shy away from the implications of an anarchist non-rapport (e.g., free association)?

Liberation, or postabyssal, psychoanalysis actualizes multiple spatiotemporal configurations of psychoanalysis and, as such, decenters Euromodernity (the here and the now) along with its conceptions of 'barbarians' (those living in the periphery or Exterior to Totality) and 'primitives' (those living in the past or in premodernity). Derrida (1991) characterized the spatiotemporal hegemony of abyssal psychoanalysis with the signifier "geopsychoanalysis." Said's (1978/2003) discussion of "imaginative geography" and "historical knowledge" as aspects of Orientalism is relevant in this context, too.

Additionally, Santos (2007) writes about the "noncontemporaneity" of what is on the Other side of the abyssal line, which gives the hegemonic I the ability to "make up pasts to make room for a single homogenous future" (p. 50). The postabyssal alternative is what Santos (2007) calls "radical copresence," that is, equating "simultaneity with contemporaneity, which can only be accomplished if the linear conception of time is abandoned" (p. 66). Luckily, psychoanalysis presupposes a nonlinear conception of time, as evidenced by the concept of *Nachträglichkeit* (*après-coup*). However, are the analyst and the analysand "contemporary in equal terms" (p. 66)? In other words, can we characterize their non-rapport in terms of radical copresence, particularly given "the impossibility of the copresence of the two sides of the line" (p. 45)?

This impossibility of copresence is what I term "colonial difference" (see Beshara, 2021a), hence, we can assert: *il n'y a pas de rapport colonial.*

Is psychoanalysis open to "the epistemological diversity of the world" (p. 67)? In other words, are we able to delink psychoanalysis from modern (abyssal) thinking? Situating psychoanalysis within an ecology of knowledges entails a commitment to "counterhegemonic globalization" (p. 68), which is a postabyssal praxis of anticapitalism, antiracism, antifascism, antisexism, decoloniality, transmodernity, liberation, etc. To put it differently, counter-hegemonic globalization involves "transcalar" resistance (p. 72) against racial capitalism. Santos (2001) writes:

> *Transcaling* presupposes a certain unlearning of current criteria of relevance determination. It invites us to consult social reality through different cognitive maps operating at different scales. The learning process consists in raising the consciousness of the limits—contrasting representation with orientation, position with movement—without getting paralyzed. A higher consciousness of limits is at the core of the kind of prudent knowledge I am proposing here, a form of knowledge that teaches us how to keep consequences under the control and within the sight of the actions that cause them.
>
> (p. 274, emphasis added)

In psychoanalytic terms, transcalar resistance is none other than the ethico-political link between the singularity of being (the microcosm of the psyche) and the ecology of knowledges (the macrocosm of the social). Transcalar resistance, or *critical unconsciousness*, is the basis for cosmopolitan solidarity among the subaltern. This subaltern cosmopolitanism will necessitate "intercultural translation" (p. 74), which is not without contention, as Santos (2007) shows.

In the clinic, transcalar resistance is at work when the analyst refuses to treat the microcosm of the psyche as if it exists in a vacuum. The analyst embodies a critical unconsciousness that allows them to recognize that the analysand's singularity of being is always linked to the macrocosm of the social. Transcalar resistence is an intervention that brackets the hegemonic I and instead fosters a cosmopolitan solidarity that acknowledges the analysand's material and ideological struggle within racial capitalism as part of their analytic work.

Furthermore, psychoanalytic interventions must be pragmatically and ethically assessed using "an epistemology of consequences," which follows "the principle of precaution" (Santos, 2007, p. 72). According to the principle of precaution, "preference must be given to the form of knowledge that guarantees the greatest level of participation to the social groups involved in its design, execution, and control, and in the benefits of the intervention" (p. 72). In other words, there is no such a thing as a neutral psychoanalyst; neutrality is an ideological position, for it signifies being uncritical of Totality. Neutrality is a fantasy that covers over the Real of coloniality.

Given the beginnings of psychoanalysis (with Freud) and the developments (since Freud) on the Euromodern side of the abyssal line, these are some of the questions that we must wrestle with if we are to move beyond abyssal thinking and towards ecological thinking, particularly since the universality of knowledge and Law is never applicable to the damned, who are rendered disposable and fungible (Curry, 2017, p. 34), given their Exterior or 'savage' status *vis-à-vis* 'civil' society.

The abyssal line structurally blinds the 'civilized' masters to their bloody savagery (see Figure 8.1). If the modern subject of metropolitan societies is barred, as Santos (2007, p. 46) asserts, by the 'universal' socio-political paradigm of regulation (the community, the state, the market) vs. emancipation (the aesthetic-expressive rationality of the arts and literature, the cognitive-instrumental rationality of science and technology, and the moral-practical rationality of ethics and the rule of Law), then the ~~colonial subject~~ of the Exterior territories is doubly-barred ($) by that visible social reality (the Symbolic-Imaginary order as a common global order) along with an invisible dichotomy: appropriation (incorporation, cooptation, assimilation) vs. violence (physical, material, cultural, and human destruction).

The subject of psychoanalysis is the modern 'civilized' subject; hence, the ~~colonial subject~~ does not exist, except as either a spectral $ or a commodified *objet a*. For this reason, we must superimpose the four discourses with four more discourses, their uncanny doubles, to account for both modernity and its ~~colonial Other~~, that is, the Other of the Other. This Other of the Other is Exterior to the modern Other of knowledge (i.e., scientific, philosophical, and religious truths) and Law (i.e., legal v. illegal); A^2 represents *Other forms of knowledge* (popular, lay, plebeian, peasant, Indigenous) as well as the *Other as nonlaw* (lawless, alegal, nonlegal, nonofficially recognized law)—see Santos (2007, pp. 47–48).

The Other of the Other, in this sense, signifies pluriversality (an ecology of languages) and does not signal the existence of a universal "metalanguage" (Lacan, 1966/2006)—incidentally, mathematics is the metalanguage of modern science, which is interesting to think about in view of Lacan's attempts at formalizing psychoanalysis. Moreover, both Others are barred (for no Other can say it all), but while the modern Other is visible, the ~~colonial Other~~ is invisible, so it is doubly barred like the ~~colonial subject~~.

The ~~colonial Other~~, as the ghost in the machine, is the logical foundation for the rhetoric of the modern Other; however, this colonial logic, as a product of the historical imperial process, is invisible because of how modern discursive-fantasies, particularly regarding the universality of knowledge and Law, unconsciously suture the specter of the colonial Real. Unlike the visible rhetoric of regulation/emancipation, which acknowledges the law of persons (i.e., European = hu*man*], the invisible "logic of appropriation/violence only recognizes the law of things [e.g., non-European = thing]" (Santos, 2007, p. 52). For this reason, we must pay attention to the *jouissance* of *jouissance*, that is, the meta- or surplus-*jouissance* of racial capitalism (the extraction of value, knowledge, and enjoyment *vis-à-vis* racialized bodies).

In sum, postabyssal psychoanalysis, as situated within an ecology of knowledges, is driven by what Santos (2007) calls "action-with-*clinamen*" (p. 76, emphasis in original). Clinamen signifies neither revolutionary action nor a dramatic break; rather, it refers to "a slight swerve or deviation whose cumulative effects render possible the complex and creative combinations among … living beings and social groups" (p. 77). Postabyssal psychoanalysis does not refuse abyssal psychoanalysis; "on the contrary, it assumes and redeems the past by the way it swerves from it. Its possibility for postabyssal thinking lies in its capacity to cross [i.e., traverse the fantasy of] the abyssal lines" (p. 77). The cosmopolitan subject of postabyssal psychoanalysis is "endowed with a special capacity, energy, and will to act with *clinamen*" (p. 77, emphasis in original)—Du Bois's gift of second sight. He or she is driven to swerve from the Totality of Euromodernity toward the Exteriority of transmodernity, as an ecology of knowledge and legal practices.

To end on a concrete note rather than an abstract one, I shall reference three further interventions that exemplify what I have been calling postabyssal psychoanalysis throughout this chapter: Sheldon George's (2016) *Trauma and Race: A Lacanian Study of African American Racial Identity*; Patricia Gherovici and Christopher Christian's (2018) *Psychoanalysis in the Barrios: Race, Class, and the Unconscious*; and Daniel José Gaztambide's (2019) *A People's History of Psychoanalysis: From Freud to Liberation Psychology*. These interventions, and other ones I reference later, typify postabyssal thinking as liberation praxis, for they critically engage psychoanalysis through what Santos (2014) calls an "epistemology of seeing," which "inquires into the validity of a form of knowledge [e.g., psychoanalysis] whose point of ignorance is colonialism and whose point of knowing is solidarity" (p. 156). In other words, my transmodern/decolonial argument in this chapter has basically been: *don't throw the baby (psychoanalysis) out with the bathwater (coloniality).*

Chapter 9

Analectical Psychology as a Transmodern Praxis: Three Theoretico-Practical Resources from the Underside of Modernity

Having established the need for a 'transcalar' approach to decoloniality, this chapter now explores the philosophical and psychological framework that enables such a project: a transmodern praxis based on analectical psychology. If we accept Erica Burman's (2008) thesis that "psychoanalysis is the repressed other of psychology" (p. 176), then we may deduce that critical, or analectical, psychology is essentially a form of psychoanalysis of the liberatory variety (cf. Parker & Pavón-Cuéllar, 2021). Undergraduate students in any Introduction to Psychology course are introduced to this oft-repeated story about the so-called birth of psychology, as a modern scientific discipline, in 1879 with Wilhelm Wundt's establishment of the first experimental psychology laboratory in Leipzig, Germany—for one counter-narrative see, for instance, the contributions of Muslim scientists (e.g., al-Razi, Ibn Sina, al-Ghazali, Ibn Tufayl, and Ibn Rushd) to psychology between the 9th and 13th centuries CE (Haque, 2004).

This hegemonic story has a dual purpose: (1) confirming psychology as a natural science and, therefore, cutting its centuries-long connection with philosophy and (2) instituting psychology as a chiefly Euromodern discipline and, subsequently, deemphasizing non-European contributions from ancient times to the present day. The story of psychology, however, is complicated by a bifurcation within the history of the discipline itself: psychology as a natural science vs. psychology as a human science (Walsh, Teo, & Baydala, 2014). The former camp attempts to align itself with natural philosophy or science (*qua* physics, biology, chemistry) and objectivity; consequently, it lays stress on experimental research and mathematization. The latter camp strives to reconnect psychology with its humanistic roots through philosophy, history, and theory; it seeks to know subjectivity via qualitative research methodologies. Both approaches recognize empiricism and rationalism or induction and deduction, but while qualitative research begins from subjectivity, the analectical method specifically begins with an ethical choice to align with the oppressed. In practice, this means moving beyond theory to a concrete historical praxis where the researcher does not just recognize the Other, but references them as a source of truth that is Exterior to Totality.

Critical psychologists clearly belong to the second camp, but, as human scientists, their critiques of naturalistic (Euromodern) psychology tend to be from

DOI: 10.4324/9781003768104-9

the perspectives of critical modernism and postmodernism. In other words, their critiques, while valuable, remain Eurocentric. In this essay, I will argue for an eco-centric transmodern praxis, which Burton and Osorio (2011) qualify as "analectical psychology" based on Dussel's (1985) philosophy of liberation—another name for analectical psychology is "decolonial psychology" (Maldonado-Torres, 2017).

Lest I be misunderstood, this transmodern praxis is meant to extend—as opposed to cancel—the already established critiques within critical psychology. Before I unpack these terms and other ones, which may be unfamiliar to some readers, I shall first address both *the coloniality of psychology as a modern scientific discipline* and *the silence of critical psychology*, in the face of this coloniality. I then end with an argument for the importance of centering radical work by Indigenous, Black, and Global Southern theorists before recommending three theoretico-practical resources that are neglected in critical psychology and which should be central in analectical psychology as a transmodern praxis. By radical, I mean specifically anticapitalist (socialist) and antiracist (humanist); in other words, to be radical is to materially struggle for collective liberation and against colonial oppression (and, by extension, postcolonial sub-oppression).

Throughout the chapter, I frame the discipline of psychology as an ideological modern/colonial project that is situated within the apparatus of racial capitalism. Therefore, my historicization of modernity/coloniality is not meant to suggest that racial capitalism is an event; rather, my aim is to contextualize the emergence of psychology as a scientific discipline in late 19th century Europe and to document some of the ideological effects of this emergence: namely, *psychologization* and *universalization*. To neutralize these effects, I employ decoloniality and materiality as radical tools of psychosocial analysis.

The Coloniality of Psychology as a Modern Scientific Discipline

Coloniality, as opposed to the material practice of colonialism, is a relevant theoretical term for analectical psychology because it signifies an unconscious style of thought (e.g., *not thinking* that the U.S. is a settler colonial society or *not knowing* that the territory of Puerto Rico is a franchise colony). To understand the significance of psychology's emergence as a modernist science in the late 19th century, one must first understand the invention of modernity in the 15th century and how it was, and continues to be, dialectically linked with coloniality, for "while modernity is undoubtedly a European occurrence, it also originates in a dialectical relation with non-Europe" (Dussel, 1995, p. 9).

In other words, Euromodernity is only intelligible in relation to a negated non-European alterity, for the rhetoric of modernity has always been, and continues to be, ideologically and materially sustained by a "coloniality of power" (Quijano, 2000) structured around two fundamental axes: a racial axis (p. 533) and a labor axis (p. 539). However, this coloniality of power is usually occluded by what Dussel (1995) calls "the myth of modernity," which, he writes, "perpetrates a gigantic *inversion*: the innocent victim becomes culpable and the culpable victimizer becomes innocent" (p. 67, emphasis in original).

We must bear this relationship, between the culpable victimizer and the innocent victim, in mind when thinking about the modern psychologist *vis-à-vis* the psychologized/colonized, which is the ethical question of psychological harm (or torture[1]) in experimental and applied research (e.g., the little Albert experiment, the Milgram experiments on obedience, and the Stanford prison experiment). Of course, none of these 'experiments' represent the minimum acceptable standards of ethical, or even scientific, research, yet the latter two in particular are often taught as "classic studies" in Social Psychology courses (Smith & Haslam, 2017). Tod Sloan (1996), drawing on Jürgen Habermas, qualified this precise relationship, between the objective psychologist and the psychologized subject, as the "colonization of the lifeworld" (for a definition see p. 62).

The coloniality of psychology becomes clear when one looks at how psychology furthers the two fundamental axes of 'race' and labor. Psychology, or the psy-complex (Ingleby, 1985; Rose, 1979) more generally, is in service to capital through at least two abstractions: (1) *psychologization*, which "has served, directly or indirectly, to strengthen the oppressive structures, by drawing attention away from them and toward individual and subjective factors" (Martín-Baró, 1996, p. 19) and (2) an idealist, and *universalizing*, emphasis on the primacy of *consciousness*, which is a function of *commodity fetishism* that "does not so much dispense with philosophical contemplation as it grants such contemplation a scientific status" (Arfken, 2017, p. 50).

Put differently, psychologists often reduce, and depoliticize, complex psychosocial phenomena to the abstract level of the psyche *qua* behavior, brain, and/or cognition; they do so in a positivistic fashion, which entails ignoring the uncontrollable negativism (the materiality) of the social world beyond the experimental laboratory (Martín-Baró, 1994, pp. 21–22). This psychologizing tendency, which undoubtedly aligns with the current neoliberal ethos of racial capitalism, is paradoxically accompanied by a universalizing tendency that can be demonstrated with a quick survey of psychological experiments since the beginning of the discipline, wherein the 'universal' subject of psychology was often bourgeois, male, and of European descent.

This chauvinistic trend has changed over the last 50 years, particularly since the crisis in social psychology debates that took place in the 1970s (Moghaddam, 1987; Parker, 1989), which explored questions of ethics, methodology, and diversity. For example, the National Research Act was passed into law in 1974, one year after the ethico-methodological scandal known as the Stanford prison experiment—a non-experiment that was never even published in a peer-reviewed journal. Critical psychology and qualitative research rose like a phoenix out of the ashes of this crisis, but Marxist critiques of the discipline's naturalism (e.g., Politzer, 1928/1994) as well as human scientific alternatives (e.g., Brentano, 1874/2015) can be traced back to the late 19th and early 20th centuries.

While the reality of psychological studies today is quite different and reflects the diversity of the worlds in which the studies are situated, the colonial logics of the discipline continue to plague our research as a function of the myth of modernity. These psychologizing/universalizing tendencies, however, have been resisted by liberation psychologists, who do not confuse bias with objectivity (Martín-Baró, 1996, p. 29), and radical psychoanalysts, who privilege the sociability of the unconscious. Psychology is a master, an ego formation, which explains the discipline's obsession with objectivity. The illusion of mastering the psyche through experimentation or quantification is a function of phallogocentrism, after all psychology is *the Logos of psyche*, a phallic Logos *par excellence* to overcompensate for its physics envy. Whereas Logos is typically translated as *science* by orthodox psychologists, I define psychology, from a critical perspective, as *the discourse of psyche*. We can account for this discourse and even analyze it, but it is neither measurable nor quantifiable in my view. Lacanian Discourse Analysis grounds the discourse of psyche in ideological fantasy, which sutures the traumatic Real.

Being neutral in the face of oppression is neither objective nor ethical, which is why reflexivity and bias, on the part of the analectical psychologist, are important first steps toward psychosocial analyses that are grounded in decoloniality and materiality. For example, Parker (2011) argues that the current medical model—with its bonanza of so-called mental disorders that function via the DSM as the basis for (mis-/over-) diagnosis and treatment in Euro-America—essentially pathologizes *distress under racial capitalism* through psychologization and universalization. Parker (2011) frames distress, from a psychoanalytic perspective, not as a neurocognitive substance but as a psychosocial process (p. 40).

Consequently, the globalization of psychology—with its management of distress through medicalization (reducing a psychosocial process causally to a biological substance)—mirrors the structure of global racial capitalism itself, which (re)produces distress via exploitation and alienation. Moving from the labor axis to the racial one, the reader is encouraged to check out the excellent text, *'Race', Racism and Psychology: Towards a Reflexive History* (Richards, 1997), which provides an overview of the history of racism within the discipline of psychology (see p. 294 in particular).

Psychology's so-called objective or neutral analyses of psyche occlude the material conditions, in racial capitalist societies, which position us as certain social beings within the division of labor (Arfken, 2017). Our social being is specifically determined by what Quijano (2000) calls the "[c]oloniality of labor" (see p. 539), which sheds light on the primacy of "racial capitalism" (Burden-Stelly, 2020) in our decolonial psychosocial analyses.

Modernity/coloniality, as inspired by the work of Quijano (2007), signifies the historical, and ongoing, colonial relationship between Totality and Exteriority, which mirrors the psychoanalytic dialectic between consciousness and the unconscious, respectively. To put it another way, modernity is a conscious rhetoric, which is premised on an unconscious colonial logic (e.g., Afrika[2] as the dark continent or

Latin America as the U.S.'s backyard). The colonial unconscious, which sustains the rhetoric of modernity, is none other than *the metaphorical (ideological) repression of non-European epistemologies and ontologies through the literal (material) oppression of non-European cultures and peoples* (Santos, 2014).

Duran and Duran (1995) show, from a Native American postcolonial perspective, that the solution to psychology's coloniality is not "cross-cultural psychology"—not to be confused with either "cultural psychology" (Adams, 2012) or "a cross-indigenous perspective" (Pe-Pua, 2006). For Duran and Duran (1995), "cross-cultural investigation ... is performed through the inoculated gaze of a psychology whose discourse is founded on the premise of the universal subject—the subject of a historical project of emancipation via *reason*" (p. 5, emphasis added), which is, of course, *mythic* since it excludes "the reason of the Other" (Dussel, 1995, p. 26). The problem, however, is not reasoning in psychology per se, but "the irrationality of the violence of the modern myth" (Dussel, 1995, p. 26). This irrational violence is the unconscious colonial logic, which renders Euromodernity, as a form of instrumental reasoning, mythic.

Since there is no possibility of completely decolonizing modernity, or absolutely delinking it from coloniality, the decolonial (or, even, pragmatic) answer to modernity then is neither critical modernity nor postmodernity, but, rather, *transmodernity*, which is the best of modernity and its alterity (Dussel, 1995). I must note that when I used the value-laden term 'best' I am thinking of Dussel's (2013) ethics of liberation along with Galtung's (1969) conception of social justice as "positive peace" or as the "absence of structural violence" (p. 183). I am also invoking the Maatian principle of truth and justice, which is why my conception of libertarian socialist politics is inherently tied to the human sciences. In deconstructing the myth of modernity, Dussel (1995) writes:

> The birthdate of modernity is 1492, even though its gestation, like that of the fetus, required a period of intrauterine growth. Whereas modernity gestated in the free, creative medieval European cities, it came to birth in Europe's confrontation with the Other. By controlling, conquering, and violating the Other, Europe defined itself as discoverer, conquistador, and colonizer of an alterity likewise constitutive of modernity. Europe never discovered (*des-cubierto*) this Other as Other but covered over (*encubierto*) the Other as part of the Same: i.e., Europe. Modernity dawned in 1492 and with it the myth of a special kind of sacrificial violence which eventually eclipsed whatever was non-European.
>
> (p. 12, emphasis in original)

Conversely, Sunil Bhatia (2018), who has pioneered a postcolonial line of research within critical psychology over the past two decades, is more optimistic about decolonizing psychology, which for him "entails examining both how Euro-American scientific psychology becomes the standard-bearer of psychology throughout the world and how specific local cultural flows and ideas play an important role in shaping identities across the world" (pp. xx–xxi).

The emergence of psychology, as a modern scientific discipline in the late 19th century, coincides with the Scramble for Africa. This co-occurrence did not go unnoticed by the new imperialists, for psychology was put to use by colonial administrators as a management tool in the so-called civilizing mission (Mannoni, 1950/1990). To the colonizers, psychology was/is "yet another tool with which to mold minds" (Martín-Baró, 1996, p. 20). This was the case in Africa when European imperialists colonized it; the situation was similar in India (Nandy, 1983), in Latin America (Martín-Baró, 1994), and among Indigenous peoples on Turtle Island (Duran & Duran, 1995). Furthermore, psychology can be regarded as a secularist ideology. For example, Slife, Smith, and Burchfield (2003), drawing on the work of Paul Meehl, write about psychotherapists as "crypto-missionaries" who "attempt to convert their clients to their own value system" (p. 56).

The coloniality of psychology—not mentioning "the laws of the psychology of colonization" (Fanon, 1959/1965, p. 47)—has been explored most lucidly by a certain Martiniquais revolutionary psychiatrist in the context of the Algerian war of independence (1954–1962). In *A Dying Colonialism*, Fanon (1959/1965) writes, "The native [Algerian] doctor, because of the operation of the complex psychological laws that govern colonial society, frequently finds himself [sic] in a difficult position" (p. 132). For Fanon (1959/1965), non-European psychologists, particularly in franchise and settler colonial societies, are "colonized intellectuals" (p. 132) because of their "scientistic mimicry" (Martín-Baró, 1996, p. 20) and subsequent collusion with the colonial system (cf. Hoffman, 2015), which are effects of the psy-complex as a "technology of the colonizing power" (Gendzier, 1976, p. 513). To resist scientistic mimicry, the analectical psychologist must adopt a stance of psychosocial non-alignment to modernity. This involves rejecting the myth of modernity—which blames the colonized and excuses the colonized—and instead centering the reason of the Other as a primary source of psychological knowledge.

The transmodern corrective to the coloniality of psychology entails embracing "both modernity and its alterity" (Dussel, 1995, p. 139). It would be irrational to both reject everything produced by Euromodern psychologists as colonial and accept all of the contributions of Euromodern psychology as inherently good or universally applicable. Similarly, I am not arguing that non-European psychologies are *ipso facto* truthful or just, but simply that these subaltern psychologies—given their Exteriority *vis-à-vis* Totality—shed light on Other (doubly negated) epistemologies, ontologies, and methodologies.

Transmodernity, then, means subsuming the liberatory aspects of psychology, as a modern scientific discipline, in a "world horizon" (Dussel, 1995, p. 139), which entails rejecting psychology's "mythic-sacrificial behavior toward its *Others*" (p. 139, emphasis in original). Those doubly negated Others are namely non-Europeans; therefore, centering Indigenous, Black, and Global Southern psychologies constitutes an important feature of transmodern praxis.

What is called 'psychology'—without qualifying it as Euro-American—was never, and can never be, universal. Even though it is a provincial psychology, since it is essentially of an Anglo-Saxon variety, it established itself as *the* hegemonic

Psychology as opposed to being one significant approach among many. The hegemony of Euro-American psychology is a function, therefore, of cultural/linguistic imperialism,[3] which was only possible due to the First World's politico-economic hegemony after 1945. This post-Second World War context sheds light on the materiality of (post)colonialism, which can also be paradoxically characterized as *(neo)colonialism without colonies* (Nkrumah, 1965). Transmodernity rejects psychology's false universality and advocates instead for pluriversality or parallel universalities, which is akin to cultural pluralism as opposed to multiculturalism.

At this juncture, Bassam Tibi's (2013) controversial notion of *Leitkultur* (guiding culture) comes to mind since the assumption within multiculturalism is that subaltern cultures must assimilate into the hegemonic (guiding) culture, which is assumed to be more civilized. While I wholeheartedly agree with Tibi (2013) on societies having "a consensually accepted value system," I find it, however, highly problematic when he ethnocentrically equates said system with "a European value system" (p. 49). I think it is crucial—for the survival of all forms of life on this planet—that we seriously think and act in terms of an ecocentric (or worldcentric) value system. In my view, Dussel (2013) provides us with *a* compelling blueprint—and it is not the only one—for such an ecocentric value system with his magnum opus: *Ethics of Liberation*. An ecocentric value system moves away from the psychologization that reduces psychosocial distress to a behavioral, neurological, or cognitive explanation. Instead of treating a disorder within the individual, analectical praxis treats distress as a psychosocial process reflecting the lack of positive peace as a result of a severed kinship with the land.

In sum, mainstream (Euro-American) psychology, that is, psychology as a modern scientific discipline, or as a natural science, "is the dominant paradigm, which pretends to universality but actually generalises from a particular situation at the heart of *the state–capital–colonial nexus*, hence experimental psychology, psychometrics, therapy and management of the individual as the dominant approaches" (Burton & Osorio, 2011, p. 30, emphasis added).

The Silence of Critical Psychology *vis-à-vis* the Coloniality of Psychology

To begin, I theoretically and practically position myself as an analectical psychologist, who is not attempting to either save or improve the discipline of psychology. I critique psychology because I am interested in actualizing a transmodern praxis grounded in decolonial materiality. In other words, I am trying to not only denaturalize psychology by reclaiming its human scientific roots (Adams, Dobles, Gómez, Kurtiş, & Molina, 2015), but also to un-discipline psychology through radical "epistemologies of the South" (de Sousa Santos, 2014), which I address towards the end of the chapter when discussing three theoretico-practical resources from the underside of modernity. Un-disciplining psychology involves using critical tools to build a world that functions without coloniality. This requires the analectical psychologist to act as a radical subject—materially struggling for collective liberation—rather than serving as a crypto-missionary, who interpellates individuals into the oppressive state apparatus.

In this section, I will critique critical psychology's silence in the face of psychology's coloniality building on, but stretching, Parker's (2009) argument that "what is called 'critical psychology' in the English-speaking world is already starting to colonize and sanitize what they [critical psychologists] have been doing" (p. 74). Parker (2009) is writing from a revolutionary Marxist perspective, and he views psychology as an Ideological State Apparatus within racial capitalism, which is ultimately in the service of the Repressive State Apparatus (Althusser, 1970/2014).

In other words, psychology's primary function, as an Ideological State Apparatus, is to interpellate us (concrete individuals), through psychologization, into concrete subjects of the oppressive and violent state–capital–colonial nexus (Althusser, 1970/2014). For this reason, like Parker (2009), I do not regard critical psychology as an ideological sub-discipline of psychology (p. 78), but instead as a material form of ideology critique (a praxis) *vis-à-vis* psychology *qua* ideology. I extend Parker's (2009) Marxist critique, from a decolonial perspective, in order to emphasize the primacy of both the racial and labor axes in the coloniality of power.

Building on Said's engagement with critical theory, Bruce Baum (2015) writes, "the Frankfurt School failed to engage adequately colonial racism and anti-colonial resistance. The critical theorists' account of racism was Eurocentric and too narrowly focused on anti-Semitism" (pp. 420–421). I diagnose a similar problem in critical psychology, which is that its critiques of psychology as a modern science are valid but they tend to be Eurocentric (i.e., citing mostly, if not only, European theorists) and they fail to engage adequately the coloniality of psychology, let alone the question of decolonial liberation.

Perhaps, following Robert Nichols (2020), *dispossession* ought to be reconstructed as a category of critical psychology, "one that may serve to mediate between critiques of capitalism and colonialism, with a particular focus on the late modern and contemporary Anglo settler world" (p. 4)? Dispossession, according to Nichols (2020), is "a broad macrohistorical process related to the specific territorial acquisition logic of settler colonization" (p. 5)

Critical psychology owes a great deal of debt to the early Euromodern tradition of theorizing and practicing psychology as a human science, which can be traced back to the works of Wilhelm Dilthey, Franz Brentano, Edmund Husserl, and Sigmund Freud, among others (Walsh, Teo, & Baydala, 2014). These works are also the theoretical roots of radical qualitative research approaches (Wertz, Charmaz, McMullen, Josselson, Anderson, & McSpadden, 2011). In addition to hermeneutics, phenomenology, and psychoanalysis, the Frankfurt School's critical theoretical approach, which was mostly Freudo–Marxist, is another key influence on critical psychology (Stewart, 2007). Not mentioning the legacy of Marxist psychologists (e.g., Lev Vygotsky and Henri Wallon) and other European radicals: philosophers (e.g., Ludwig Wittgenstein, Maurice Merleau-Ponty, Michel Foucault, Gilles Deleuze, Jacques Derrida, etc.), psychoanalysts (e.g., Melanie Klein,

Jacques Lacan, Félix Guattari, etc.), and anti-psychiatrists (e.g., Thomas Szasz, R. D. Laing, David Cooper, etc.).

The previous paragraph demonstrates the Eurocentrism of critical psychology, which neglects, through its history and ongoing citational practices, non-European points of reference. Now, of course, there are exceptions to this rule, which I address in the next section. For instance, the *Annual Review of Critical Psychology* has included two special issues (2006, 2013) on critical psychologies from around the world (e.g., Turkey, Iran, Japan, South Africa, India, Venezuela, Chile, Brazil, Kenya, Colombia, China, Cuba, Mexico, Nigeria, the Philippines, and Sri Lanka).

However, it is not a question of tokenism; these critical psychological interventions, particularly the ones from the Global South, should be normalized in critical psychology (Adams et al., 2015). In other words, they are not simply a peripheral element to be included merely to demonstrate the diversity of our critics or to validate the inclusivity of critical psychology, especially when the key points of reference remain Eurocentric. Furthermore, our critiques of psychology need not be situated within the European intellectual tradition mentioned in the previous paragraph. We can begin our decolonial critiques from Other traditions (e.g., Dussel, Fanon, Said, Martín-Baró, Freire, etc.), be in critical dialogue with the European tradition, while grounding our transmodern praxis in the ongoing material reality of colonial dispossession. This is how we remain focused on the fact that our ideology critiques of psychology are simultaneously a material dismantling of racial capitalism.

While psychology as a human science may sound emancipatory to the ears of most critical psychologists, the Eurocentric conceptions of *the human*—the subject of psychological science—are highly problematic in the eyes of non-Europeans. Sylvia Wynter (2003) shows, for example, the genealogy of the human from "the theocentric conception of the human, Christian" to "the new humanist and ratiocentric conception of the human, Man (i.e., as homo politicus, or the political subject of the state)" (p. 269). This modern/colonial category of "the human" never included those 'primitives' and 'barbarians' who were regarded by the European bourgeoisie as subhuman. As Wynter (2003) shows, the coloniality of being was "enacted by the dynamics of the relation between man—overrepresented as the generic, ostensibly supracultural human—and its subjugated Human Others (i.e., Indians and Negroes)" (pp. 287–288).

In other words, the universal subject of psychology is none other than this Man, or overrepresented human. This, however, does not mean that the category of the human ought to be abandoned *in toto* in the name of anti-/post-/trans-humanism. On the contrary, the category must be radicalized, via Fanon's (1961/2004) "new humanism" (p. 178), to specifically include, and be overrepresented by, non-Christians, women, and non-Europeans since affirming "the reason of the Other" is "a step toward a transmodern *worldhood*" (Dussel, 1995, p. 26, emphasis in original).

Following Dussel, Burton and Osorio (2011) renounce the two European paradigms for critiquing psychology as a modern science, namely: critical modernism and postmodernism. The former "recognizes some of the problems inherent in the modernist paradigm but retains a commitment to the emancipatory elements of rational (enlightenment) methods" (p. 30), and the latter not only throws out "the erroneous universalism of the modernist-colonial model it also rejects the advances in reason produced through the development of that system" (p. 31). Transmodernity, on the other hand, "moves beyond the alternatives of critical modernity and postmodernity, promising to overcome the shortcomings of each, constructing a more adequate and super-ordinate orientation invigorated by the critical perspective of the oppressed other" (Burton & Osorio, 2011, p. 23).

Analectical Psychology as a Transmodern Praxis

According to Dussel (1995), critical modernity and postmodernity, which are the two dominant paradigms in critical psychology, are Eurocentric critiques of Totality from within. Transmodernity, conversely, surpasses this Eurocentrism while upholding "negated alterity, the dignity and identity of other cultures, and the covered-over (*en-cubierto*) Other" (p. 66, emphasis in original). In other words, transmodernity is a decolonial critique from the underside of modernity, which

> might in effect be the ana-dialectical solution to psychology's paradigm wars – transcending them with this positive dialectic extended from the underside (the analectic), and underpinning the method of psychology not just epistemologically and ontologically but in the first place ethically.
>
> (Burton & Osorio, 2011, p. 34)

Here is what Dussel (1985) means by ana-dialectic or analectic:

> Dialectic in its positive sense or "ana-dialectic" permits us to open ourselves to methods that not only are not scientific but are not even theoretical (because analectic is a method whose point of departure is an *ethical choice* and a *concrete historical praxis*). This is of great importance because without it one would not be able to describe the epistemological level of the human sciences (which retain analogies with the factual sciences but are distinct because natural beings are not human beings—beings with history, culture, and freedom).
>
> (p. 160, emphasis added)

Analectical psychology then, as Burton and Osorio (2011) show, is ecocentric, worldcentric, pluriversal, critical realist, liberatory, human scientific, and ana-dialectical with its foundational point of reference being liberation praxis (e.g., Frantz Fanon, Paulo Freire, Ignacio Martín-Baró, and Maritz Montero). Analectical psychology can also be qualified as "a really social psychology" (Burton & Kagan, 2009), a "decolonial psychology" (Adams et al., 2015; Kessi, 2019; Maldonado-Torres, 2017; Pickren, 2020), a "transmodern psychology" (Burton & Osorio, 2011), a "pluriversal psychology" (Beshara, 2019), or a "border psychology" (Beshara, 2021).

According to Walter Mignolo (2000), pluriversality, or pluriversal epistemology, is a form of ecocentric critical thinking, which can also be characterized—following Gloria Anzaldúa—as *border thinking*. Analectical psychology entails transdisciplinary border thinking, which is directed "toward 'using' the disciplines [e.g., psychology] beyond the disciplines themselves, aiming and building a world without modernity/coloniality. Border thinking is actional" (Mignolo, 2000, p. xviii); hence, the centrality of *praxis*. Pluriversal epistemology "emerges from diverse local experiences through time and around the world, between local Western histories and non-Western local histories" and "interconnects the plurality and diversity of decolonial projects" (Mignolo, 2000, p. xxii).

Furthermore, de Sousa Santos (2014) addresses pluriversality in terms of *epistemologies of the South*, which he defines as "ways of knowing born in the struggle against capitalism, colonialism, and patriarchy" (p. 238). Raewyn Connell (2007) explores the same topic using the phrase Southern Theory, which for her "calls attention to periphery-centre relations in the realm of knowledge" (p. viii). Yet another important nomenclature is Global Social Theory, which refers to concepts, topics, and "thinkers from around the world" (Bhambra, Last, Mayblin, & Tilley, 2018, p. 2).

Transmodernity is an ethics-based praxis, which

> re-founds the project of human emancipation that had been conceived within the totality of the dominant world system as one of *liberation* from exploitation that can only be finally achieved by reaching, on equal terms, to those beyond that system.
>
> (Burton & Osorio, 2011, p. 23, emphasis added)

This section is titled *analectical psychology as a transmodern praxis* because the aim of decolonial materialist critiques is to reflect on critical psychology in order to act upon the capitalist-colonial world. For this reason, Dussel (1995) qualifies transmodernity as "a practico-political program … characterized by ecological civilization, popular democracy, and economic justice" (p. 117). In sum, analectical psychology does not cancel critical psychology, rather, it materially grounds it in a transmodern/decolonial praxis (cf. Beshara, 2021b).

Three Theoretico-Practical Resources from the Underside of Modernity

According to Freire (1970), liberation is a revolutionary process, which must be led by the oppressed for the humanization of all (the oppressed and oppressors). Consequently, it is important for analectical psychologists to not only cite but also center radical work by Indigenous, Black, and Global Southern theorists in their transmodern praxis. I would further emphasize being in dialogue in our research with marginalized *living scholars–activists–practitioners*, who are on the frontlines of the struggle for collective liberation. This ethos is inspired by initiatives, such as Cite Black Women (citeblackwomencollective.org), and scholars like Sara Ahmed (2017), who is reflexive about her "citational practice" (p. 148), for citation as a praxis is inherently a political act.

Ahmed (2017) writes that citations "are the materials through which, from which, we create our dwellings" (p. 16); therefore, in closing I will recommend three theoretico-practical resources from the underside of modernity that can facilitate for our dwelling to become "a transmodern *worldhood*" (Dussel, 1995, p. 26, emphasis in original). On this note, it is worth highlighting the contributions of decolonial feminists, such as María Lugones (2007), who articulated how the colonial unconscious is a gendered space. This final section is not meant to be exhaustive; rather my effort is to provide a selective bibliography as a source of inspiration for analectical psychologists who dream of living in a liberated world, wherein Exteriority is affirmed on its own terms.

Indigenous praxis

Indigenous praxis refers to radical Indigenous theories and practices developed by Native folks both before and after the colonization of the Americas in 1492. As far as psychology is concerned, Indigenous works typically emphasize the centrality of historical trauma and attempt to ground their accounts in an Indigenous perspective, which is inherently pluriversal given the heterogeneity of First Nations. An excellent example here is the overlooked text, *Native American Postcolonial Psychology* (Duran & Duran, 1995).

As we continue to experience modernity-induced environmental disasters, Indigenous ecopsychology (e.g., Estes, 2019; Gray, 1995; Parry, 2016) as both a tradition and an ongoing way of life, particularly with its emphasis on kinship or the interdependence between humans and the non-human world, becomes the obvious path forward through the crisis. Nick Estes (2019) qualifies Indigenous praxis using a nonlinear approach to historical materialism: *history as the future*. As such, Indigenous praxis provides us with the tools for decolonizing Euromodern histories (Dunbar-Ortiz, 2014) and methodologies (Smith, 2012). By employing Estes's concept of *history as the future*, analectical psychology treats the colonial unconscious not as a static past event, but as an ongoing covering over of non-European ontologies and epistemologies. This nonlinear approach allows for a decolonial materialist analysis that treats Indigenous kinship as a living tool for future survival.

Adams et al. (2015), for instance, write about Indigenization as "a strategy whereby locally grounded researchers and practitioners re-claim local or Indigenous wisdom to produce forms of knowledge that resonate with local realities and better serve local communities" (p. 223). For them, it is one of "three approaches to decolonizing psychological science" (p. 221), the other two being: accompaniment and denaturalization.

Finally, Indigenization has an international dimension, which Steven Salaita (2016) highlights when he writes about the revolutionary links between the

Palestinian struggle for liberation and the struggles of Indigenous folks on Turtle Island and elsewhere. Additionally, Estes (2019) grounds the socialist notion of solidarity or comradeship in "kinship relations," an ecosocialist model of interdependence between humans, non-human animals, and the land. Furthermore, The Red Nation, a coalition co-founded by Estes, indexes the signifier 'red' to link "Redskins" with the "Red Scare" as a practical effort at cultural appropriation that reframes *solidarity as kinship.*

Black praxis

Black praxis refers to radical theories and practices developed by members of the African Diaspora, particularly descendants of slaves. Cedric J. Robinson's (1983/2000) term for this praxis is the "Black Radical Tradition"—that is, "the continuing development of a collective consciousness informed by the historical struggles for liberation and motivated by the shared sense of obligation to preserve the collective being, the ontological totality" (p. 171). His examples of Black radicals include: W. E. B. Du Bois, C. L. R. James, and Richard Wright. But the list obviously includes other Black men (e.g., Eric Williams, Oliver Cox, Walter Rodney, etc.) and many Black women (e.g., Claudia Jones, Angela Davis, Sylvia Wynter, etc.).

Robinson (1983/2000) adds, "Black radicalism is a negation of Western civilization, but not in the direct sense of a simple dialectical negation" (p. 73). Here Robinson is arguing that Black radicalism is a different (perhaps, even anarchist) program for revolutionary change, adjacent to but distinguishable from Western Marxism (cf. Losurdo, 2024). He writes:

> the record of resistance for four centuries or more, from Nueva Espana to Nyasaland, leaves in no doubt the specifically African character of those struggles. Resistances were formed through the meanings that Africans brought to the New World as their cultural possession; meanings sufficiently distinct from the foundations of Western ideas as to be remarked upon over and over by the European witnesses of their manifestations; meanings enduring and powerful enough to survive slavery to become the basis of an opposition to it. With Western society as a condition, that tradition almost naturally assumed a theoretical aspect as well.
>
> (Robinson, 1983/2000, p. 5)

In other words, Black radicalism must be understood on its own terms (not through a Eurocentric lens) as a distinct praxis, without reducing it to slavery—that "critical foundation for capitalism" (Robinson, 1983/2000, p. 116). Robinson's (1983/2000) most important theoretical innovation in *Black Marxism* is perhaps that of "racial capitalism" (p. 2). Here is his account: "The development, organization, and expansion of capitalist society pursued essentially racial directions, so too did social ideology. As a material force, then, it could be expected that racialism would inevitably permeate the social structures emergent from capitalism" (p. 2). For Robinson, racialism predated the Atlantic slave trade, given the history of Europe's racism toward its own internal Others, like the Irish or Slavs.

To clarify, racial capitalism is not a sub-type of capitalism. Robinson's point—also echoed by Quijano—is that capitalism has always been, and will always be, racial, as a function of both colonialism and coloniality. In other words, there is a direct link between the colonization of the non-European world—along with the enslavement of non-European peoples—and the 'primitive' accumulation of wealth by the European bourgeoisie, which then provided the necessary fertile ground for a modern discipline like psychology (and psychoanalysis) to emerge as a science in late 19th century Germany (and Austria).

To highlight a few more resources, the reader is encouraged to explore Black psychology (e.g., Azibo, 1996; Bynum, 2012; Wilson, 1993) and the Association of Black Psychologists, which publishes the *Journal of Black Psychology*. For instance, whenever I teach Social Psychology, I find myself returning to Clark and Clark's (1947) *Racial Identification and Preference in Negro Children*, which is informally known as the 'doll study.'

The influential study was cited as evidence in the United States Supreme Court's (1954) *Brown v. Board of Education* decision, since it indisputably showed the harmful effects of segregated schools on racialized children, who identified with the "colored doll" that they were shown by the researchers, and yet perceived said doll as uglier than the "white doll" (Clark & Clark, 1947). Clark and Clark (1947) empirically demonstrated that this (mis)perception can be explained in terms of the racialized children's *internalization of racism*, which is a radical psychosocial insight that analectical psychologists must take note of.

Bynum (2012) argues that because modern humanity originated in Africa, the unconscious is structurally and historically African. Two theses, in particular, stand out: (1) the nonlocality of the (African) unconscious and (2) the Osirian complex. Bynum writes, "The ego is a local and boundary-setting process. The unconscious or the ancient Kemetic Amenta [underworld] is a nonlocal phenomenon" (p. 84). The series editor, Allen Ivey, connects Bynum's quantum thesis about the nonlocality of the (African) unconscious to Lacan's formulation of *the unconscious as the discourse of the Other*: "First, the nonlocality of the unconscious. Bynum reminds us that we do not 'own' our unconscious experience, but rather we have the whole of history within us … Lacan suggests that we do not speak, but are spoken [through the discourse of the Other]" (pp. xiii–xiv). In other words, nonlocality refers to the idea that the unconscious is not an interiority, but the exterior expression of historical reason.

Subsequently, the colonial unconscious of modernity may be understood as a negation of Africanness, for if the unconscious is fundamentally African, then the modern/colonial ego must actively negate that Otherness to maintain its European identity. This is an Afrocentric argument, which prefigures Afropessimism. Bynum's *pièce de résistance*, however, is his second thesis, which displaces the Oedipus complex by shifting the focus from the family to cosmic metamorphosis. For Bynum, while Oedipus is trapped in a tragic, circular logic of the nuclear family—doomed by the acting out of an incestuous and parricidal prophecy—Osiris represents a transpersonal process of fragmentation, recollection, and spiritual rebirth that integrates the somatic, familial, and universal levels of existence:

> the Osirian complex is an all-encompassing myth, model, and spiritual metamorphosis that touches each level of the human life cycle. Unlike other myths, such as the Oedipal myth or even the myth of Job, the Osirian myth covers issues concerning every level. These include the somatic level of embodiment itself and the woes and terrors that are inherent in physical embodiment. It covers the individual psychological principles and conflicts of an intrapsychic and interpersonal nature. It encompasses the familial unconscious and the dynamics that play out in family processes, as seen in the dynamics of Osiris, Isis, Horus, and their various encounters with other gods and forces. It incorporates the heroic myths of courage and flight up and beyond one's source … Osiris replaces Oedipus in the great drama.
>
> (pp. 168–169)

The anthology *African Psychology in Historical Perspective and Related Commentary* (1996), edited by Daudi Ajani ya Azibo, articulates the origin, essence, and destiny of African psychology *vis-à-vis* Eurocentric psychology. Azibo argues that African psychology originates in Ancient Egypt circa 3200 BCE. Whereas the essence of African psychology is cultivating the human soul, its destiny is building "a technologically advanced and morally upright society" (pp. 3–6). The destiny of African psychology supports my thesis regarding modernity not being an event that began in the 15th century, but is, rather, a structure of thinking as old as human civilization itself. The 15th century start date for modernity serves as a gatekeeping mechanism. By claiming modernity started in 1492 (or thereabouts), western historiography effectively marginalizes the alter-modernity of Africa, Asia, and the (Indigenous) Americas.

In a similar vein, Amos N. Wilson (1993) writes about the falsification of Afrikan-centered consciousness by Eurocentric historiography:

> Consequently, when the European makes us unconscious of our own history, we not only become unconscious of our history as knowledge, we become unconscious of the sources of our behavior as persons and as a people; and our behavior becomes a mystery.
>
> (p. 37)

By negating non-European historical reason, Eurocentric historiography ensures that the decolonial unconscious is no longer rooted in the logic of alter-modernity, but is, instead, populated by the myths of Euromodernity (e.g., Oedipus). Therefore, the colonial unconscious operates through a *double negation*—a simultaneous lie of commission (telling a wrong story) and omission (pretending there is no story)—that effectively severs the Afrikan subject from their historical reason. This severance ensures that when the Afrikan acts, they do so through an unconscious that is no longer their own, rendering their cultural and political formations unintelligible to themselves. The antidote to this alienating twoness, for Wilson, is writing an Afrikan-centered historiography, which would be "healing of the wounds of African peoples" (p. 2). African psychology, therefore, aligns with the Indigenous framework of healing the "soul wound" (Duran & Duran, 1995)—or the wounding of the environment and the psyche as a result of colonial trauma (p. 195).

Critical Race Theory (CRT), which recently some conservative legislators in the Global North identified as a threat to whiteness, rose out of Critical Legal Studies. Derrick Bell is the originator of the movement; CRT currently includes many figures, such as Richard Delgado and Jean Stefancic (2012) as well as Tommy J. Curry (2009), to name a few.

The basic tenets of CRT include: (1) "racism is ordinary, not aberrational"; (2) "our system of white-over-color ascendancy serves important purposes, both psychic and material, for the dominant group"; (3) "the 'social construction' thesis, holds that race and races are products of social thought and relations"; (4) "the dominant society racializes different minority groups at different times, in response to shifting needs such as the labor market"; (5) "Closely related to differential racialization—the idea that each race has its own origins and ever-evolving history—is the notion of intersectionality and antiessentialism"; (6)

> the voice-of-color thesis holds that because of their different histories and experiences with oppression, [B]lack, American Indian, Asian, and Latino writers and thinkers may be able to communicate to their white counterparts matters that the whites are unlikely to know.
>
> (Delgado & Stefancic, 2012, pp. 7–10)

In closing, it is important to mention that a fecund project has been outlined over the last decade or so on the basis of CRT: Critical Race Psychology (Adams & Salter, 2010; Salter & Adams, 2013).

Global southern praxis

The phrase *the Global South* has a history that can be traced back to the Haitian Revolution (1791–1804) and the League Against Imperialism (1928), but its official beginning is in 1955 with the Bandung Conference in Indonesia, an Afro-Asian conference in which 29 countries participated—representing more than half of the world's population at the time. This conference took place in the context of the decolonization of Africa and Asia (1945–1960), and eventually led to the establishment of the Non-Aligned Movement (NAM)—a forum of 120 countries that are not formally aligned with or against any major power bloc—in 1961 at the

Conference of Heads of State or Government of Non-Aligned Countries in Serbia, Yugoslavia. Vijay Prashad (2012) writes:

> The central concept for the new nations was the Third World. The Third World was not a place; it was a project. Galvanized by the mass movements and by the failures of capitalist mal-development, the leaderships in the darker nations looked to each other for another agenda. Politically they wanted more planetary democracy. No more the serfs of their colonial masters, they wanted to have a voice and power on the world stage.
>
> (pp. 20–21)

Similarly, the Global South is not a place; it is a *project* of South–South cooperation that refers to a "concatenation of protests against the theft of the commons, against the theft of human dignity and rights, against the undermining of democratic institutions and the promises of modernity" (Prashad, 2012, p. 64). Prashad (2012) adds, "The global South is this: a world of protest, a whirlwind of creative activity" (pp. 64–65).

To put it in Dusselian terms, the Global South is Totality's alterity, which is not only geographically Exterior to the Global North, as is the case with the Tricontinent of Africa, Latin America, and Asia, but also culturally, politically, and libidinally Exterior, even when geographically interior, as is the case with non-European sub-cultures in the Global North. To be clear, I will never argue for any cultural supremacy. My bias is for transmodernity, as the best of modernity and its alterity, which is an ethico-political question of truth and justice; however, this transmodernity, as Freire (1970) argues, can only be realized through the revolutionary leadership of the oppressed given the historical and ongoing violence caused by modernity/coloniality since 1492. Recent efforts in this direction include the edited volume, *Critical Psychology Praxis: Psychosocial Non-Alignment to Modernity/Coloniality* (Beshara, 2021b), and the forum: Afro-Asian Critical Psychology.[4]

Africa

Here I am referring to radical theories and practices developed by continental Africans (e.g., Manganyi, 2019; Ratele, 2019). South Africans are leaders in this context given the important conference that was organized in 2019 at the University of Western Cape in Cape Town, which was titled, *Toward a Decolonial Psychology: Theories from the Global South*. Keynote speakers at that conference included Nelson Maldonado-Torres, Shose Kessi, and Sabelo J. Ndlovu-Gatsheni, as reported by Glenn Adams (2019). This conference challenged the WEIRD (Western, Educated, Industrialized, Rich, and Democratic) bias inherent in Eurocentric psychology. According to Arnett (2008), while Americans represent less than 5% of the world's population, they make up 68% of psychological research participants and 100% of journal editors-in-chief. When including other western and English-speaking countries, these regions account for 95% of research samples, but represent only 12% of the global population.

Analectical psychologists can deepen their practice by engaging also with Africana philosophy (Gordon, 2008; Hord & Lee, 2016), which offers a critical phenomenology of the oppressed that traditional clinical models often ignore. Furthermore, the writings of pan-African revolutionaries—such as Thomas Sankara, Amílcar Cabral, Patrice Lumumba, Kwame Nkrumah, and Steve Biko—provide a roadmap for psychic decolonization (cf. Adi, 2018; Thiong'o, 1986). Their work suggests that healing is not merely a cognitive or behavioral process of individual adjustment, but a sociogenic reconstitution of subjectivity in the aftermath of colonial trauma. By integrating these pan-African perspectives, analectical psychology moves beyond adapting to a sick society or coping with distress and toward a transformative psychosocial healing rooted in collective liberation.

Latin America

The key reference here is, of course, not only liberation psychology (Martín-Baró, 1996), but also liberation philosophy (Dussel, 1985). A recent book titled, *A People's History of Psychoanalysis: From Freud to Liberation Psychology* (Gaztambide, 2019) provides an erudite account of the links between radical psychoanalysis and liberation psychology. Because I have written extensively about Latin American liberation praxis in the book's introduction, I shall not repeat myself here.

Nevertheless, I highly recommend the modernity/coloniality research program (MCRP), as led by Dussel, Quijano, and Mignolo, for it has had the most influence on my theorization of decolonial psychoanalysis since 2017—but I have also critiqued aspects of decoloniality (cf. Beshara, 2024b). Arturo Escobar (2007) summarizes the MCRP program as follows:

> The conceptualization of modernity/coloniality is grounded in a series of operations that distinguish it from established theories of modernity. Succinctly put, these include the following: (1) an emphasis on locating the origins of modernity with the Conquest of America and the control of the Atlantic after 1492, rather than in the most commonly accepted landmarks such as the Enlightenment or the end of the eighteenth century; (2) a persistent attention to colonialism and the making of the capitalist world system as constitutive of modernity; this includes a determination not to overlook the economy and its concomitant forms of exploitation; (3) consequently, the adoption of a world perspective in the explanation of modernity, in lieu of a view of modernity as an intra-European phenomenon; (4) the identification of the domination of others outside the European core as a necessary dimension of modernity, with the concomitant subalternization of the knowledge and cultures of these other groups; (5) a conception of eurocentrism as the knowledge form of modernity/coloniality – a hegemonic representation and mode of knowing that claims universality for itself, and that relies on "a confusion between abstract universality and the concrete world hegemony derived from Europe's position as center."
>
> (p. 184)

Asia

Finally, in terms of radical theories and practices developed by continental Asians—e.g., "Asia as method" (Chen, 2010)—I have particularly drawn on Engaged Buddhism, as developed by Vietnamese Zen master Thích Nhất Hạnh, and I have related his radical approach to critical psychology (e.g., Beshara, 2016, 2017, 2024a). Hạnh (1998) is most known perhaps for his notion of "interbeing," which signifies a relational ontology that resonates with the Indigenous praxis of "kinship networks" (Hau'ofa, 1994, p. 155). However, to avoid spiritualizing Asian praxis, it is important to mention *Sikolohiyang Pilipino* (Pe-Pua & Protacio-Marcelino, 2000), specifically the work of Virgilio Enriquez (1986). The Tagalog concept of *kapwa* as "the unity of 'self' and 'others'," for example, is a powerful theoretico-practical resource that is as relational as interbeing, for it is "a recognition of shared identity" (Enriquez, 1986, p. 11). It also resonates with my theory of non-identity politics, as a politics of difference, wherein our collective enjoyment of desiring the commons is driven by the Otherness of historical reason.

Buddhist psychology (*abhidharma*) is thought-provoking because it is framed as a "contemplative science" (Wallace, 2007), which is distinct from both natural science and human science, and dates back thousands of years. Buddhist psychology is grounded in empiricism or direct experience—therefore, should not be confused with introspection—since meditation is a rigorous qualitative method of sorts. Buddhist psychology (like psychoanalysis) is also critical psychological because of how it decenters the ego. Most significantly, the "cosmic unconscious" of Zen Buddhism (Odin, 2025) decentered the ego millennia before Freud's invention of the Euromodern unconscious (cf. Beshara, 2024a).

I will end my chapter on analectical psychology as a transmodern praxis with another compelling intervention from Asia, by way of Hong Kong, namely Fu Wai's (2013) *Critical Psychology is not Psychology*. In this witty piece, Fu Wai (2013) draws on a paradox by ancient Chinese philosopher Gongsun Long, which reads, "white horse is not horse."

Analectical psychology—which indexes Confucius's *Analects*—is a "non-psychology" (Wai, 2013, p. 278), for it is neither a "reformist counterpart" nor a subdiscipline, but a transmodern praxis, that is, a radical negation of the negation (cf. Samir Amin's delinking). In other words, the transmodern praxis of analectical psychology constitutes a radical humanist and libertarian socialist negation of a modern/colonial discipline that has historically doubly negated the humanity of non-Europeans. To put it differently, our ana-dialectical negation is a praxis, which materially affirms the ethico-political significance of our transmodern subjectivities along with their decolonial epistemologies, ontologies, and methodologies.

Finally, Wai's (2021) intervention regarding the Name-of-the-Grandfather provides the theoretical grounding for the Exteriority of the Other of the Other (A^2), precisely because it recovers the nonlinear dimension of ancestorship—a complex structure of collective human experience that is missing from western, individualistic psychology. By shifting the focus from the immediate father to the ancestral grandfather, Wai affirms an ontology of interdependency common to non-European cultures, wherein the subject is not an autonomous unit but a relational being, whose humanity is materially animated via their connection to divine ancestors. This transmodern subjectivity replaces the *colonial I* with an *ancestral we*—a metaphorical substitution radicalized through Freud's (1939) notion of "archaic inheritance," which Wai repurposes to affirm a lineage-based discourse over an individualistic one. The Name-of-the-Grandfather represents lineage and historical reason rather than authoritarian rule, and certainly implies the *desire of the grandm(O)ther*.

Notes

1 cf. the American Psychological Association's collusion with the US government to torture, via "enhanced interrogation techniques" that include waterboarding, "enemy combatants" who are not protected as prisoners of war under the Geneva Conventions (Hoffman, 2015).
2 For reasons as to why Africa should be spelled with a K (see Madhubuti, 1973, p. 13).
3 I write this essay in English, for example, when my native tongue is Arabic because English is the dominant language of science, particularly as a function of US hegemony post-Second World War.
4 https://afroasiancriticalpsychology.wordpress.com/

Chapter 10

Critique of Postcolonial Unreason

Building on our discussion of transmodern praxis, we must now turn to a critical assessment of certain trends within postcolonial thought that, while well-intentioned, risk replicating the very dynamics of oppression they seek to dismantle. Over the past five years, exacerbated by the universal anxiety surrounding the COVID-19 pandemic, liberals and conservatives in North America have published numerous books on the most recent culture war: 'woke'—an empty signifier in essence, which functions as an umbrella term for anything from cancel culture to identity politics.

In this chapter, I wish to evaluate whether *woke being* and *decolonial thinking* are structural elements of *radical subjectivity*. While cancel culture (like woke) is difficult to define (cf. Clark, 2020; Ng, 2022), identity politics is often conflated with the concept of intersectionality, as developed by Kimberlé Crenshaw (1989), when, in fact, its genealogy can be traced back to a revolutionary statement from 1977 by the Combahee River Collective. Radical identity politics stemmed not only from a Black feminist standpoint but also from a Marxist perspective:

> Although we are in essential agreement with Marx's theory as it applied to the very specific economic relationships he analyzed, we know that his analysis must be extended further for us to understand our specific economic situation as Black women.
>
> (Combahee River Collective, 1977)

Barbara Smith, the leading author of the Combahee River Collective statement, famously endorsed Bernie Sanders in 2020 and wrote an article about it for the *Guardian* to make the case that radical identity politics is not reducible to Imaginary identifications with charismatic and diverse 'masters.' *Radical identity politics*, which I also consider *non-identity politics*, arises from a Real identification with the symptom of (post)leftism: the failure of radicalism or socialist politics and the success of liberalism/conservatism or cultural politics. Cultural politics affords all sorts of postmodern criticisms within capitalism, but lacks a meta-critique of capital itself. Olúfẹ́mi O. Táíwò (2022) gets into the history of how the liberal elite captured (and deradicalized) identity politics, which maps onto the genealogy of leftism I unpack below.

DOI: 10.4324/9781003768104-10

The Genealogy of Leftism in the U.S.

In essence, this chapter traces the genealogy of leftism in the U.S. (old left → new left → post-left) and how *post-leftism*—a concept broader than post-left anarchism—today realizes itself through *performative* politics centered around the *affective* (as opposed to *intellectual*) hystericization of master signifiers. *Master signifiers* are signifiers that are often repeated and taken for granted as to their signification. Examples in the context of U.S. culture include signifiers like 'democracy' and 'freedom,' which can be invoked to justify humanitarian imperialism. *Hystericizing* master signifiers amounts to questioning them, or showing that their meaning is unstable or context-dependent. As such, meaning (the signified) is not as self-evident or commonsensical as ideology would like us to think. Master signifiers draw their power from this ideological mechanism.

As we shall see, according to post-leftists, postcoloniality is affirmed, and psychoanalysis is negated, but this is done undialectically or without reason. As Kwame Nkrumah (1965) demonstrated, postcolonialism amounts in practice to neocolonialism (economic colonization), and he regarded it as the last stage of imperialism—the latter being the highest stage of capitalism according to Lenin (1917). In other words, we can consider the *material decolonization* of Asia and Africa between 1945 and 1960 as incomplete, for it is *political decolonization* without *economic decolonization*. Consequently, postcolonial criticism in the academy, particularly in the Global North, is mostly focused on questions of culture, or *ideological decolonization*, which is important, too, for it involves the work of *psychic decolonization* that must be complemented with *social decolonization*. The problem, of course, is how these phenomena are shaped by the political economy of global capitalism. These are the postmodern conditions that transform postcolonial criticism into postcolonial unreason.

Wokeism is a symptom of the irrational regression from new leftism to post-leftism, a postmodern retreat from modernity. The new left's sense of defeat has been increasing exponentially since the collapse of the Soviet Union, or what right Hegelian thinker Francis Fukuyama (1989) called "the end of history … the universalization of Western liberal democracy as the final form of human government." Post-leftism, in my view, is *pseudo-leftism*. I also consider it *faux radicalism* because *wokeism is the liberal emperor's new clothes*. The solution is not a nostalgic return to old or new leftism but a sublation of both. Perhaps #altwoke leftism is the answer to wokeist post-leftism? I ask this question tongue in cheek. According to the #altwoke manifesto (Anon, 2017):

> AltWoke injects planning back into left-wing politics. AltWoke supports universal basic income, biotechnology, and radical energy reforms to combat climate change, open borders, new forms of urban planning and the liquidation of Western hegemony. AltWoke sees opportunity in disaster. AltWoke is the Left taking futurism away from fascism. David Harvey is #altwoke. Situationist International

> is #altwoke. Lil B is #altwoke. Jean Baudrillard is #altwoke. Kodwo Eshun is #altwoke, Mark Fisher is #altwoke, Roberto Mangabeira Unger is #altwoke. Edward Snowden is #altwoke.

What Is Left?

To begin with a polemic, Neiman (2023) bluntly titles her provocative book, "Left is not woke" or "Left ≠ woke," to facetiously display her central argument on the cover. But what are 'left' and 'woke,' and how do they relate to my 'critique' of "postcolonial unreason"? For Neiman, leftism is an umbrella term encompassing socialism, a radical politico-economic position to the left of liberalism (centrism) and conservatism (rightism)—the two key ideologies of global capitalism since the French Revolution. Today, it is hard to know what one means by the term 'left' since, in the U.S., for example, conservatives consider liberals leftists when in reality, both liberals and conservatives are ruthless capitalists.

Still, conservatives are currently identifying as *anti-woke capitalists*. In contrast, the liberals are supposedly *woke capitalists*. Given this infighting among racial capitalists, what can we (radicals) contribute to this debate on 'woke' through ideology critique? What is the analectical materialist move here? Before I answer these questions, we must unpack the signifier 'left' since it is doing a lot of heavy lifting for Neiman and should not be taken for granted among radicals.

Leszek Kolakowski (1968) defines the Left as "a movement of negation toward the existing world" (p. 146). He then adds, "The Left is defined by its negation, *but not only by this*; it is also defined by the direction of this negation, in fact, by the nature of its utopia" (p. 146, emphasis in original). Neiman, however, distances herself from Kolakowski's utopianism when she writes that political and social rights, or human rights, are not utopian aspirations. Perhaps the difference between them lies in this statement from Kolakowski, "A utopia is a necessary component of the revolutionary Left" (p. 148).

In other words, while Neiman may identify as a *social leftist*, she may be weary of *revolutionary leftism*; hence, her use of a vague signifier like 'left' instead of 'socialist.' It is worth noting that Marx and Engels were both critical of utopian socialism and in favor of scientific socialism. In the words of Frederick Engels (1880/2020), "To make a science of socialism, it had first to be placed on a real [economic or material] basis" (p. 53) as opposed to an ideological one, as in the case of both capitalism and utopianism. However, we should not give up on concrete utopias, as Ernst Bloch reminds us, or confuse them for abstract utopias. For Bloch (1986), a concrete utopia is

> of an anticipatory kind which by no means coincides with abstract utopian dreaminess, nor is directed by the immaturity of merely abstract utopian socialism. The very power and truth of Marxism consists in the fact that it has driven the cloud in our dreams further forward, but has not extinguished the pillar of fire in those dreams, rather strengthened it with concreteness.
>
> (p. 146)

Radicalism

Immanuel Wallerstein (2004) contributes to this debate through the lens of his world-systems analysis by qualifying leftism as *radicalism*, which he defines as "the third of the great ideologies of the nineteenth and twentieth centuries" premised on a collective desire for fast "progressive social change" (p. 96). Radicals (i.e., authoritarian and libertarian socialists) were the leaders of proletarian "antisystemic movements" until 1967, when a paradigm shift occurred, displacing the old left. To get a sense of the infighting that resulted from this displacement: new leftists consider old leftists to be class reductionists, and old leftists regard new leftists as anti-Marxists.

The spectacle

Guy Debord (1967/2018) captured this displacement of the old left with his concept of *the spectacle*, which remains relevant today since we are dealing, in essence, with questions of mediated representations, or "a social relation among people, mediated by images." It is worth noting that representations need not be reducible to fantasies or Imaginary identifications. In other words, Symbolic representation is a radical possibility against the lure of the spectacle, and this was precisely Said's (1994) central argument in *Representations of the Intellectual*:

> Intellectual representations are the *activity* itself, dependent on a kind of consciousness that is skeptical, engaged, unremittingly devoted to rational investigation and moral judgment; and this puts the individual on record and on the line. Knowing how to use language well and knowing when to intervene in language are two essential features of intellectual action.
>
> (pp. 27–28, emphasis in original)

1967: New Leftism

In the Global North, 1967 indexes the accumulation of three student movements (the sit-in movement in 1960, the free speech movement in 1964, and the anti-Vietnam war movement in 1965) and prefigures the international student movement in 1968, but in the Global South, particularly in the Arab world, it is a year of anti-colonial defeat remembered with shame as *al-naksa* (setback). When Egypt, Syria, and Jordan under the leadership of Gamal Abdel Nasser lost the Six-Day War, Israel came out not only victorious, it rubbed its triumph in the faces of its Arab enemies by occupying large swaths of their territories: the Gaza Strip and the West Bank (Palestine), the Sinai Peninsula (Egypt), and the Golan Heights (Syria). Therefore, the metaphorical displacement of the proletariat coincided with the literal displacement of Palestinians.

As such, 1967 announced the death of not only old leftism in Euro-America (and, by extension, the vacuousness of Soviet communism), but also that anti-imperialist socialism (e.g., Arab socialism) in the Global South had no legs to stand on. Che Guevara was captured and executed by the Bolivian military the same year. It is within this worldwide context that we can interpret the terror tactics used by new left groups, such as the Red Army Faction and the Palestine Liberation Organization. These were desperate (and, perhaps, counterproductive) attempts at resuscitating the non-existent spirit of revolution. The revolution was not televised; however, what was televised as a 'counterculture'—between the Detroit riots and the so-called "summer of love"—was the spectacle of the hippie movement, which, as time shows, was nothing but a spectacle by the bohemian bourgeoisie. For new left radicals, primarily university professors and students, class was no longer the central fulcrum of antisystemic movements. In the face of the above-mentioned defeats, class was strategically decentered and ostensibly complexified by an intersectional emphasis on race and sex (i.e., culture).

1991: Post-Leftism

The post-left moment began in 1991 with the collapse of the Soviet Union, an event that put an already defeated left into an identity crisis. This post-left identity crisis is responsible for wokeness decaying into wokeism and for leftism being conflated with liberalism. The post-left moment also marks the ideological shift from the red scare (Communism) to the green peril (Islamism). Socialism was no longer seen as a worthy enemy of global capitalism; hence, the full-throttle shift toward culture war epitomized by Samuel P. Huntington's (1993) "clash of civilizations" thesis: the west vs. the rest.

The new proletariat

The displacement of old leftism amounts to the displacement of the proletariat, thereby inverting the division of labor: intellectual labor displacing manual labor as the new site of exploitation—or oppression—under new and post leftism. The new proletariat consisted of racialized and sexually oppressed students, who would later become the Professional-Managerial Class (PMC). This inversion was central to the development of wokeism, the irrational or anti-intellectual version of wokeness, which is compatible with liberal capitalism. The error, of course, is assuming that workers are mostly 'white' and, therefore, 'evil' (i.e., racist, patriarchal, colonial, settler, etc.); or that 'white' = 'evil.' This error conflates the ideology of whiteness—an invention by the U.S. elite in the 17th century to divide and conquer a diverse proletariat—with the Euro-American working class (cf. Allen, 2012). One of the theoretical sources for this error is J. Sakai's (1983) *Settlers: The Mythology of the White Proletariat.*

Colonialism vs. coloniality

The traumatic legacies of genocide and slavery in the U.S., of course, must be wrestled with today, particularly in terms of their colonial afterlives. Hence, I distinguish *colonialism* (the material practice of over-exploiting non-European peoples and their resources) from *coloniality* (the psychic remainder of that material practice, which functions as the instrumental logic of modernization).

In my view, rejecting colonialism and coloniality in the name of wokeness is legitimate. However, rejecting modernity (European or otherwise) *in toto* is an irrational and anti-intellectual feature of wokeism. The antimodern retreat from historical reason and the romanticization of a fantasmatic premodernity characterizes the fascistic dangers of wokeist ideology, particularly when its perfect compatibility with liberal capitalism is never questioned. This is why the (post)left is divided and conquered by the liberal status quo—cf. Chris Cutrone's (2023) *The Death of the Millennial Left*.

Cultural Marxism and anti-CRT hysteria

The problem with conservatives is that they conflate wokeness with wokeism and leftism with liberalism, thereby flattening the political field. Their hysteria is fascist through and through. They claim that there is a cultural Marxist conspiracy and believe that the origin of this conspiracy is Frankfurt School scholars (e.g., Max Horkheimer, Theodor Adorno, Herbert Marcuse, etc.) who infiltrated the U.S. higher education system to destroy America (and the west, by extension) through their critical theoretical attacks on Christianity, capitalism, and traditional family values.

The latest target in their delusional conspiracy is Critical Race Theory (CRT), which conservative politicians are successfully banning from K-12 curricula in Republican states based on the claim that CRT teaches children that America is inherently racist. Of course, it does not help that Nikole Hannah-Jones (2019) stated in her *1619 Project*: "Anti-black racism runs in the very DNA of this country" (p. 21). Nonetheless, the anti-CRT conspiracy repeats an older Nazi conspiracy by the name of cultural (or Jewish) Bolshevism, wherein Jews and Communists are conflated and scapegoated as the enemy of Western civilization. While wokeism must be critiqued, anti-wokeness must be rejected for its anti-Semitism, anti-Blackness, and anti-radicalism.

Collective liberation and unconscious wokeness

Conservatives are fighting windmills because liberals are Imaginary or faux radicals. Our fight, as radicals, must be on the lines of the Symbolic and the Real, which concerns the question of collective liberation. After all, Lyotard (1993) reminds us, "political economy is a libidinal economy" (p. 104). What do we, as comrades, want? Is our desire aligned with our politics? Also, what is it that we enjoy together? In liberalism, these questions are hyper-individualized, but hyper-individualism is false because it replaces the complex subject's singularity of being with a narcissistic illusion.

When woke being is a substitute for social being, the outcome is false consciousness. For liberal capitalists, the unconscious is negated and overstuffed with ideological fantasies that drive us to consume while believing that we are unique. The ideal liberal consumer today is a faux radical individual, who believes that they are 'woke' without any reflection on their social being and how this lack of reflection determines their subjectivity: their consciousness as well as their unconscious. As such, both the liberal ideology of wokeism and the conservative ideology of anti-wokeness produce false consciousness—the kind of consciousness needed for global capitalism to continue operating without interruption. Unconscious wokeness, a revolutionary meta-consciousness engaged in decolonial thinking, is the missing third.

Herbert Marcuse and Angela Davis

One of the most prominent leaders in the new left movement was Herbert Marcuse (1969), who envisioned students as the new proletariat: "a considerable part of the student population is prospective working class–'new working class'" (p. 43). One of his students was a former affiliate of the Black Panther Party (BPP) and an ex-member of the Communist Party USA (CPUSA), Angela Davis. Davis is a brilliant scholar and activist, but in many ways, she embodies, in her social being, a major coordinate in the "matrix of domination" (Collins, 1990/2000), as a Black woman from the South (Alabama) with humble yet radical roots. Embodying, in other words, an intersectionality of two struggles: racism and sexism. As such, if Marcuse were the mastermind of new leftism, Davis was the poster child of new leftism in the U.S.

To get a sense of the decay of new leftism into post-leftism, one must study the dissolution of the BPP as a function of the Repressive State Apparatus (i.e., the FBI's COINTELPRO), and the deterioration of the CPUSA into the American Communist Party (ACP), a red-brown alliance for "MAGA communism." The ACP's so-called patriotic socialism is a symptom of the Ideological State Apparatus of Trumpism. Defenders of the ACP's controversial strategy will claim that "MAGA communism" is a dialectical sublation of conservatism with communism; however, *if it looks like fascism, then it probably is fascism.*

Oppression Olympics

What makes Davis brilliant, in my view, is that she never overlooks the centrality of class in her analyses, as a Marxist feminist, and she does not reduce intersectionality to an Oppression Olympics of competing marginalized identities—a liberal error *par excellence* and may even be considered as the kernel of wokeist ideology. Oppression Olympics was introduced by Elisabeth Martínez in 1993 during a public conversation with Davis (Davis & Martínez, 1993). Martínez prefaced her rejection of Oppression Olympics with the following statement: "no competition of hierarchies should prevail." Davis agreed and added, "we need to be more flexible in our thinking about various ways of working together across differences." Davis (2015) would later characterize her position as an "intersectionality of struggles," a radical framework of solidarity across class, race, and sex.

The Personal Is Political?

At this point, I must mention an incident that occurred years ago during a conference on Islamophobia—a topic that I wrote my doctoral dissertation on. After presenting my paper on Islamophobia as a fundamental fantasy, a conference participant was very angry with me during the Q&A for citing the work of Slavoj Žižek. This was in 2016, around the time of the Left Forum controversy, when some post-leftist activists attempted (unsuccessfully) to deplatform Žižek.

Žižek faced sharp criticism from the Left for his commentary on the European refugee crisis, particularly in *In These Times*. Critics argued his defense of European cultural values bordered on racism, as he prioritized liberal norms over the lived realities of non-European migrants. Furthermore, he was accused of failing to account for the darker side of Euromodernity: the fact that the Syrian exodus was exacerbated by a Western-backed proxy war where, in the pursuit of regime change, the lines between "moderate rebels" and terrorist groups were often strategically blurred.

Since then, Žižek has been criticized for his writings on transgender people and the Gaza genocide. I was unsure how to respond during the Q&A since the attack was very emotional and boiled down to a demand that I apologize for citing the master signifier 'Žižek,' which I did not do. In 2017, I wrote my response to the conference participant in the form of a critique of Žižek. My essay was published as a book chapter a year later. The title of the chapter was 'Decolonizing Psychoanalysis/Psychoanalyzing Islamophobia' (Beshara, 2018). This research led to my doctoral dissertation and first book.

In short, I do not think that Žižek was or is racist, but a number of his political analyses were sloppy as a function of his Eurocentrism, which he proudly embraces—cf. Žižek's (1998b) "A Leftist Plea for 'Eurocentrism.'" Islamophobia is under-theorized in Žižek's political commentaries, even though he wrote excellent accounts of anti-Semitism in a number of his books, particularly *The Plague of Fantasies* (Žižek, 1997).

This was my first experience with cancel culture, which one scholar defines as "*collective strategies by activists using social pressures to achieve cultural ostracism of targets (someone or something) accused of offensive words or deeds*" (Norris, 2021, p. 148, emphasis in original). I was expected to cancel Žižek; otherwise, the implication was I would be *canceled by association.*

Years later, I would experience similar emotional responses at conferences, particularly when the topic was controversial, such as Ye (formerly known as Kanye West). I see such affective responses as a function of *wokeism* and do not regard them as decolonial interventions because the latter is a praxis grounded in historical reason. That is not to say that affect is useless or has no place in radical politics. Freire (1970/2000), for example, conceives of *liberation as an act of love* (p. 45). However, when I refer to affect, I think of its relationship to transference in particular, which is legitimate in a clinical setting, but should not be the basis for how we relate to one another in the social sphere. Transference outside of the clinic is dehumanizing because the Other is reduced to an object, a fantasy-screen for all sorts of projections.

Parasitic Criticism vs. Mutualist Critique

Postmodernity/postcoloniality is a parasitic criticism of modernity/coloniality from within Totality. Transmodernity/decoloniality is a mutualist critique from without—that is, Exteriority. Let us consider the works of Enrique Dussel and Aníbal Quijano as two important representatives of decoloniality. They are rigorous scholars in philosophy and sociology, respectively; their decolonial projects aim to negate coloniality and affirm alter-modernity–i.e., non-European modernity, which is Exterior to the Totality of Euromodernity. Dussel's concept of transmodernity sublates Euromodernity and stretches it to include alter-modernity. In other words, decoloniality is not a pre-modern fantasy. This essay defends *decolonial thinking* against its destruction by wokeist ideology.

Wokeness vs. Wokeism

For clarification, Michael Karson (2021) distinguishes between wokeness and wokeism. According to Karson, "Awareness of unfairness in the treatment of others [i.e., wokeness] … makes the world a better place and us better people." In liberalism, wokeness is translated through an *ethics of equity*, which is realized through Diversity, Equity, and Inclusion (DEI) initiatives. The conservative Jungian polemicist Jordan Peterson (2019) characterizes such a liberal approach "equality of outcome" and argues instead for what he prefers to call "equality of opportunity." For him, there is no distinction between liberalism and radicalism; the two political groups are lumped together as "the left"—a mysterious representative of Symbolic authority behind numerous conspiracies in Euro-America that the right is obsessed with. Peterson does not seem to recognize that the leftist Other (like the leftist subject) is lacking.

At a crass level, the rejection of wokeness/wokeism ranges from an aversion toward anti-racism, particularly in the aftermath of the Black Lives Matter (BLM) movement and the 1619 Project, to the gender-critical feminist criticism of (trans) gender ideology. Gender-critical feminism is often considered transphobic and labeled by trans activists as Trans-Exclusionary Radical Feminism (TERF). Aside from the obvious stance of white supremacists against anti-racism, some social justice advocates (e.g., Finkelstein, 2023a) regard the business of anti-racism to be "an extortion racket" (p. 62), particularly in light of reports about the BLM foundation's accusations of fraud. Adolph Reed Jr.'s (2022) critique of anti-racism is more compelling:

> The contemporary discourse of 'anti-racism' is focused much more on taxonomy than politics … This view, however, is mistaken. The post-war activism that reached its crescendo in the South as the 'Civil Rights movement' wasn't a

> movement against a generic 'racism'; it was specifically and explicitly directed toward full citizenship rights for black Americans and against the system of racial segregation that defined a specific regime of explicitly racial subordination in the South.
>
> (pp. 45–46)

At a more nuanced level, there is, of course, the now infamous Harper Magazine's "Letter on Justice and Open Debate," which was published in 2020 and had 153 signatories, a list that most notably included Noam Chomsky—now disgraced because of his association with elite pimp Jeffrey Epstein. Several authors wrote the letter, but the representative of the group has to be Thomas Chatterton Williams, who regards cancel culture—in an interview for the New Yorker (as cited in Chotiner, 2020)—as a bad faith and mob-driven practice of rendering folks with normative identities (i.e., straight white men) insecure.

Williams, the son of a southern Black man, is making a liberal argument for free speech (and against the politicization of identities). For Williams, the cancel culture mob exists for the most part on Twitter (X). Similarly, in her resignation letter from the *New York Times*, Bari Weiss (2020) blamed the social media platform now owned by tech tycoon Elon Musk: "Twitter [X] is not on the masthead of The New York Times. But Twitter [X] has become its ultimate editor."

Reducing cancel culture to discourses on Twitter (X) does not take into account the material effects of cancel culture on society beyond the Internet or social media specifically. As an educator, my paramount concern is how cancel culture manifests in the classroom and whether it has any relation to critical pedagogy. Williams and Weiss also do not see the fantasmatic dimension of cancel culture, which I am curious about as a radical psychoanalyst committed to ideology critique.

A Lacanian Discourse Analysis of Wokeism

Karson (2021) continues, in a way echoing Peterson's (2019) paranoid delusional sentiment in "Equity: When the Left Goes Too Far": "On the political left, wokeness sometimes drifts into *wokeism*—a system of thought and behavior characterized by intolerance, policing the speech of others, and proving one's own superiority by denouncing others" (emphasis in original). While I find Karson's distinction between wokeness and wokeism helpful, I disagree with his political analysis, which folds liberalism into radicalism.

If anti-woke is the conservative master's discourse, then wokeism is the liberal university's discourse. Wokeness, however, is the hysteric's discourse. For Lacan (2007), "discourse is bound up with the interests of the subject" (p. 92). See Figure 10.1, the Four Discourses and Figure 10.2, the Four Subject Positions. *Intellectual hystericization*, according to Lacanian discourse theory, produces critical knowledge (e.g., Marxism and psychoanalysis), or the science of dialectics: the political economy of the social and the libidinal economy of the psychic. Analysis and hysteria are radical (anticapitalist or socialist) positions from which we can scientifically

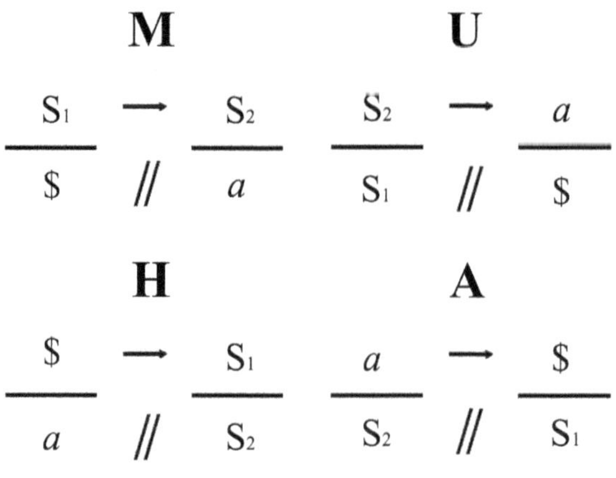

Figure 10.1 The four discourses

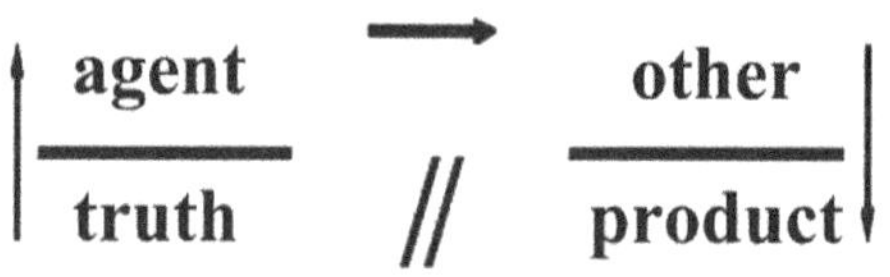

Figure 10.2 The four subject positions

critique ideology. It is no coincidence that Lacan (2007) says the following in Seminar XVII: "What is characteristic of the two of them, Freud and Marx, is that they don't bullshit" (p. 71).

On the other hand, the university manufactures the ideology (e.g., wokeism) necessary for sustaining the mastery of global capitalists (S_1). After all, culture war is of benefit to the ruling class since it is a distraction from class conflict. Hystericization ($) is a means (a praxis) but not an end: it is not a substitute for the revolutionary politics of class struggle. In the aftermath of the May 1968 student movement, Lacan (2007) famously said, "What you aspire to as revolutionaries is a master. You will get one" (p. 207). This is what happens when *performative* or *affective hystericization* (S_2) becomes a political end in itself, as is the case with liberal identity politics, wherein identity is fetishized *à la* the commodity form (*a*). Lacan's statement is an apt observation on the shift from old leftism to new leftism, predicting the regressive future of post-leftism. According to wokeism, it is considered 'radical' to *affectively hystericize* Freud by performatively canceling him and replacing him with a new charismatic and diverse 'master.' This, of course, assumes that Freud himself was European, a question that Said (2003) found to be far from straightforward.

Intellectually hystericizing (or critiquing) Freudian psychoanalysis would conversely amount to challenging some of the field's master signifiers (e.g., the phallus), which has been taking place a great deal since Freud's time, and that is part of the scientific process (i.e., dialectics). Illustrative examples include *Black Skin, White Masks* (Fanon, 1952/1967), *Psychoanalysis and Feminism* (Mitchell, 1974/2000), and *Freudianism: A Marxist Critique* (Voloshinov, 1976/2014).

Hystericization is a praxis that challenges master signifiers (e.g., capital or the phallus); it is not the business of canceling 'masters' (e.g., Marx or Freud). Affective hystericization conflates Imaginary masters with Symbolic signifiers. Intellectual hystericization critiques master signifiers through sublation; affective hystericization is the negation (disavowal) of 'masters' through cancelation. The postcolonial unreason of liberals is very close to what Žižek (1989) terms "cynical reason"—a form of ideological bad faith, which is ultimately aligned with the instrumental reason of global capitalism.

The Irrational Epistemology of Postcolonial Unreason

By framing the postcolonial unreason of liberal wokeism as an irrationalism, I am invoking Georg Lukács's (1952/1981) point about how irrationalism comes about in capitalist society as the bourgeoisie's reactionary answer to material problems that arise from the class struggle (p. 9). So what is the irrational (or reactionary) epistemology of postcolonial unreason? First, there is Judith Butler's (1990/1999) claim "that identity is performatively constituted" (p. 33), which implies not only an identity politics, but also *a performative aesthetics of melancholic identification*. For Butler, identification is "crucial to a notion of performativity that emphasizes the way minority identities are produced and riven at the same time under conditions of domination" (p. 192).

In psychoanalysis, identification (with the analyst) is an impediment that must be overcome. In ego psychology, that kind of identification is the goal of therapy. Butler's account of identification aligns with ego psychology's: "it must be possible to enact an identification that displays its phantasmatic structure" (p. 41). Butler finds the Imaginary fantasy of wholeness guaranteed by what she terms "melancholic identification" more compelling than the sense of subjective loss (unconscious desire) afforded by the Symbolic order of language and Law. Butler writes,

> The mask [i.e., the performative persona, ego, or being] thus conceals this loss, but preserves (and negates) this loss through its concealment. The mask has a double function which is the double function of melancholy. The mask is taken on through the process of incorporation which is a way of inscribing and then wearing a melancholic identification in and on the body.
>
> (p. 63)

Second, this performative aesthetics of melancholic identification is not a view from nowhere, but from a specific standpoint: *the new proletariat*, that is, "marginalized lives" in the words of Sandra Harding (1993). Harding argues,

> Hegel was not a slave, though he argued that the master/slave relationship could better be understood from the perspective of slaves' activities. Marx, Engels, and Lukacs were not engaged in the kind of labor that they argued provided the starting point for developing their theories about class society.
>
> (p. 59)

Class struggle stems from an objective social problem (exploitation) and cannot be reduced to being considered merely the subjective standpoint of the proletariat.

A liberated, or classless, society implies the humanization of all, and not the humanization of a select group of people. The proletariat is not a special interest group, they represent the pluriversal category of alienated subjectivity. The psychoanalytic imperative is for us to traverse our Imaginary fantasies, which are alienating us, as opposed to wearing them as performative masks of melancholic identification.

Third, the performative aesthetics of melancholic identification from a marginalized standpoint is translated through affect theory as cultural politics. Sara Ahmed (2004/2014) distances herself from Marx's critique of capital to develop her *cultural politics of emotion*. She writes,

> emotions work as a form of capital: affect does not reside positively in the sign or commodity, but is produced as an effect of its circulation. I am using 'the economic' to suggest that objects of emotions circulate or are distributed across a social as well as psychic field.
>
> (p. 45)

Later in the book, Ahmed notes, "To think of emotions as a cultural politics is to attend to *what comes up*" (p. 212, emphasis in original). These are some of the postmodern coordinates of postcolonial unreason's irrational epistemology, which can be contrasted with the historical reason of decolonial thinking, whose rational epistemology is grounded in the critical method of analectical materialism.

Instead of celebrating the idealism of cultural politics, we ought to critique the materiality of political (and libidinal) economy. Affects do matter, but they should not be substitutes for dialogue and critique. They can, however, drive both on our collective quest for truth and justice. Affects are not a stand-in for the Real either because affects are deceiving—anxiety being the only exception. As Lacan (2014) notes in Seminar X, anxiety is "*that which does not deceive*" (p. 116, emphasis in original). Ahmed (2004/2014) is interested in the "the object of feeling," but for Lacan, the object-cause of anxiety is, of course, the object-cause of desire (*a*)—that bit of the Real, which the subject fantasizes about *vis-à-vis* the Other.

From (Post)colonial Unreason to Unconscious Wokeness

Conservatives engage in affective hystericization, too, but foreclosure is their form of negation. Their brand of irrationalism is *colonial unreason*: Bruce Gilley's (2023) *The Case for Colonialism* being the most concrete example. The outcome of the conservative anti-CRT hysteria is the banning (or foreclosure) of CRT from K-12 school curricula in several Republican states, such as Idaho, Texas, Oklahoma, Iowa, and Tennessee. This is, of course, reminiscent of Nazi book burnings in 1933. "Postcolonial unreason" is a provocative misnomer, a paradox that points to the Real symptom of (post)leftism today: the failure of socialism and the success of colonialism. Decoloniality is embracing and working through this failure via historical reason toward the concrete utopian horizon of transmodernity. We must prefigure our overcoming of capitalism and coloniality.

Lacan (2007) considered mastery to be the other side of psychoanalysis, which implies that analysts and hysterics are both revolutionary positions from which one can critique the Totality of modernity/coloniality: the global apparatus of racial capitalism. By apparatus, I mean that racial capitalism is not only an oppressive ideology comprising liberal/conservative discursive-fantasies, but also a violent materiality expressed through exploitative means and relations of production. In other words, analysts and analysands are comrades. As such, we may speak of transmodernity/decoloniality as *an unconscious wokeness*—a revolutionary critique of coloniality and antimodernity. Unconscious wokeness (i.e., decolonial thinking) sublates historical reason: Euromodernity and non-European alterity.

However, Marco Malaguti (2023), a research fellow at the Machiavelli Center, would disagree with me and insist:

> Wokeism is therefore configured, in Hegelian terms, as the synthesis of the opposition between liberalism and Marxism, which inherits from the former the individualistic-solipsistic Lockean and Stirnerian utopia of the Subject as an autopoietic entity and builder of itself, and from the other the praxis of superstructural revolution to be implemented with targeted interventions within the structure.

Criticisms of the Discourse of Wokeism

In my view, leftists (a term I use interchangeably with radicals, socialists, or anticapitalists) should embrace wokeness—defined as critical consciousness or decolonial thinking. Furthermore, leftists should critique wokeism as the current liberal ideology of racial capitalism. Books critical of wokeism on the liberal side include John McWhorter's (2021) *Woke Racism*, Norman Finkelstein's (2023a) *I'll Burn That Bridge When I Get To It!*, and Susan Neiman's (2023) *Left Is Not Woke*.

On the conservative end, there are Helen Pluckrose and James Lindsay's (2020) *Cynical Theories*, Alan Dershowitz's (2020) *Cancel Culture*, Mark Levin's (2021) *American Marxism*, Gad Saad's (2020) *The Parasitic Mind*, Christopher Rufo's (2023)

America's Cultural Revolution, and Xi Van Fleet's (2023a) *Mao's America*. Interestingly, Fleet (2023b) argues, in an interview for Fox News, that "wokeism is … Maoism with American characteristics."

As I will explain later, liberal authors tend to focus on criticizing (as opposed to critiquing) wokeism. Therefore, they fail to see how wokeist ideology is part and parcel of liberalism. In other words, liberal criticism does not go far enough because capitalism is the limit of bourgeois criticism, which is why the class struggle is negated or, more precisely, disavowed in liberal analyses. Furthermore, we can say that liberals are critical of the discourse of wokeism, but their criticism has no material (or economic) basis. This is because liberals are ideologically invested in the fantasy of wokeism; this investment becomes concrete in the form of false (or alienated) consciousness: "I know very well that wokeism is an ideology, yet nevertheless I am captured by the fantasies of liberal capitalism and will therefore focus my criticism on the discourse of wokeism." The Harper's Letter is a case in point here.

Their conservative counterparts—for the situation can only be described as *a narcissism of minor differences among racial capitalists*—lean on the side of rejecting wokeness *in toto* as a cultural Marxist conspiracy, thereby justifying their anti-Semitism, anti-Blackness, and anti-radicalism. The conservatives' negation of historical and ongoing forms of oppression amounts to the foreclosure of ~~the Other of the Other~~.

It is worth noting that Gad, a Canadian marketing professor with Lebanese Jewish roots, is a former Mossad agent. That is not to say that all conservatives in North America are pro-Israel to the extent of becoming spies, for there are numerous anti-Zionists on the Christian right (e.g., Candace Owens and Nick Fuentes); however, it is fair to characterize anti-woke conservatives as *antisemitic Zionists* since most of them support the State of Israel and its colonial policies against the Palestinians while also believing that wokeness is a Judeo-Bolshevik plot engineered by Frankfurt School scholars since the mid-1930s. Echoing the scholarship of historian Paul Hanebrink, Samuel Moyn (2018) writes for the *New York Times*:

> The wider discourse around cultural Marxism today resembles nothing so much as a version of the Judeobolshevik myth updated for a new age. In the years after the Russian Revolution, fantasists took advantage of the fact that many of its instigators were Jewish to suggest that people could save time by equating Judaism and communism—and kill off both with one blow … according to the Judeobolshevik myth, the instigators of communism were the Jews as a whole, not some tiny band of thinkers, conniving as a people to bring communist irreligion and revolution worldwide … As in Judeobolshevism, cultural Marxism homogenizes vast groups of shadowy enemies and assigns them a secret design to upend society. As in Judeobolshevism, those supposedly under threat are invited to identify themselves with "the Christian West" and surge in self-defense before it is too late.

In a June 2024 episode of InfoWars, Alex Jones claimed, "*The global banking cartel* [which is often code for the Rothschild family] has used one tried and true process to create wars, rob us of our currency, and eat away at *our substance* [Ripper's "precious bodily fluids"?]. This process of control over the masses is called [drum roll] *the Hegelian dialectic*" (emphasis added). Consequently, right-wing paranoid delusions are not worth considering for scholarly examination since one of the conservatives' main theses for proving the cultural Marxism conspiracy is that *Critical Race Theory is nothing but a racial variation on the "cultural Marxism" of the Frankfurt School's Critical Theory*; in Lindsay's words (2022): "Critical Race Theory is race Marxism" (p. 6).

In essence, for conservatives, woke is Marxist, Jewish, and Black as opposed to capitalist, Christian, and white. As such, I will focus in this essay on the liberals' bourgeois criticism of wokeist discourse and the radical alternative (the critique of wokeist ideology), which includes publications such as Niles Niemuth, Tom Mackaman, and David North's (2019) "The New York Times' 1619 Project", adrienne maree brown's (2020) *We Will Not Cancel Us*, and Adolph Reed Jr.'s (2022) *No Politics but Class Politics*.

Woke Being or Social Being?

So what is the problem with staying or being 'woke' then, in our so-called new (or post) leftist context? For Neiman, the problem is not with staying or being 'woke' *per se*, but, rather, with woke capitalism (i.e., wokeist ideology), "which hijacks demands for diversity in order to increase profit" (p. 7). In other words, for Neiman, liberal capitalism has been capitalizing on diversity through Oppression Olympics to maintain the liberal status quo—a post-leftist strategy of flirting with the spectacle of radical aesthetics without any ethical commitment to socialist politics. In other words, post-leftism is a performative politics of affects—or, to use contemporary slang, *a politics of vibes*. It is vital now to distinguish between two forms of woke: (1) wokeness as an analectical materialist praxis and (2) wokeism (or woke capitalism) as a liberal ideology.

A genealogy of wokeness

In the history of the U.S., wokeness is an antiracist praxis developed primarily within the African American community as a way of resisting racial segregation after the Emancipation Proclamation. Jamaican activist, Black nationalist, and Pan-Africanist Marcus Garvey (2004) is often credited with popularizing this praxis in his speeches, such as when he said the following in 1917, "The Negroes of the West Indies have been sleeping for seventy-eight years … These people want a terrific sensation to awaken them to their racial consciousness" (p. 43), or this statement in 1922,

> I come to the people in the role of the reformer and say to them, 'Awake! the day is upon you, go forth in the name of the race and build yourselves a nation,

> redeem your country Africa, the land from whence you came and prove yourselves men worthy of the recognition of others.'
>
> (p. 108)

As such, the praxis of wokeness informed the antiracist efforts of civil rights activists, notwithstanding the diversity of their political approaches, from the nonviolent resistance of the Southern Christian Leadership Conference to the militancy of the BPP. The adjective 'woke' had a resurgence recently in popular culture, particularly in the context of the BLM movement, with the release of Childish Gambino's (Cambino & Göransson, 2016) song "Redbone," which was used in the opening scene of Jordan Peele's (2017) film *Get Out*. The chorus of the song begins with the phrase, "But stay woke," a variation on Martin Luther King Jr.'s (2010) words in his "World House" speech given in 1968: "today our survival depends on our ability to stay awake … to remain vigilant and to face the challenge of change" (p. 181).

King (2010) asks his listeners "to remain awake through great periods of social change" (p. 181). King's message is radical; his vision is of an internationalist "world house" free of the "triple evils" of "racism, materialism, and militarism" (pp. 196–197). King later qualifies this vision by adding, "This revolution of values must go beyond traditional capitalism and Communism" (p. 197). When he indexes 'Communism,' King is referring to the Soviet Union, an authoritarian socialist regime run through a state capitalist economy.

The materialism King negates can be understood as a form of *colonial idealism*, an unconscious drive to colonize nature and exploit 'savages' in the name of modernization. He says, "Violence has been the inseparable twin of materialism, the hallmark of its grandeur and misery. This is the one thing about modern civilization that I do not care to imitate" (p. 68). As such, I would argue that King's rejection of materialism negates the instrumental reason of modernization: colonial idealism. This opens up the possibility for analectical materialism as a decolonial method for critiquing capitalist ideology (wokeist or otherwise). I say more on this in the conclusion.

Therefore, wokeness, as an internationalist praxis of solidarity among the proletariat, the racialized, and the sexually oppressed of the world, is essentially anticapitalist, antiracist, and antisexist—in other words, socialist and humanist. It is also antimilitarist, which is not to say that it is necessarily pacifist or nonviolent. However, the question of revolutionary violence is complex and requires justification:

> Power needs no justification as it is inherent in the very existence of political communities; what, however, it does need is legitimacy … Violence needs justification and it can be justifiable, but its justification loses in plausibility the farther away its intended end recedes into the future.
>
> (Arendt, 1969)

Critical consciousness

Wokeness is also related to a key neo-Marxist conception: critical consciousness—similarly, consciousness-raising was a praxis pioneered by U.S. feminists (e.g., New York Radical Women) toward the end of the 1960s. In his preface to "A contribution to the critique of political economy," Marx (1859/1978) famously stated, "It is not the consciousness of men [or women] that determines their being, but on the contrary it is their social being that determines their consciousness." The primacy of social being points to the fact that the human subject is essentially both psychosocial (because they are interdependent with the Other, that is, any representative of Symbolic authority) and divided (between ego and unconscious); in other words, the materiality of the human subject's social existence determines their psychic division.

As such, wokeness *qua* critical consciousness or decolonial thinking is, in a way, a meta-consciousness of social being. This meta-consciousness is *radical subjectivity*, a negativity contra ideology, that is, discursive-fantasies that justify any oppressive system (e.g., exploitation under capitalism, racism under white supremacy, or sexism under patriarchy). Therefore, whereas woke being is a function of wokeist ideology, an ego identification, decolonial thinking is an unconscious wokeness stemming from this meta-consciousness of psychosocial dialectics: divided subjectivity (ego vs. unconscious) and the class struggle (bourgeoisie vs. proletariat).

The concept of critical consciousness (or *conscientização*) is attributed to Brazilian pedagogue Paulo Freire. Freire's new leftist intervention, particularly with his publication of *Pedagogy of the Oppressed* in 1970, was meant to theorize the dynamics of oppression in a general sense beyond capitalist exploitation. The classroom, especially the relationship between the teacher and the student, became a microcosm of how oppression operates in society, thereby mirroring the oppressor–oppressed dynamic, which were positions that used to be occupied by the bourgeoisie and the proletariat under old leftism. Freire's goal was to theorize this oppression in an effort to practice liberation from the bottom up, in the classroom and beyond. We see an echo of Marcuse's thesis that students are the new proletariat.

The wokeist distortion of critical pedagogy

The wokeist distortion of critical pedagogy is that the student (like the customer) is always right. According to this decadent logic, the Great Books of the Western World must be burned since they are written mostly by "dead white men." Also, the oppressed, in wokeist ideology, are assumed to be inherently pure or morally superior, which can sometimes justify cruelty against anyone who is perceived as an 'oppressor.' However, upon carefully reading Freire, his thesis is that *liberation is for all*: oppressors and the oppressed. As such, liberation praxis must be driven by historical reason, or truth and justice.

The problem of oppression is that it dehumanizes everyone; the solution cannot be sub-oppression or Oppression Olympics. The solution is *radical humanism*, and the path is *critical dialogue*. Radical humanism is a Freudo–Marxist conception of the human subject as negativity: a divided subject. The desire for liberation arises from the stifling alienation of our social being by language and labor. Through dialogue and critique, the subject can separate from the alienating demands of the Other (the Symbolic order of exchange) to explore the negativity of their unconscious desire—that which is lacking and may never be fulfilled.

Wokeness as divine enjoyment

Traversing the ideological fantasies of racial capitalism (i.e., those of liberalism and conservatism) opens up the possibility for the *radical-subject-as-drive*: wokeness as divine enjoyment or the enjoyment of comrades in solidarity against untruth and injustice. Walter Benjamin's (1921/1996) example is that of the general strike. Wokeism, conversely, is mythic enjoyment, a sadomasochistic enjoyment (*ressentiment*) that disavows the materiality of oppression and violence under racial capitalism. Capitalism, imperialism, and neocolonialism are increasingly obscured by neoliberal woke fantasies. Through tokenism, homonationalism, and pinkwashing, rainbow capitalist mechanisms suture the Real pain of the oppressed—concealing the raw exploitation and systemic violence felt across both the core and the periphery.

Wokeness is not about canceling the Great Books; rather, the analectical approach is to critique the Eurocentrism of the Great Books to stretch the list toward *the Great Books of the World*. Greatness must be sublated wherever we find it; in other words, (Euro)modernity is not the problem and must be affirmed. What must be negated is Eurocentrism and its colonial idealism as opposed to modernity. One should be able to read Freud generously yet hold him accountable for any racist or sexist views. One should not stop there, and this is why it was important for me to read Freud alongside Said (Beshara, 2021a), for example.

Wokeness is an analectical materialist praxis; it sublates the best of modernity and its alterity in the pluriversal quest for truth and justice. The praxis is *collective liberation through radical humanism and libertarian socialism*. Historical reason drives this praxis, which is why we must be wary of the faux radicalism of wokeist anti-intellectuals along with their antimodern discourses and regressive fantasies. Deplatforming racists is legitimate, but judging everyone as guilty of racism until proven innocent is absurd (i.e., dehumanizing). This is the absurdity of wokeism as a liberal ideology within racial capitalism—what we can also call "the destruction of reason" following Lukács (1952/1981).

A Critique of the Wokeist Ideology

In *The German Ideology*, Marx and Engels (1846) define ideology with this powerful statement: "The ideas of the ruling class are in every epoch the ruling ideas, i.e. the class which is the ruling material force of society, is at the same time its ruling intellectual force." Wokeism is currently a ruling idea in the U.S., an idea of the liberal elite, for it is a way of dividing and conquering the working-class. But, as I argued before, wokeism is not only an alienating discourse; it is also an ideological fantasy. We can even call it "the new American dream," and it works as a liberal fantasy because it is about reinforcing our identity as individual consumers away from any collective political movement. It plays on the narcissism of the American consumer, who disavows the material reality of exploitation and imperialism and desires to see diversity fetishized and represented in the commodity form, as an aesthetic token of 'progress.' In this sense, woke capitalism is a variation on American exceptionalism. U.S. liberals feel exceptional in their wokeism.

So, we must ask ourselves: What is the Real contradiction sutured by the wokeist ideological fantasy? Class struggle. The rallying cry, "Workers of the world, unite!" from *The Communist Manifesto* (Marx & Engels, 1848), is crucial to invoke here because, contrary to wokeist nationalism, socialism is about *proletarian internationalism*. However, there is no proletarian internationalism without *unconscious wokeness*. The international proletariat must first realize the commonality of their social being as workers before developing the critical consciousness necessary for their unity as divided but pluriversal subjects of Totality and Exteriority.

Criticism vs. critique

To move beyond the liberals' bourgeois criticism of wokeism as a discourse, we first must distinguish between criticism and critique. Citing Reinhard Koselle's *Critique and Crisis*, Wendy Brown (as cited in Asad, Brown, Butler, & Mahmood, 2009) writes, "critique emerges in ancient Athens as the jurisprudential term *krisis* ... [which] integrates polis, rupture, tribunal, knowledge, judgment, and repair at the same time that it links subject and object in practice" (p. 9, emphasis in original). As such, the genealogy of critique reveals it to be a dialectical methodology.

Brown adds that Marx distinguished "criticism [particularly of religion as illusory or false consciousness], 'mere criticism' or 'critical criticism,' from critique" (p. 11). She argues, "This is the move that really secures the conviction that critique is secular in the Western critical theory tradition" (p. 11). Brown continues, "For Marx, then, there was a great difference between criticism of religion as illusory and *a critique* of the *conditions* that produce religious consciousness and that religion can be seen to express" (p. 12, emphasis in original).

With Immanuel Kant (1781/1998), who inspired the title for my essay along with Gayatri Spivak (1999), we can also think about the dogmatic metaphysics of wokeism. However, wokeism is far from pure reason, for while it constitutes *a priori* judgments (e.g., judging Marxism or psychoanalysis based on no experience with the literature), it does not deserve to be considered a form of reasoning. Wokeism is a counter-Enlightenment and postmodernist symptom of Totality. Wokeism is mostly irrelevant in the non-European world; it is very much a Euro-American phenomenon that correlates with the identity crisis of (post)leftism after the supposed end of the Cold War.

Therefore, it is not enough to criticize the discourse of wokeism, which functions as a religious illusion today (cf. McWhorter, 2021), from a liberal bourgeois position. We must also critique the wokeist ideology to "(1) apprehend the real order of things, (2) explain why this real order is not manifest but requires critique to be revealed, and (3) explain what kind of human future is adumbrated in religious illusion" (Brown, 2009, as cited in Asad, et al., p. 12). This order of things is Real in a Lacanian sense, too. It is the libidinal order of surplus enjoyment, made possible by the capitalist generation of surplus value.

In other words, the kind of enjoyment afforded by the wokeist ideology is sustained by liberal capitalist exploitation. This Real order of things is not manifest because it is the political unconscious, the level of the wokeist fantasy, which sutures the enjoyment of the wokeist consumer, who is more interested in aesthetic representations of diversity *vis-à-vis* the commodity form (the spectacle) over ethical and political commitments (e.g., intellectual representations). This is precisely what I mean by wokeism as faux radicalism.

I must share a personal example here to illustrate the material conditions that lead to the performativity of wokeist consciousness and the actualization of its central affect: *ressentiment*. According to Butler (1990/1999), "performativity is not a singular act, but a repetition and a ritual, which achieves its effects through its naturalization in the context of a body, understood, in part, as a cultural sustained temporal duration" (p. xv).

The Person Is Political: Part Deux

In 2023, I was invited to teach a graduate-level course on psychoanalysis at a private institute of higher education on the West Coast. My syllabus included readings from Freud, Fromm, Marcuse, Lacan, Fink, Žižek, Danto, Khan, Gherovici, Webster, and Zupančič. The course was organized around the issues of social justice, ideology critique, and sexual difference to address Marxist and feminist critiques of psychoanalysis as well as relevant topics today, such as racism and sexist oppression.

I suffer from degenerative disk disease, osteoarthritis, and scoliosis, and I traveled to teach this course even though my physical condition was sub-optimal. One day I shall write about the skeletal unconscious and the spinal drive, for the spine protects the spinal cord, which is part of the central nervous system, among other crucial roles (e.g., providing structural support, facilitating flexibility and movement, shock absorption, weight distribution, posture maintenance, bone marrow production, and nerve transmission) that we take for granted.

I mention my chronic back condition because, as will become apparent, the students were cruel to me, and when I told them about my excruciating pain, they said, "Maybe that was a sign that you shouldn't have come here in the first place." Here I am, a racialized subject from the Global South working at an underfunded public institution in the U.S. and the author of a book on *Decolonial Psychoanalysis*, and yet I was treated with so much contempt. So what exactly happened?

The class had around a dozen students. There was tension in the air from the beginning, which was confusing. Still, I later learned from the department chair that rebellions at this liberal institution are common because the students are hystericized by wokeist ideology to be suspicious of 'masters.' Not to mention that the students also pay a hefty sum to attend this private institution, which treats them as righteous consumers, wherein the student (customer) is always right. Within the first half an hour of class, one of the students started crying. This immediately shifted the energy in the room from anxiety to anger. I asked the student why they were crying. Then they said they had not done the readings and refused to do them, claiming the material was 'poison' for their body.

The premise of this 'decolonization' metaphor is that Freud, Fromm, and Marcuse are "dead white men," and therefore, psychoanalysis is 'colonial' and 'poisonous.' Psychoanalysis indeed has colonial features, which I and other scholars have critiqued, but to think that the praxis of psychoanalysis is ontologically colonial is irrational. I found the student's attitude fascinating because it was an *a priori* judgment based on crass ignorance.

When addressing the passion for ignorance, Lacan distinguished between crass and learned ignorance—the latter stems from the Socratic axiom: "I know that I do not know." Subsequently, the other students identified with the crying student and turned against me as the enemy (a 'master') since my syllabus caused a student to cry. I realized later from conversations with another instructor that the students at this institute expect group process, and they prefer affective exercises, such as sitting in a circle outside of class to have some sort of metaphysical experience. The students accepted this other instructor after they cried in front of them and became openly vulnerable. As someone who practices psychoanalysis and is an academic, I uphold the boundary between the clinic and the classroom. I was hired to teach a course on psychoanalysis and not to facilitate a group analysis session.

The students refused to learn about psychoanalysis and associated it with evil, and that was the negative transference I had to work with, this projection of evil onto me—the evil of whiteness and patriarchy as master-signifiers. I felt dehumanized as an Egyptian with indigenous roots on my father's side and as a sexual trauma survivor. In other words, I do not identify with either whiteness or patriarchy. Perhaps this is what Finkelstein (2023a) means when he defines cancel culture "as the turning of a person into a non-person" (p. 355). I was considered a non-person because I was perceived to be contagious, a thing infected with the 'poison' of psychoanalysis. Interestingly, in 1909, Freud referred to psychoanalysis, in conversation with Jung on their way to the U.S., as 'the plague.'

I reiterated to the students that psychoanalysis must be *critiqued from a place of love*, but to do so, we must engage directly with the texts. The modernity of psychoanalysis (a dialectical science of the unconscious) must be delinked from its coloniality (its scientific racism/sexism). After all, one should not throw the baby out with the bathwater. The students felt impatient. They wanted to learn about decolonial psychoanalysis from me, but they were not interested in how I got there, and I kept insisting that we must begin with Freud. I was shocked by the students' anti-intellectualism. This is the sort of faux radicalism that wokeist ideology produces, an irrational attitude invested in liberal capitalism through the surplus-enjoyment of spectacular commodities that 'look' or 'feel' radical.

An excellent illustration of the wokeist idealism that underlies the affective death drive of identity politics is the following critique of the "1619 Project":

> The methodology that underlies the 1619 Project is idealist (i.e., it derives social being from thought, rather than the other way around) and, in the most fundamental sense of the word, irrationalist. All of history is to be explained from the existence of a supra-historical emotional impulse. Slavery is viewed and analyzed not as a specific economically rooted form of the exploitation of labor, but, rather, as the manifestation of white racism. But where does this racism come from? It is embedded, claims Hannah-Jones, in the historical DNA of American "white people." Thus, it must persist independently of any change in political or economic conditions.
>
> (Niemuth, Mackaman, & North, 2019, p. 8)

At one point, I invoked Marxism, and one student (who is also a yoga instructor) defended capitalism as a system within which individuals can do 'radical' or 'decolonial' things *à la* interstitial politics. At another point, I tried to argue that Freud was not 'white,' but an Eastern European Jew, then I explained the anti-Semitic milieu of Vienna at the time, yet the students did not seem to care about Freud's experience with anti-Semitism as a racialized subject. Critique involves serious intellectual work. The students' performative refusal of psychoanalysis (as a radical act, in and of itself) was completely founded in *ressentiment* vibes. This faux radicalism is what I also call *postcolonial unreason.*

In her critique of wokeist ideology, Ayishat Akanbi (2018) explains the cruelty that results from death-driven affective politics of *ressentiment*:

> Wokeness has robbed many a people of compassion and replaced it with moral superiority. Compassion and empathy is paramount to any social movement and to any form of progress. Once you have compassion and empathy you can often see that you have a lot more in common with people than you do apart and it's the system under which we live in that forcefully tries to group us on our differences. What is radical is kindness. What is radical is understanding … wokeness does run the risk sometimes in reducing very complex issues. Wokeness tends to be quite reactionary instead of responsive.

Akanbi uses the word wokeness, but her critique aligns with what I call *wokeism* in this chapter. She refers to "wokeness 2.0" as "the second stage of the anger," wherein "the focus is a lot more inward." This is crucial, particularly since wokeism often manifests as group identification followed by negative transference against the one who must be canceled. For Akanbi, "the root cause as to why [wokeists] act in the ways that [they] act often is insecurity." The projection of insecurity is the source of wokeist dehumanization, wherein the Other is merely a virtual punching bag.

Compare this West Coast experience with my place of work, a public institution in the Southwest dedicated to underserved (working-class) students, primarily from Indigenous and Hispanic backgrounds. In contrast to the bourgeois students on the West Coast, my students are very curious to learn and work hard to advance themselves. This is because their social being is rooted in the materiality of class struggle as opposed to the liberal ideology of wokeism. Freire drew a parallel between the oppressor–oppressed and teacher–student relationships, not to say that this is a universal (and unchanging) truth inherent to social reality and critical pedagogy. Rather, his point was that the classroom should not repeat these dehumanizing and oppressive dynamics that exist under global capitalism. Instead, teachers and students can work together critically and dialogically to solve material and ideological problems and, thereby, transform social reality.

Decolonial Thinking vs. Postcolonial Unreason

Decolonization is not a metaphor, as Tuck and Yang (2012) argue; however, decolonization is a metonym. To metaphorically consider psychoanalysis as a form of 'poison' is not a decolonial position but an irrational one: a tearful student's Imaginary 'poison' garnered empathy, but my Real back pain was ignored; this is an ideological function of idealism being valued over materialism. Decoloniality is rational, for it is not the negation of modernity. That is a gross misreading, which animates Olúfẹ́mi Táíwò's (2022) critique of postcolonial unreason in *Against Decolonisation*. Decoloniality sublates modernity, delinks it from coloniality, and integrates Euromodernity with non-European alterity.

Decolonization is a metonym because it must displace both coloniality and antimodernity; it is not supposed to condense modernity with antimodernity, which is the error of the wokeist approach. Just as coloniality is the unconscious of modernity, antimodernity is the unconscious of postmodernity. Decolonization is a move beyond the instrumental reason of modernization and the irrationalism of antimodernity.

Decolonial thinking embraces historical reason, which is the use of reason in the service of liberation. Psychoanalysis is an important tool for decolonial thinking because its method of interpretation is grounded in a form of unconscious reason. The experience I shared above made me appreciate the Great Books tradition, of which I am still critical, in a newfound way because reading will always be better than not reading. The Eurocentrism of the Great Books must be challenged, which is easy to do by expanding its reading list to include masterpieces of literature from the non-European world. Let us remember that it was the Nazis who burned (or canceled) books that were considered too dangerous to read.

Whereas conservatives are banning books that argue the U.S. is inherently racist, liberals (faux radicals) refuse any book not written according to the guidelines of wokeist ideology. This is postcolonial unreason, which is irrational, faux-radical, and essentially authoritarian (cf. Wolin, 2004). As such, conservatism and liberalism are two sides of the same capitalist coin; the difference between them is that one side is anti-woke (fascist) while the other is wokeist (totalitarian). The solution to the authoritarianism of anti-woke and wokeist irrationalism is wokeness as the authority of critical consciousness, that is, decolonial thinking.

Wokeness as an Analectical Materialist Praxis

Wokeness, as decolonial thinking, has the potential to be revolutionary. As critical consciousness, wokeness is an awareness of the exploitation that drives capitalist ideology in its liberal and conservative guises. Wokeness also strives to end this distress through analectical materialism, a liberatory praxis grounded in truth and justice. Comrades desire a classless society—a libidinal economy not premised on surplus-enjoyment or the enjoyment of the few (the bourgeoisie). Wokeness names the possibility of an enjoyment-to-come: the divine enjoyment of the many (the proletariat).

Wokeness is analectical in its awareness of the interdependent relationship between theory and practice, ideology and materiality, subject and Other, ego and unconscious, Totality and Exteriority, etc. Wokeness is material in its traversal of the capitalist fantasy. It is not enough to criticize wokeism, as a discourse, from a liberal standpoint. A radical critique of wokeist ideology entails traversing the capitalist fantasy of liberalism. Wokeness, as an analectical materialist praxis, theorizes wokeism while practicing critical consciousness—a revolutionary meta-consciousness of our social being.

Non-identity politics

We must heed Mignolo's (2007) advice and move from a politics based on identity to *an identity based on politics*. Liberal/conservative identity politics can never be radical because they are an Imaginary politics of sameness, essentially an authoritarian politics grounded in ego identifications. For conservatives, it is MAGA, wherein 'greatness' is a substitute for bourgeois whiteness. For liberals, it is tokenism and rainbow capitalism. But what of the proletariat, regardless of their race and sex? They have been thrown under the bus by liberals and deceived by conservatives. Finkelstein (2023a), who has been canceled by the powers that be for his scholarship on Palestine, states it clearly:

> The cancel culture of my childhood targeted, in the name of anticommunism, popular leftist movements rooted primarily in class politics. The new cancel culture still targets class politics but this time round in the pseudo-radical name of identity politics … Whereas class politics has historically focused on a massive redistribution of wealth from the haves to the have nots, identity politics focuses on the proportional inclusion of ever-multiplying identities (racial, sexual, etc.) in the uppermost tier of a social structure left largely intact in all its

> steep gradations. The primary vehicle of this politics is the Democratic Party, the mass base of which was once the white working class, but which is now in transition to becoming an identity-based party, in which identity displaces class as its organizing principle and base constituency.
>
> (p. 369)

Non-identity politics is grounded in desire and enjoyment instead of identification. As comrades in solidarity, we can ask ourselves: What do we commonly desire—despite our differences—that would drive our collective enjoyment? Davis (2015) means this by *the intersectionality of struggles*: comradeship and solidarity. We have different identities, but how do our struggles intersect? Non-identity politics is a libertarian socialist politics of difference, wherein the goal is the humanization of all: oppressors and the oppressed—the classless society as a liberated society. Two caveats remain: (1) beware false generosity and (2) beware sub-oppression.

False generosity

According to Freire (1970/2000):

> Only power that springs from the weakness of the oppressed will be sufficiently strong to free both. Any attempt to "soften" the power of the oppressor in deference to the weakness of the oppressed almost always manifests itself in the form of false generosity; indeed, the attempt never goes beyond this. In order to have the continued opportunity to express their "generosity," the oppressors must perpetuate injustice as well. An unjust social order is the permanent fount of this "generosity," which is nourished by death, despair, and poverty.
>
> (p. 44)

The above quote can be easily applied to any settler colonial context, whether in Israel or the U.S., wherein Palestinians or Indigenous and Black folks are the oppressed, respectively. The solution to this problem is not to say that the oppressed are morally superior or pure humans and that the oppressors are simply evil. "True solidarity with the oppressed" (p. 49) is possible for Freire (1970/2000). It is a radical act of love. True solidarity "means fighting at [the] side [of the oppressed] to transform the objective reality which has made them these 'beings for another'" (p. 49). The American abolitionist John Brown is a great example of someone who practiced true solidarity with the oppressed.

Sub-oppression

The second caveat is the problem of sub-oppression (Freire, 1970/2000, p. 45), which results from the oppressed internalizing oppression, thereby becoming sub-oppressors in the Oppression Olympics. For Freire, this results from an undialectical mistake: identification with the oppressor. Our praxis must be more ethically sound than the status quo: socialism is not worth its weight in gold until the contradictions of capitalist exploitation have been traversed.

In other words, liberation is not the upside down of oppression. The revolutionary move is not to replace the oppressors in power with the oppressed in power, which is the error of state capitalism under the USSR; rather, what is revolutionary is ending oppressive systems and actualizing a liberatory model of power through free associations. I believe that how we self-organize—as subjects or civilization—should be informed by systems theory because resilient complex systems are more sustainable in the long run (Capra, 1996).

Sublation culture

For Finkelstein (2023a), "The *woke politics* underpinning cancel culture is a reinvention of what used to be called *political correctness* or p.c." (p. 28, emphasis in original) or "political correctness 2.0" (p. 60). Furthermore, Finkelstein (2023a) adds, "Cancel culture is the civic form of McCarthyism" (p. 60). This is a curious statement in light of the essence of McCarthyism: anti-radicalism.

In her MA thesis on the topic, Loydie Solange Burmah (2021) defines cancel culture as "a socio-cultural phenomenon that features diverse, complex communication processes whereby individuals create and assert forms of punitive justice against others whose behaviors, attitudes, characters, etc., are deemed problematic" (p. 3). Burmah relates the concept of cancel culture with wokeism by stating, "Intertwined with authentic objectives of restorative justice (or radical activism) are acts of *performative 'wokeness'* in which individuals capitalize their social media platforms by creating posts meant to provoke user engagement" (p. 5, emphasis added).

Performative 'wokeness' is a helpful way of thinking about wokeism, particularly because, as Burmah argues, "it pays to act woke" (p. 52). She continues, "many individuals are capitalizing on mass engagement to advance their agendas for financial gain and high social status" (p. 52). So, there is an element of bad faith at work in wokeism, which speaks to the link between the libidinal and political economies of global capitalism and the forms of performative and affective enjoyments they afford.

In her critiques of cancel (or call out) culture, brown (2020) encourages us to shift our critical consciousness toward community accountability and transformative justice. brown regards cancel culture as socially destructive. For brown, "Call outs elicit both a consistent negative and dismissive energy, and a pleasurable takedown activation, regardless of what the call out is addressing" (p. 12). She continues, "Call outs don't work for addressing misunderstandings, issuing critiques, or resolving contradictions" (p. 30). brown argues that "call outs need to be used specifically for harm and abuse, and within movement spaces they should be deployed as a last option" (p. 34).

The kind of cancel culture I would support would be a *sublation culture*: for example, canceling student debt, canceling U.S. military aid to foreign countries engaged in crimes against humanity, or even negating Freud's false beliefs (e.g., on race) while affirming the truth of the unconscious. Revolution is not about the cancelation of individuals; it is about the cancelation of a socially unjust system. We all internalize this system, which is why fantasmatic purity is an illusion. Otherwise, we would all be canceling ourselves *à la* the Great Purge.

According to brown, the offensive person should participate in "community accountability processes" (p. 34), wherein they can acknowledge any harm they may have caused and authentically apologize for it. In essence, brown is advocating, like Freire, for dialogue. To provide an absurd example, I organized an academic conference in 2019, and one of the participants anxiously asked me on the second day of the gathering to kick out all white attendees and limit the conference to BIPOC people only. Of course, I refused, but this is the sort of irrationalism that masquerades as radicalism. Wokeism is faux radicalism. It pretends to be radical through performative wokeness when it is liberal through and through. Radicals must reject this (post)leftist irrationalism. brown writes, "Transformative justice is relational, it happens at the scale of community" (2020, p. 34).

With Marx and Freire, I would add that transformative justice is analectical—a negation of the negation—and dialogical, that is, problem-solving. For Freire, the problem to be solved dialogically through critical pedagogy is, of course, *oppression*. For Marx, the negation that must be negated is *exploitation*. In sum, a liberated society is a radical humanistic one free from oppression (exploitation, racism, sexism, etc.). But this freedom entails an analectical and dialogical praxis, particularly among the oppressed: "to liberate themselves and their oppressors as well" (Freire, 1970/2000, p. 44).

The oppressed, or the proletariat, are not special. Historical and material conditions determined their social being as oppressed. The key is for them to use their critical consciousness to revolt against the dehumanizing forces of oppression instead of celebrating the diversity of their oppressed social being. To stay woke (and not merely be a wokeist ideologue), we must engage in decolonial thinking as an analectical materialist praxis whose key coordinates are dialogue, critique, radical humanism, libertarian socialism, and historical reason.

Chapter 11

A Lacanian Discourse Analysis of Anti-CRT Ideology

The questions of ideology and ideology critique are relevant to unpack, particularly *vis-à-vis* the recent anti-Critical Race Theory (CRT) discourse. The notion of ideology can be traced back to Marx and Engels (1846) and their understanding of it as *the ruling ideas of the ruling class*. Ideology is dialectically related to the material base of any given society—i.e., the means and relations of production. As such, ideology is not something to be dismissed; we must consider the dialectical relationship between ideology and materiality—*apparatus* links those two notions together. Racial capitalism is an apparatus that is very much tied to the historical materialism of European colonization, particularly of the Americas since 1492. That year is a starting point for decolonial analysis because it was an *event*—in the philosophical sense of the word—that changed the world. The modern/colonial world system that we live in today (i.e., Totality) is essentially a long-term *structural* effect of that traumatic or earth-shattering *event*.

Ancient and modern forms of colonialism are distinguished in terms of conquest vs. colonization. There was, we can say, premodern conquest, such as the Muslim conquest of the Iberian Peninsula. Decolonial scholars, such as Dussel (1985), trace 1492 as the beginning of modernity, which is a contentious statement because different scholars will locate modernity at different points in time: the Renaissance, the Age of Reason, or the Enlightenment. Still, Dussel's argument is that 1492 marks the beginning of the modern/colonial world system, wherein before that event and structure, there were contestations of power between different interregional systems; however, the so-called "discovery of the new world" facilitated the hegemony of European empires through the apparatus of racial capitalism.

Their establishment as powerful empires was not just political but also economic, so after 1492, the Totality of modernity/coloniality was established as a world system through instrumental forms of oppression and violence never before seen, particularly in terms of genocide and enslavement. The transatlantic slave trade is often described as the most significant forced displacement of around 12.5 million Africans. There is no comparable event before 1492 whether in terms of scale or scope.

The question is: What is the beginning of capitalism? Do we connect it with industrialization in the United Kingdom? Racial capitalism as an apparatus, but also

DOI: 10.4324/9781003768104-11

as a concept, captures the accumulation that took place under colonialism (cf. Luxemburg, 1913/2003). No nation-state would have been able to accumulate capital the way European empires of Portugal, Spain, Britain, France, and the Netherlands did without the colonization of non-European lands and the enslavement of non-European peoples, so we cannot just index industrialization without addressing this accumulation, which is referred to as "primitive accumulation," a problematic term that reveals the racism at the core of capitalism.

This accumulation of capital was possible as a result of settlement, extraction, and forced labor on a mass scale, which eventually led to the possibility of industrialization in Europe in the 18th century. To invoke the notion of racial capitalism suggests that *capitalism has always been racial* or *essentially racist* from the beginning. In other words, we cannot consider over-exploitation without factoring in genocide and enslavement as conditions. We cannot analyze class struggle and labor relations without also addressing this racializing and racist dimension of the racial capitalist apparatus: Quijano's racial axis.

So, what is the genealogy of racism? Racism started as religious racism. Pre-modern xenophobia arose from the experience of ethnic differences; however, with the establishment of the modern/colonial world system in the 15th century, Christianity as a religion (ideology) became a racial marker. 1492 is an important event because not only was it the year when the colonization of the Americas began, but also the year of the expulsion of Muslims and Jews from the Iberian Peninsula. Christianity was not just perceived as a religion; it was an ideology, so if a Spanish subject was not Christian back then, they did not have "purity of blood" in the eyes of the Spanish Crown.

Iberian Muslims and Jews were alienated between two choices: to either leave the Iberian Peninsula or stay and convert. In my first book, which is on Islamophobia, I wanted to understand the genealogy of the Islamophobic fantasy (Beshara, 2019a). A lot of scholars were writing about Islamophobia only as a reaction to the "war on terror" discourse and the tragedy of 9/11. Still, I wanted to trace the genealogy of Islamophobia as a fantasy. In my literature review, I went back to sources from the 15th century to look at this displacement that took place in the psyche of the Spanish conquistadors, where the kind of racism (Islamophobia and anti-Semitism) that they had experienced *vis-à-vis* Muslims and Jews in Spain was projected onto Native Americans, and this is actually documented in their writings.

I looked at the letters that the Spanish conquistadors were writing about their perceptions of Native Americans, whom they saw as infidels in relation to Spanish Muslims and Jews. The way the Conquistadors were looking at Native Americans was through the lens of the non-European Other *qua* infidel (Muslim and Jew); that was their frame of reference or schema. That is the beginning of religious racism with its basis in anti-Semitism and Islamophobia, which then gets projected onto any kind of non-European (*qua* non-Christian) Other. The Conquistadors were not able to understand Indigenous peoples on their own terms, so they racialized them, based on their (mis)perception of the Other.

Over time, religious racism morphed into scientific racism. The pseudoscience of social Darwinism and phrenology, in the 19th century, were used to explain differences between humans and why some ethnic groups were supposedly more intelligent or innately superior. The kind of racism that is hegemonic today combines those two forms together under the umbrella of cultural racism, wherein cultural markers end up functioning as markers of difference in an ideological hierarchy; as such, these markers form the basis for racialization today. The historical materialist logic goes something like this: racism → racialization → 'race.'

Let us return to the question of ideology, an important concept for radical scholars, practitioners, and activists committed to ideology critique. The Marxist notion was revised later on by Lacan and Žižek, and what they inject into it is the problem of fantasy, which is so central, particularly in Žižek's (1989) work, but it is also there in Lacan (1991). What I show in *Decolonial Psychoanalysis* is the ideological relationship between the "war on terror" discourse on the one hand and the Islamophobia/Islamophilia fantasy on the other hand, or how the two are theoretically and practically linked. Before my book, scholars always suggested that there was a connection. Still, it was never theorized, so I attempted to *theorize* this relationship through the lens of ideology critique via Lacan, Žižek, Said, and Dussel. The Islamophobia/Islamophilia fantasy ideologically sustains the "war on terror" discourse, and I link this ideological relationship to Lacan's notion of the master's discourse.

In Seminar XVII, *The Other Side of Psychoanalysis*, Lacan (2007) talks about four important discourses. They are not the only discourses in the world, but he highlights them as important discourses for humans since we shift between them, and they position us as subjects in different ways. The most popular one—which is connected to racial capitalism as an apparatus—is the discourse of the master. Lacan loved using *mathemes* (algebraic symbols), and he did that not to be overly complicated; in fact, his intention was to formalize psychoanalysis so that regardless of cultural or linguistic differences, we would look at these mathemes and know what the symbols refer to.

There are four elements (see M in Figure 11.1): at the bottom left (*the truth* of the master's discourse), there is the barred subject ($) of psychoanalysis, divided between ego and unconscious; a subject divided by language and Law, or since their entry into the Symbolic order. Above that, you have S_1 or master-signifier. Master-signifiers are any kind of signifiers that are used without the need to explain them. They usually function ideologically, so I like to use 'freedom' and 'democracy' as examples of signifiers that are repeated *ad nauseam* in the context of humanitarian imperialism, for instance. You do not have to analyze or break them down, one simply repeats them, and that is how they become ideologically cathected. They unconsciously elicit a certain affective response. S_2 signifies knowledge or the idea that once you begin any signifying chain with the master-signifier, you will then create a series of signifiers based on that first one, which is how discourse is born. Therefore, the discourse of freedom and democracy is generated this way. It is no coincidence that masters—those who are politically and economically

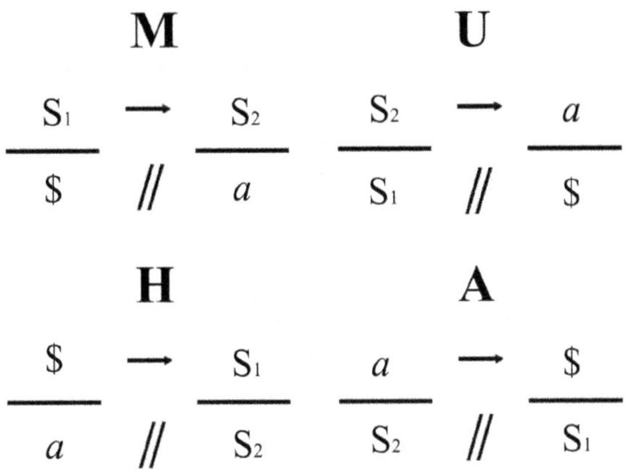

Figure 11.1 The four discourses (M: Master; U: University; H: Hysteric; A: Analyst)

powerful—repeat master-signifiers. They themselves are nothing but repetitions of previous masters, the way Trump repeats Reagan *à la* infinite regress.

At the top of the master's discourse, there is an arrow going from the left to the right, and this signifies that the master-signifier is *the agent* speaking to *the other* as knowledge, but it is a unidirectional relationship (see Figure 11.2). It is not bidirectional because there is miscommunication, wherein we are being spoken to without the chance to respond. Consider how master discourses function in society; we are constantly exposed to them in mediated cultural products without the possibility of a response; they are monological. Master discourses reproduce themselves through repetition. But something has to make the master's discourse stick, and that something is *ideological fantasy*.

Asking, "What is freedom?" or "What is democracy?" is a hysterical act, for it disrupts the master's discourse by challenging or questioning master signifiers. So, if we were to imagine the barred subject ($) being in the position of the agent by moving the four mathemes clockwise, they would be questioning the S_1. In that case, that would be the discourse of the hysteric (see H in Figure 11.1). It took hysteric (Anna O, or Bertha Pappenheim) to invent psychoanalysis, not Freud, by questioning what he and Breuer were doing; therefore, this idea of questioning or being critical–bracketing the negative connotations of hysteria as a Victorian diagnosis of sexually repressed European bourgeois women—is a radical human

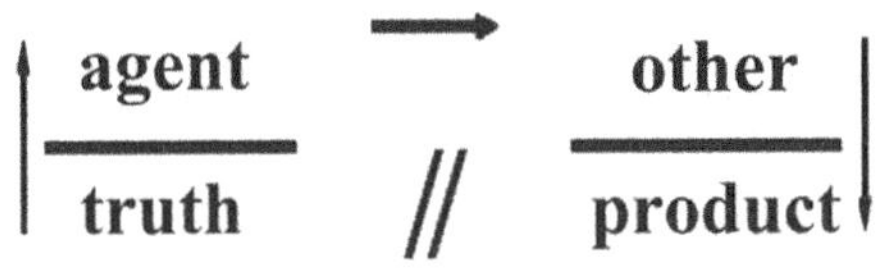

Figure 11.2 The four subject positions

scientific act *vis-à-vis* truth. Hysteria is the position that produces critical knowledge, such as Marxism or psychoanalysis. Hysteric discourses challenge master discourses, or ideologies, in general.

Whenever we hear any kind of discourse where certain words are repeated without any criticality or reflexivity, we know that we are dealing with the master's discourse, and that is why I located the "war on terror" discourse there, for (counter) terrorism is a discourse where you do not have to think about what is going on, you merely have to repeat the T-word *ad nauseam* in relation to Muslims, for example. It is a racist discourse that is meant to ontologically frame Muslims as terrorists, but I also went further by looking at the Islamophobic/Islamophilic fantasy ideologically sustaining said discourse.

Back to the master's discourse. At the bottom right, we have *a*, which is *the product* of this discourse. The *objet a* is referred to as the object-cause of desire or sometimes as surplus-*jouissance*. The master's discourse is producing this *a*. If you look at the bottom, there is no relation between the barred subject ($\$$) and *a*. There is miscommunication at the top, which is fundamental in psychoanalysis. When we communicate as two egos or little others, the outcome will always be semblance or misunderstanding because each ego will imagine what the other ego is saying and then talk across one another in the spirit of 'understanding.'

Psychoanalysis is not interested in (mis)communication but in what is happening at the level of the unconscious, wherein we encounter not-knowing or things that we do not understand and do not seem to make sense, such as tongue slips, symptoms, or dreams. George W. Bush recently slipped and said 'Iraq' instead of 'Ukraine.' His unconscious was owning up to what he did, but at the same time, his ego defensively distanced himself from his war crimes as encouraged by the audience's laughter, which implicates them as complicit, too. Everyone is in on it, they all accept the master's discourse, and Bush Jr. (like Trump) is another good example of a mini-master, a repetition of another master (Bush Sr.).

The relationship between the barred subject ($\$$) and *a* is impossible because there is no direct relationship between the two, so that relationship is characterized by fantasy (or sexual non-rapport). Lacan uses the matheme of the lozenge $\lozenge$ to symbolize the fantasy relationship or the four kinds of relation in fantasy: alienation ($\vee$), separation ($\wedge$), greater than ($>$), and less than ($<$).

In *Decolonial Psychoanalysis*, I employ the master's discourse as a template for ideology critique. If we want to analyze how ideology works, especially not just from a Marxist perspective, but also from a Lacano–Žižekian one, we have to invoke the discourse of the master to interpret how ideology is supported by fantasy through the relationship between the barred subject ($\$$) and the object-cause of desire (*a*).

My analysis so far may seem abstract, so I wish to make it more concrete by analyzing the recent anti-CRT discourse, which we can locate at the top of the master's discourse. Anti-woke subjects who index this discourse are saying that there is a connection between critical theory and critical *race* theory, which is their ur-thesis. It is not a very sophisticated thesis because all they did essentially was equate two different theories that have two signifiers in common (*critical theory* → *critical* race *theory*); therefore, they assumed that the two theories must be inherently equivalent. The entire "cultural Marxism" conspiracy is based on this faulty logic.

Now, of course, at the bottom, we have the barred subject ($), which we can think of, in this context, as white, Christian, conservative, pro-capitalist, male, heteronormative, etc. This is the kind of conservative subject who experiences anxiety upon coming across the discourses of critical theory or critical race theory, which are essentially hysterical discourses. We can subsume *incels* (involuntary celibates) under this category as well because they are part and parcel of this conservative ideological world.

The barred subject ($), by default, is castrated or lacking, but incels cannot deal with the anxiety stemming from that structural negativity. One of the things we learn from psychoanalysis is how to accept lack (Symbolic castration) and deal with it as opposed to denying it or pretending it is not there at the core of our being. Therefore, lack is constitutive, and incels are not the only lacking subjects in the world, but in their narcissism—or 'white' fragility—they fatalistically position themselves as 'blackpilled' victims at the center of a feminist or 'gynocentric' universe designed for alpha males (Chads) and alpha 'femoids' (Stacys).

Incels feel melancholic in the face of their growing sense of irrelevance since they believe that 80% of women are attracted to 20% of men, which is a paradoxical position since they are genetic determinists, yet blame society for their 'weaponized subordination.' This paradoxical position reveals a Real symptom sutured by a specific ideological fantasy. The ideological functioning of the anti-CRT discourse points toward fascism because the fantasy beneath the incels' anti-woke *faux hysteria* (Reed, 2024)—mastery in the guise of hysteria—is *the great replacement* fantasy, which requires further analysis. A true hysteric questions master-signifiers to produce critical knowledge (like Marxism or psychoanalysis), whereas a faux hysteric performs victimhood only to reinforce existing power structures.

Fantasy has two functions, psychoanalytically speaking. A fantasy is like a screen—and the word screen is apt here because it has two meanings, which capture the two functions of fantasy: (1) a fantasy-screen conceals, so the great replacement fantasy is concealing something, and what it is concealing is desire; (2) a fantasy-screen is like a movie screen onto which one can project things, so fantasy can also reveal desire through metonymic displacement. Ideological fantasy functions as a contradiction, and its logic follows the paradoxical logic of the dream. Freud defined a dream as *wish fulfillment*. However, the wish is always *disguised* or *distorted*, so we need psychoanalytic interpretation to unravel the unconscious desire at work in the dream, the task is translating the dream-work to reveal the latent dream-thoughts in the manifest content of the dream.

Going back to the nightmarish great replacement fantasy, anti-woke subjects will claim that racialized Others (e.g., "Hispanic peoples") are virtually replacing them, but what they are, in fact, desiring is being their replacement, and that is the fascist function of the anti-CRT ideology. Let us recall that "Hispanic peoples" have lived on what is now U.S. soil for centuries, when many parts of this land belonged to first the Viceroyalty of New Spain and then Mexico. Of course, this whole conservative effort to ban (or negate) CRT in K-12 curricula is meant to overwrite the actual history of the *ungreat displacement*, which is the genocide against Native Americans, the enslavement of African peoples, and the racism toward immigrants from the Global South. The great replacement fantasy ideologically supports the anti-CRT discourse: critical theory (S_1) → critical *race* theory (S_2). Criticality and theorizing are suspicious master-signifiers within this ideology because of their spurious connection with 'race,' a knowledge that threatens the uncritical, atheoretical, and 'race'-less ideology of whiteness.

In the position of *a*, I put what I would call *the conceptual woke* because anti-woke subjects always refer to their enemies as woke, which is an interesting term. After all, if the other side is woke, then that means anti-woke subjects are asleep, and that would support my thesis that they are dreaming of this nightmarish great replacement fantasy, which disguises their unconscious desire as descendants of settlers *qua* ungreat displacers. The nightmare scenario, of course, is that they are sleepwalking, too, and the 2022 Buffalo shooting is an example of acting out the great replacement fantasy in a violent way.

The *conceptual woke* is meant to capture this ideological fantasy figure, this *objet a* that is causing anti-woke subjects great anxiety; this fantasy object is an amalgam of many things. On the one hand, it is non-white (or non-European) people in general, but it is specifically Jewish and Black people. The reason is the spurious connection between Frankfurt School *critical theory*—Jewish scholars who escaped from Nazi Germany and moved to the U.S.—and, of course, *critical race theory*, which was mostly theorized by Black scholars in critical legal studies. In addition to those two fantasmatic figures of Otherness, who are the main objects of anti-woke racism, there are also radicals in general: communists, socialists, anarchists, or leftists; all these Imaginary figures are combined together in the form of *the conceptual woke*, through metaphorical condensation. This is the political unconscious of the anti-woke subject.

The knowledge or S_2 of the anti-CRT discourse is the conspiracy of "cultural Marxism" or "race Marxism": the kind of 'knowledge' that will reveal the 'truth' about CRT. This ideological form of knowledge is meant to drive fascists to believe in this ideology and to act upon it, and this is the latent danger behind their reactionary dream-work. Anti-CRT ideology is masking or covering over the traumatic Real of colonization: genocide, slavery, and racism.

The 'great' replacement fantasy sustains the anti-CRT discourse. Note the signifier 'great' and consider Trump's presidential campaign slogan: "Make America Great Again." What is 'great' about the replacement fantasy? What is this fantasmatic return to 'greatness' all about? Fascist ideology is premised on a nationalist fantasy of sameness, so this greatness is a Totality where we are all the same; it is the end of difference through the negation of the Other of the Other.

The purpose of ideological fantasy is to suture social antagonisms and material contradictions, that is, the traumatic Real of colonization (genocide, slavery, and racism). The question is: How will racial capitalist society deal with this Real? Is it going to cover it up ideologically through a master's discourse like anti-CRT and banning CRT from public schools? Or is this society going to face the Real directly and deal with it, knowing that it is impossible yet still our ethico-political responsibility, if we are interested in the radical potential of collective liberation: the humanization of all? Facing the Real implies that we must work through that traumatic colonial legacy instead of negating it (cf. Comas-Díaz, Hall, & Neville, 2019; Saketopoulou, 2023; Viego, 2007) with the awareness that the Real of coloniality cannot be represented, for it resists symbolization.

The interesting thing about anti-woke subjects is, of course, that they are masters, but they are too anxious about the fact that they are becoming irrelevant, which is a form of Symbolic castration, so instead they are pretending to be victims. They are *faux hysterics*: Masters who are pretending to be oppressed. What I am trying to show here is that *their fantasy about a great replacement reveals their unconscious desire for ungreat displacement*. This fantasy acts as a screen to prevent the anti-woke subject from confronting the actual, irreconcilable traumatic Real of coloniality: the afterlives of genocide and slavery. The anti-woke subject's fear of being replaced reveals their desire for displacing the Other of the Other. As such, they are over-identifying with the Hispanic subjects, who will virtually replace them one day and are subsequently pre-mourning losing their official status as ungreat displacers—being descendants of the settlers, who displaced millions of Indigenous, Black, and Brown people. In the words of conservative Charlie Kirk: "We are not a nation of immigrants. We are a nation of settlers."

Anti-woke subjects are masters pretending to be hysterics, but they are not true hysterics because the whole point of hysteria is to question master-signifiers. Critical race theory and critical theory are not master-signifiers and positioning them as such is nonsensical and shows that we are now living in a topsy-turvy reality; true hysterics question master-signifiers like "racial capitalism" and reveal how these master-signifiers function not only as an ideology but also as an apparatus. Who is critical of modernity/coloniality? Hysterics. Who is sustaining Totality? Masters. The fascist anti-CRT ideology has a structural function within the apparatus of racial capitalism. The position from which to critique hysterics—because that is a possibility also within psychoanalysis—is the analyst's position (see A in Figure 11.1). Infinite hystericization is destructive and leads to nothing but new master-signifiers. Analysis is the limit of infinite hystericization, which affords us interpretation and (re)construction.

If we move the $ in the position of S_1, that would be the discourse of the hysteric. Now move it one more time, and you get *a* in the position of *agent*—the analyst as an object causing the desire of the analysand, who is doing the grueling work of analysis. The challenge of analysis is to produce new master-signifiers when the old ones do not work anymore. In a sense, the analyst is the one who challenges the hysteric, not the master. The analyst is in an ethical position, which involves less speaking and more listening.

The Analytic Act in a political context is not just passive listening, but a cut that disrupts ideological fantasy. While the hysteric asks what the master wants, the analyst forces the subject to confront their own desire. For example, instead of just arguing against anti-CRT claims, the analytic position would involve questioning the *jouissance* that anti-woke subjects get from their "ungreat displacement" fantasy. The end of analysis should produce master-signifiers that are desacralized—meaning they are recognized as tools for organization rather than absolute truths to be worshipped. If racial capitalism is the master-signifier the hysteric critiques, the analyst helps the analysand construct a new signifier, such as "the commons," as a way to organize desire toward collective liberation.

Ideology is structural: We perceive reality through fantasy because we often have unrealized and unrealizable unconscious desires. In ideology, we fantasize about a sense of mastery—organic unity or wholeness—as a source of enjoyment, and there is no way to get rid of that fundamental fantasy, but it speaks to the current crisis of a divided left: the failure of resistance in the face of capitalism. Lacan addressed that aporia in the aftermath of the May 68 movement, when the students were challenging him as a representative of psychoanalytic mastery. There is a video on YouTube of a Situationist student (Anatole Atlas), who interrupts and disrupts one of Lacan's lectures. That is a concrete instance of a hysterical subject having an intervention, but Lacan raises the question: *Che Vuoi?* (What do you want?)

The answer is that hysterics desire new masters, and that is quite disturbing in the context of how analysis works: The hysteric produces new master-signifiers, which means that those new master-signifiers are going to potentially be the basis for new master discourses, especially if there is a revolutionary shift in power (e.g., the dictatorship of the proletariat). The problem with any revolution in human history is that we literally have these elements in the discourse shifting and moving around all the time, and they end up reproducing different kinds of ideologies, but the discursive/fantasmatic structures remain the same. We always end up with a master's discourse, as *the* discourse of power, which is ideologically sustained by fantasy. The university discourse is the discourse of knowledge legitimizing the power of the master.

When I concluded my book *Decolonial Psychoanalysis*, after I went through the revolution of the four discourses, I realized that even if we challenge the "war on terror" discourse or the anti-CRT discourse, what we will eventually produce are new master discourses. Hence, the cycle never stops; in a way, the symptom is an apt poetic metaphor here because it speaks to the driven *jouissance* of the human spirit, which is never stagnant, but always dialectical and analectical. However, the symptom also points to the structural effect of language, that is, how desire is a never-ending process.

There is a need to face up to the fact that any new master discourse that we come up with, as a libertarian socialist left, will always have unconscious fantasy elements, which means it will structurally produce new forms of Othering. And that has to do with the way that the Real functions, given that it cannot be represented. Think, for instance, about the traumatic Real of coloniality (genocide, enslavement, and racism). We can talk or write about its effects, but we will always fail to linguistically or even visually capture the kernel of that traumatic experience. This is ultimately the traumatic legacy we have to work through. Liberatory discourses can lead to a shift in power, especially when revolutionary hysterics end up in the position of mastery, as was the case with Stalin, Nasser, and Castro, for example.

As revolutionary masters, they are tasked with solving material (politico–libidinal–economic) problems in society, such as the class struggle, racism, and sexist oppression. However, these revolutionary masters are always going to come face to face with this traumatic Real, which cannot be represented in a Symbolic or Imaginary way, and they will revert to using ideological fantasy to cover it up, which points to the spectral dimension of the libidinal economy that always accompanies the political economy as a shadow or apparition. That is what fantasy does, it plugs in the ideology and hides any inconsistency resulting from the traumatic Real. As the point of impossibility in ideology, the Real shows us the incoherence of the Symbolic, where it fails. In the final analysis, liberation entails working through inconsistency, impossibility, incoherence, trauma, failure, etc.

What is the political question—and I write about this in *Freud and Said* (2021a)—from a Lacanian perspective? First of all, we have to resist authoritarian politics based on Imaginary identification, or populist politics where there is a charismatic leader, whom we feel we identify with. These Imaginary politics of sameness exist on the left as totalitarianism and on the right as fascism. We must then consider these follow-up questions: (1) What do we desire as a collective? Do we have common desires? What do we want from a truthful and just society? We are going to get different answers, but to have solidarity or to build a coalition, we will need to have a list of questions (rather than answers) that we can agree on. The second set of questions related to the first set is: (2) What would we collectively enjoy together? We can think about the commons here as an example of public goods. While the first set of questions is ethical, the second is aesthetic.

In sum, these are the two fundamental political questions: (1) What commons do we collectively desire? (2) What commons would we collectively enjoy? They are basic questions, but they are not often asked because we tend to fall into the trap of Imaginary politics, the spectacle, wherein we are suddenly charmed by a charismatic leader, who appears on the left or the right. We think that the solution lies with this person or their party. However, this person is a flawed human being, a divided subject like the rest of us. We must build a movement, however flawed, that outlives us, as a gift for future generations and for the rest of the planet.

We do not wish to have a politics of answers but *a politics of questions*, wherein we generate incomplete answers together, which will be revised according to historical reason. This politics is about embracing complexity *vis-à-vis* psychosocial problems. Complexity means that I may not have the solution, but that through

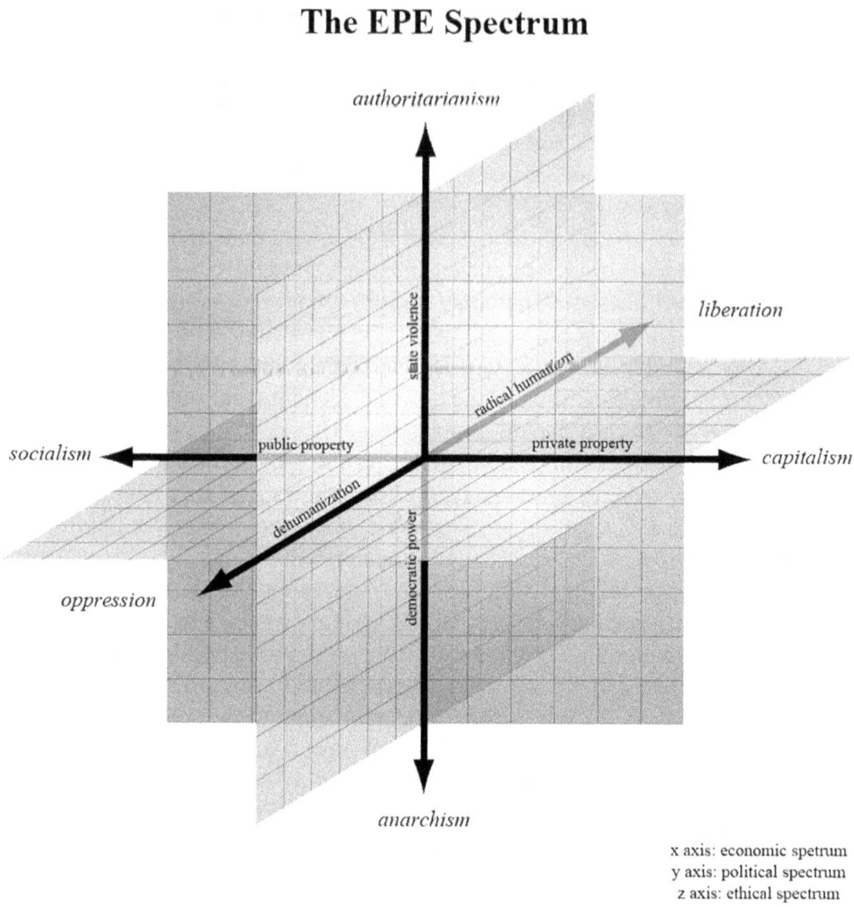

Figure 11.3 The economic–political–ethical spectrum

collective questioning we can come together to problem-solve. This entails putting our minds and bodies together, for politics is a collective effort of thinking and being. *A politics of difference* acknowledges the isomorphism between the division of the subject and the division of the Other, and accounts for psychosocial complexity without translating the Real in a hierarchical fashion (see Figure 11.3). Liberation psychoanalysis exists at the intersection of libertarian socialism and radical humanism.

Chapter 12

Ye: (Anti)Christ?

In this chapter, I interpret the intensification of Ye's psychotic symptoms since 2016 as exacerbating his turn toward fascism in 2022. I also read Ye's anti-Semitism as death-driven self-hatred, which is projected outward in the form of paranoid delusional statements and fascist spectacles. This self-hatred stems from Ye's internalization of anti-Black racism within a racial capitalist society polarized between liberal and conservative factions. Ye's self-hatred manifests symptomatically as the melancholic negation, or foreclosure, of the Ray-of-the-Father (a condensation of *Ray, the Real father* and *God, the Imaginary father*). The manic solution to melancholia is: "I am a god." Because otherwise, "I am a piece of sh*t."

Ye wishes to be crucified and martyred, like Jesus, for he is Yeezus, the Radical King of the Fools. Ye's self-hatred has roots in depressed feelings of abandonment, which have gotten worse in a political world marked by extreme polarization, particularly since the 2016 U.S. Presidential election. Some of the biographical factors that structure Ye's psychotic subjectivity include (1) his father choosing his career over his family, which will drive Ye to foreclose intellectualism, Leftism, and Judeo-Christianity as radical signifiers; (2) his mOther dying and leaving him with the impossibility of her desire for giantness/nothingness, which I frame through the legacy of unconditional love—a transgenerational discursive legacy of trauma related to the afterlives of genocide, slavery, and racism under racial capitalism; (3) his ex-wife divorcing him for his "personality;" and (4) the culture canceling him for being anti-Christ.

The title of this chapter is *Ye: (Anti)Christ?* with a question mark, and anti is in parentheses to ask: Is Ye Christ or anti-Christ? And is there a difference? To answer these questions, we must consider some supernatural associations attached to Ye: starman, demigod, and monster.

Starman

Is Ye a Starman? This is a fascinating conspiracy about the connection between David Bowie and Ye (Chen, 2017). On the album cover of *The Rise and Fall of Ziggy Stardust and the Spiders from Mars* (1972), a sign reads "K. West." This concept album was very difficult for Bowie because he became the persona of Ziggy

DOI: 10.4324/9781003768104-12

Stardust to the point of almost having a psychotic break, so he eventually distanced himself from this fictional character. Bowie, who was a chameleon throughout his career, represents what the subject might look like after the end of analysis. Interestingly, the actor Gary Oldman, who was friends with Bowie, said in an interview, "Don't you feel that since he [Bowie] died, the world's gone to shit? It was like he was cosmic glue or something. When he died, everything fell apart" (as cited in Dunworth, 2025). Many users on social media ironically interpreted Oldman's words to mean that the death of Bowie in 2016 explains the decline of western culture since the rise of Trumpism.

On the album, there is a song called "Starman" that predicts the coming of a starman, who is "waiting in the sky" and "would like to come and meet us." Many believe that this starman is Ye because another reference on the album is the song "Five Years." The starman is predicted to arrive in five years. Coincidently, Ye was born five years after the release of the album. Then there is the lyric, "Let the children lose it … let the children use it … let all the children boogie," implying that the starman's spiritual purpose on Earth is to liberate the children.

Ye, at the MTV Music Video Awards 2015, announced that he was going to run for president, which he did in 2020, and he also echoed the starman's message by saying, "Listen to the kids, bro." Freud (1916) asks: "where do children come from and what has the father to do with their origin?" (pp. 50–51). This Oedipal question of the starman *qua* father—a manic father and a depressed anti-father—is crucial and occupies my thinking throughout the chapter.

Freud continues:

> Psychoanalysis has taught us the intimate connection between the father complex and belief in God, and daily demonstrate to us how youthful persons lose their religious belief as soon as *the authority of the father breaks down.* In the parental complex we thus recognize the root of religious need; the almighty, just God, and kindly nature appear to us as grand sublimations of father and mother, or rather as revivals and restorations of the infantile conceptions of both parents.
> (pp. 103–104, emphasis added)

Lacan (2006) would later on describe this psychotic breakdown of the authority of the father in terms of a cut in the signifying chain, wherein the paternal metaphor fails as a result of a foreclosure of the Name-of-the-Father. Freud's words seem to be a precise diagnosis of Ye, as we shall see later on, regarding what I am calling the Ray-of-the-Father.

Demigod

Is Ye a demigod? He said in 2013, "I am a god even though I'm a man of God," thereby contradicting himself. Contradicting oneself is a common feature of divided subjectivity, but it is a meta-feature of manic-depressive subjectivity—divided subjectivity on steroids. Ye's statements are often not only contradictory but also dialectical. Is Ye a god or a man of God? Is he a false messiah (Yeezus), or anti-Christ? Another suggestion would be to think of Ye as The Fool. The Tarot of Marseille was restored by Alejandro Jodorowsky, a Chilean artist and Tarot master, who greatly influenced Ye. I begin *A Psychoanalytic Biography of Ye* with the story of their encounter (Beshara, 2023). This story was my entry into the rabbit hole of Kanye West.

The cover art for *Vultures*, Ye's recent album, in collaboration with Ty Dolla $ign, is inspired by Jodorowsky's *The Holy Mountain* (1973), probably one of the most surreal cult films of all time. In 2014, Jodorowsky met with Ye in France, and he did a tarot reading for him. In the reading, Ye received The Fool card. Another card that Ye received was The World, so Jodorowsky's interpretation was that *Ye is The Fool walking toward The World*. I would argue that Ye is not only The Fool but *The King of the Fools*, particularly given his anti-Christ attitude, or his melancholic identification with Jesus.

Monster

Is Ye a monster? He refers to himself sometimes as such, and he said in 2010, "everybody knows I'm motherf****** monster. I'ma need to see your f****** hands at the concert." There is a promotional photo of Ye from back then showing him holding a decapitated woman's head by her hair. In 2022, Ye released the music video for "Eazy," his collaboration with The Game. In the claymation video, he is portrayed decapitating Pete Davidson, which we can interpret as a form of castration because Davidson dated Ye's ex-wife (Kim Kardashian) and taunted him about it in a text message that Ye posted a screenshot of publicly. The message shows a close-up photo of a nude Davidson, presumably in bed after or before he had sex with Kardashian, with his tongue out and signaling the V sign, which in this context of overdetermination signifies sexual provocation (i.e., V for vagina, as opposed to victory).

The monster, or (anti)Christ, is the Incarnate Son, and the connection here is made explicit by Žižek (Žižek & Milbank, 2009) in *The Monstrosity of Christ*. Is Ye "an ethical monster [anti-Christ] without empathy doing what is to be done in a weird coincidence of blind spontaneity and reflexive distance, helping others while avoiding their disgusting proximity?" (p. 303). For Žižek, "With more people like this [e.g., Ye], the world would be a pleasant place in which sentimentality would be replaced by a cold and cruel passion" (p. 303). The cold and cruel passion of anti-Christ. Whether Ye is a starman, a demigod, or a monster remains unresolved and requires further investigation.

The Shaky Ass Years

Dawn Boeck (2014) has devised three periods to make sense of the cuts in Ye's eclectic discography. Those periods are: (1) Dropout Bear (2004–2007), (2) Constructing a Fantasy (2010–2011), and (3) Commander of Culture (2011–2013). The periods are distinct in that when Ye moves between one period and another, there is a *cut* marking a shift in the structure of the signifier. In other words, Ye's discography is punctuated by ethical and aesthetic shifts in his project (Kanye West), mirroring the complex dialectics of his political subjectivity.

The period that I focus on in my book is what I term *The Shaky Ass Years* (2016–2021). On a personal level, it was a very tumultuous period for Ye, which began with a nervous breakdown in 2016 that I read as a psychotic break. I got curious about Ye's divided subjectivity because he would interrupt his performances during the St. Pablo Tour and free associate for a significant period of time. His speeches were labeled as 'rants' in the media and by the public.

As someone committed to the ethics of psychoanalysis, I was intrigued to hear him differently by listening to his unconscious. After his nervous breakdown, Ye was diagnosed with bipolar disorder. I prefer the psychoanalytic conception of manic depression. I say more on that later. It is worth noting that Lou Reed (2013) recognized the manic depressive structure of Ye's subjectivity in his review of *Yeezus*, three years before the official diagnosis.

I theorize a new period in the preface to my book: The Fascist Era. It begins in 2022. This period will be the focus of this chapter, which is an addendum to *A Psychoanalytic Biography of Ye* (2023). I will undoubtedly touch on aspects from the previous periods but will primarily analyze The Fascist Era. Now, I wish to highlight some of the *cuts* I referred to earlier to give the reader a sense of dramatic transitions and key dates, which shed light on Ye's complex subjectivity.

Psychobiography

Ye was born on June 8th, 1977, in Douglasville, Georgia. Donda and Ray West, his parents, formalized their divorce on August 28, 1980, after which Donda and Ye moved from Atlanta to Chicago. Ye is a Chicagoan through and through. In 2002, he almost died in a car crash, and a picture of him disfigured after the wreckage is immortalized in the 2004 music video for "Through the Wire."

Donda West died in 2007, which marks the first *cut* between Dropout Bear and Constructing a Fantasy. Donda was not properly mourned until 2021 with the release of *Donda*. Processing his grief for his mOther took him 14 years, for there is no direct reference to Donda's passing, in Ye's music, until 2021. In 2014, Ye married Kim Kardashian, but they filed for divorce in 2021. In 2016, Kim experienced a life-threatening hostage and robbery situation in Paris, which Ye learned about while in concert. That is when he experienced a major nervous breakdown. However, that was not the only reason, for there was also the context of the 2016 U.S. presidential election, which was extremely polarizing for a crumbling empire. These factors accumulated into an intense period (The Shaky Ass Years) characterized in the first year by his nervous breakdown, his forced hospitalization, and his diagnosis of bipolar disorder. Not mentioning the anxiety-provoking effect of being on a 'reality' tv show (*Keeping Up with the Kardashians*), as someone who struggles with 'reality.'

In 2016, when Ye experienced a psychotic break, he canceled the rest of the St. Pablo Tour. My book analyzes this period, which for most fans—and I am not referring only to hardcore ones—is probably the least interesting period, aesthetically-speaking. Most fans prefer his work before 2016, hence, the distinction between the old Kanye and the new Ye. During The Shaky Ass Years, we see Ye struggling head-on with manic depression.

Ye has been consistently saying controversial things since the beginning of his career (e.g., "George Bush doesn't care about Black people" or "I'ma let you finish, but Beyoncé had one of the best videos of all time"); however, one notices an intensification of those kinds of statements during the Shaky Ass Years, and it gets even worse from 2022 with his anti-Semitic remarks, but 2016–2021 remains a very interesting period to think about from a psychoanalytic perspective and also in relation to his creative output, which is underrated. The Shaky Ass Years is a phrase from one of his songs, "No Mistakes," wherein he makes that reference, so I try to use his own words in my analysis whenever possible. A psychoanalytic ethic informs my listening, interpretation, and reconstruction, allowing me to take seriously what his unconscious is saying.

Ye's Aristocratic Rebellion

Henceforth, I wish to explore Ye's turn toward fascism since 2022, particularly through a psychoanalytic reflection on his *anti-Christ praxis*, in an effort to unpack what that means. I juxtapose Ye with Nietzsche, both being "aristocratic rebels" (Losurdo, 2021). Ye says, "Name one genius that ain't crazy" (2016) and "no one man should have all that power" (2010). Ye's obsession with genius evinces a model of power/knowledge grounded in madness.

Eva Cybulska (2019) argues that Nietzsche also suffered from manic depression, so there are personal and theoretical overlaps between both mad geniuses, and the list includes figures, such as Lord Byron, Ludwig van Beethoven, Edgar Allan Poe, Vincent van Gogh, Edvard Munch, Virginia Woolf, Ernest Hemingway, Sylvia Plath, Jimi Hendrix, Carrie Fisher, and Kurt Cobain. There is, of course, the *Übermensch ideal*, which I explore, too. Recall, for example, the cover art for the 1979 Penguin Classics edition of Nietzsche's autobiography *Ecce Homo* (1908/1979), which was published posthumously, and how that image of an *Übermensch* was replicated in *Vultures*-era fan art depicting Ye as a "solitary rebel."

The original cover art for the album was Caspar David Friedrich's (1818) painting *Wanderer above the Sea of Fog*. According to Ana Finel Honigman (2023):

> The lone, elegant figure in *Wanderer Above the Sea of Fog* stands with his back to the viewer, a device called *Rückenfigur* that Friedrich frequently employed. The man is depicted standing on a rocky precipice gazing at a valley in which rocks, trees, and mountains appear rising above a thick, rolling mist.

In the fan art, Ye is in a similar setting, except the colors are desaturated, half a dozen vultures are flying above, and Ye seems to be wearing *Vultures*-era merchandise and a face balaclava, while a black bird of prey is sitting on his right shoulder.

Another connection that could be made is between Richard Wagner (Nietzsche's frenemy) and Ye. Wagner's name for the principle behind his aesthetics is *Gesamtkunstwerk* or total work, which is the praxis of being a total artist. People who do not know Ye think he is merely a rapper, but those who are more familiar with his work know that he is a designer, filmmaker, and has even produced an opera, which clearly impressed Leonard Cohen and moved him to write a surreal poem in 2015 titled "Kanye West is not Picasso." In the poem, which comes across as a tribute, Cohen attempts to out-do Ye's infamous braggadocio by bombastically claiming, "I am the Kanye West of Kanye West. The Kanye West of the great bogus shift of bullshit culture."

In 2012, Ye made a film called *Cruel Summer*, which was screened at the Cannes Film Festival. The film was projected, using proprietary technology, onto seven screen panels—something that had not been done before that point in time. Ye founded the Yeezy brand a year later in 2013, and it has been a fashion staple ever since. In 2019, Ye produced and directed *Nebuchadnezzar: A Kanye West Opera.* Therefore, we must think of Ye as a Wagnerian or total artist, authoritarian tendencies notwithstanding; yet, is this not precisely the problem with Totality—that it is inherently totalizing and totalitarian?

When Ye identified himself with Trump and wore the MAGA hat in 2016, it upset many of his fans. Still, according to Ye (2018), "When I put this hat on, it made me feel like Superman [Übermensch] my favorite superhero." At the White House, Ye told Trump, "You made a Superman cape for me." Ye wearing the MAGA hat, despite what everyone else thought, made him feel powerful. Is there a method to his madness?

Another interesting example is the cover art for his 2018 album *Ye*—a photo of the Teton Range mountains in Jackson Hole, Wyoming, taken by Ye with his iPhone. The album cover has the following words written in green: "I hate being bipolar its [sic] awesome." This statement essentially captures the dialectical structure of manic depression. What Ye does in this album is curious, for he reframes bipolarity, or manic depression, as *power*—a Nietzschean move *par excellence*. In a sense, we must ask: Is Ye Nietzsche's eternal return, but as difference?

Ye's bourgeois class position—with its implicit investments in white supremacy and heteropatriarchy—is complicated by the traumatic dimension of racial–sexual violence overdetermining Black male subjectivity in the U.S. (Curry, 2017). Similarly, his fascist politics post-2021 are undermined by the anti-fascist potential of his tragic aesthetics and messianic ethics pre-2022. Ye does and says many things that are a turnoff for many people, including myself. At the same time, something remains, *das Ding*, which is worth critiquing and reflecting on.

Sadly, Ye's character arc went from the tragic figure of a new messiah (Yeezus) to the farcical figure of a self-redeeming anti-Christ, which signifies a regression from the radicality of his manic unconscious (the leftist legacy of unconditional love) to fascism as depressed being. This regression is Ye's depressive defense against his mania. It coincides with the foreclosure of the Ray-of-the-Father, a melancholic negation marked by his *sinthomatic* shift from Kanye West (project/object) to Ye (subject). For a visualization of this arc, juxtapose LaChapelle's (2006) photo "The Passion of Kanye West" with *Vultures*-era Ye (2024) in a Jason Voorhees mask, which associates him with both a psychopathic killer and crucifixion on Friday the 13th.

Anti-Christ

Is Ye anti-Christ? This is not a theological question but rather a scientific (i.e., philosophical and psychoanalytic) one. Following Nietzsche (1895/1990), to be anti-Christ means to be against *décadance* values, such as nihilism, pity, and denial of life. In other words, to be against the death drive. Pity, for Nietzsche, is "*practical* nihilism … pity persuades to *nothingness*!" (p. 130, emphasis in original). To be anti-Christ is to be against *chandala*, or 'slave,' morality and to be against equal rights as a form of *ressentiment*. To be anti-Christ is to be against a cosmopolitan "God of the merely good" (p. 138), so, in a sense, to be against internationalism, or "God as God of the sick, God as spider, God as spirit" (p. 140). To be anti-Christ is to be against Jesus as a heroic or genius redeemer type and against the church, priests, or Judeo-Christianity. To be anti-Christ is to be against faith, belief, and revelation.

To be anti-Christ also means to be for the revaluation of all values, which for Nietzsche signifies going back to natural values or actuality, which could be framed as the life drive. To be anti-Christ is to be for noble, or 'master,' morality, such as life affirmation. There is a hierarchy to Nietzsche's thinking that stems from his aristocratic elitism, which again we can see in Ye as well, wherein 'self-actualized' spiritual types are at the top of the hierarchy, followed by the muscular types, who defend those spiritual types, and then at the bottom of the pyramid are the mediocre types, that is, the herd or masses. This hierarchy is the antithesis of the classless society anticipated by socialists, yet it is precisely the technocratic ideal championed by Ye's right-wing associates—from Donald Trump and Elon Musk to Candace Owens, Nick Fuentes, and Milo Yiannopoulos.

Nietzsche believed in national Gods as opposed to international Gods. National gods are expressions of the "will to power" (p. 139), which explains the manifestation of Christian nationalism for Ye and other conservative Nietzscheans (e.g., Peter Thiel, Bronze Age Pervert, Curtis Yarvin, Alexander Dugin, and Richard Spencer). To be anti-Christ also means to be for Jesus as a singular being, political criminal, and free spirit, who lived and died for "a new way of living, *not* a new belief" (p. 158, emphasis in original). To be anti-Christ is to be for science as the "wisdom of the world" and for skepticism, action, practice, and instinct. Many of the characteristics of Nietzsche's anti-Christ describe Yeezus more than Ye.

Both Nietzsche and Ye admire Jesus and identify with him to different degrees. Ye calls God his 'daddy,' which speaks to the function of the Imaginary father in the absence of the Real father (Ray). Furthermore, as a single mOther-crocodile,

Donda had to place herself in the position of the Symbolic father. Therefore, she also gets foreclosed in her role as an anxiety-provoking academic signifier, alongside the absent or abandoning Ray-of-the-Father. Ye's foreclosure of the over-present academic mOther manifested in the form of his anti-intellectualism, for the founder of Donda Academy is a self-identified college dropout, who confessed during a 2022 podcast interview: "I actually haven't read any book. Reading is like eating Brussels sprouts."

Nietzsche is undoubtedly more strongly identified with Zarathustra than Jesus. However, Ye's identification with Jesus is ambivalent because he also presents himself as an alternative redeemer through the signifier 'Yeezus': a non-castrated national god, who is beyond good and evil. Similarly, Nietzsche and Ye are both critical of Christianity as an institution, Christians as representatives of the 'herd,' and Judeo-Christian ideology understood as 'slave' morality. Their critiques are from a bourgeois class position, which affords them the privileges of aristocratic rebellion. Consequently, both have been considered not only mad geniuses and free spirits, but also bigoted monsters that must be canceled for their fascism. Interestingly, Nietzsche's Zarathustra (like Yeezus) can also be framed as a starman (*Übermensch*) for his supposed role as a visionary and a guide, who exists on a different plane of thought and being from most of humanity.

I will provide examples of Ye's critiques of Christianity, which I read as *a hystericization of paternal authority*, particularly given the unconscious associations between Ray (as a signifier of absence) and Leftism/Judeo-Christianity (as signifiers of *décadence*). Ye formed a congregation in 2019 called Sunday Service. One can, of course, find Jesusian references throughout Ye's discography, such as "Jesus Walks" from 2004, wherein he links Jesus with hustlers, killers, murderers, drug dealers, and strippers. Furthermore, in 2013, Ye released "I Am A God," where he says, "*I am a god* even though *I'm a man of God*" (emphasis added). This is a very important dialectical phrase, signifying "the split between *the enunciating subject* and *the subject of the statement*" (Lacan, 2006, p. 650, emphasis added).

However, Ye's relationship with Christianity is far from straightforward. In 2019, in the song "Hands On," Ye says, "What have you been hearin' from the Christians? They'll be the first one to judge me. Make it feel like nobody love me." And in a 2024 interview with Big Boy, Ye confesses:

> I have my issues with Jesus … there's a lot of stuff I went through that I prayed, and I didn't see Jesus show up … I'm god … I'm the god of me [i.e., self-redeemer or anti-Christ] … And you can't tell me who I am … I'm the god of me. *I don't know if I'm in heaven already*. (emphasis added)

The negation at the end of Ye's confession reveals that he unconsciously thinks he is already in heaven on Earth, probably given his status as a wealthy person uncompromisingly pursuing his cold and cruel passions. During the same interview, Ye adds, "Another thing I don't like in Christianity: the fear of God … if God is love, why should you fear Him?"

Additionally, here is Ye's double-critique, from 2018, of Leftism *qua* Christianity: "you can't bully me. Liberals can't bully me, news can't bully me, the hip-hop community, they can't bully me." Ye adopts the conservative perspective, which collapses liberalism into leftism, in an effort to reject *radical Christianity*.

According to the radical Christian perspective, Jesus was an anarcho-communist revolutionary—a Palestinian Jew. This is the opposite of the conservative Christian viewpoint, which is invested in bourgeois rebellion and hyper-individualism. In sum, Ye's Jesusian critiques amount to a foreclosure of absence in two senses: (1) the lack of paternal authority (the Ray-of-the-Father) and (2) the overpresence of *décadence*, as represented by both Leftism (e.g., socialism and liberalism) and Judeo-Christianity. Ray abandoned Ye as a child, even though he was a Leftist (a Black Panther) and a Judeo-Christian. Consequently, his absence is linked in Ye's unconscious with the *décadence* of Leftist and Judeo-Christian authority.

Spike Lee's (1989) *Do The Right Thing* ends with two quotes side by side from both Martin Luther King Jr. and Malcolm X, a juxtaposition that we can think of as *the dialectic of (non)violence*. The desire of mOther (Donda) is aligned with civil rights, which the Democratic Party hijacked. The Ray-of-the-Father is affiliated with Black Power, which the FBI's COINTELPRO defeated. In the face of this liberal–radical alienation, Ye opts for the conservative pill of fascism, which "is one of the factors in the formation of the modern spectacle," according to Guy Debord (1967/2018).

At the New York album listening party for *Vultures*, a fan was spotted watching the concert through an Apple Vision Pro headset, which is reminiscent of the 1983 cover for *The Society of Spectacle* displaying a photo by J. R. Eyerman of spectators in 1952 watching the film *Bwana Devil* through 3-D glasses. Following Debord, the fascist spectacle is "the material reconstruction of the religious illusion," that is, *racial capitalism is an anti-Christ ideology*.

The anti-Christ, a Jesusian/Zarathustrian of sorts, aspires to become a self-redeemer, hence, the motif of *baptism by fire* as a psychospiritual ritual of purification signifying ego death followed by unconscious rebirth as the *Übermensch*. There are numerous visual examples of this motif of burning in the sacred fire throughout Ye's total work that echo the chromolitho print titled *The Death of Zoroaster in the Fire Temple*.

Examples of self-immolation include the music video for "Power" (2010), the phoenix rising out of the ashes in the "Runaway" (2010) film, Ye burning a replica of the house he grew up in on the south-side of Chicago with himself in it during the 2021 Chicago listening party for *Donda*, and Sean Leon's "Burn Everything (feat. Ye)." During the Chicago listening party, Ye staged a symbolic immolation of the Kanye West project/object to liberate himself from that project's commodity form, seeking rebirth as a complex subject—one whose eventual pivot toward the reactionary right was a predictable outcome for a bourgeois subject invested in the mystical authoritarianism of instrumental reason. My claim, however, is that Ye's class position cannot entirely overdetermine a subjectivity that remains informed—albeit unconsciously—by the historical reason of the radical Black tradition.

In general, people love Kanye West (project/object), but hate Ye (subject). In an opinion poll conducted by SSRS for CNN in 2018 (n = 1,015), 23% of respondents had a favorable opinion of Ye, and they were mostly women, white, pro-Trump, 50–64 years old, and Republican. However, most respondents (53%) had an unfavorable opinion (Sparks, 2018). Kanye West refers to a project that Ye has been working on for many years; it also refers to him as an *objet a* or fantasy object for millions of fans—a commodity to be fetishized and consumed. People mostly hate Ye (subject), but that passion does not afford us with an analytic interpretation of his complex subjectivity and how it functions within the current libidinal economy.

To summarize, I am interested in this displacement from Kanye to Ye after 2016, which signifies a multi-layered *sinthome*: (1) the foreclosure of the Ray-of-the-Father as the negation of Leftism/Judeo-Christianity; (2) the movement from Kanye West as a Symbolic-Imaginary project/object to Ye as a manic-depressive subject; (3) Ye as the Letter that killed Kanye West, marking the traumatic Real; (4) Ye as one of the most commonly used words in the Bible, which means 'you'; (5) 'you' (the fans, or *we*) as the fourth ring (the *sinthome*) linking the Symbolic, Imaginary, and Real registers for Ye; (6) Ye = Yes! According to Nietzsche, "the Eternal recurrence of all things" is "the highest of all possible formulas of a Yea-saying philosophy"; (7) like Joyce, Ye produces music in such a way that the language of music no longer exists, which is "the elation that we are told lies at the root of a sort of sinthome that in psychiatry we call mania" (Lacan, 2016, p. 4); (8) Ye's manic unconscious is dialectically informed by the legacy of unconditional love, which is Donda's (and Ray's) legacy. This legacy is not only parental but also ancestral. Ye's manic unconscious is both an affirmation and a negation of this traumatic legacy; (9) finally, there is the mOther's desire for giantness/nothingness, which sheds light on Ye's polarization between life-driven giantness and death-driven nothingness. This polarization is clear to see in Ye's logic of extreme alienation: either "I am a God" or "burn everything." There is nothing in between; this is the ambivalence at the very heart of Ye's manic-depressive being.

The Libidinal Economy of Kanye West

I shall now explore the libidinal economy of Kanye West (project/object) vs. Ye (subject). Ye recently married architect and model Bianca Censori. There are many provocative—*uncensored*—photos of Censori in the media, such as her wearing a tank top and white shirt that says 'WET,' a Yeezy design. Thinking about the Borromean knot and unpacking the sinthome further, we can meditate on the Imaginary fantasy at work in Ye's subjectivity, given the foreclosure of the Ray-of-the-Father and how that fantasy plays into the fascist spectacle as an aestheticization of politics. The fascist spectacle sheds light on Ye's anti-Left/anti-Christ stance. Anti-Left, as in anti-Ray, or against the Real father who abandoned him. Anti-Christ, as in pro-Trump and pro-Jesus, because they are both perceived, by conservatives, as redeeming Imaginary fathers. There is also the fetishization of Yeezy as a commodity or brand. If Kanye West is the barred ~~Other~~, then Yeezy is the *objet a*. Christ sacrifices himself to redeem the world, and anti-Christ sacrifices themself to redeem themself; hence, Ye's statement: "I'm the god of me."

At the Symbolic level, we have the discourse of unconditional love, which is a subjectification of the mOther's desire as cause. Following Freud (1939), the legacy of unconditional love is an "archaic inheritance," a transgenerational trauma in the form of a discourse passed on from generation to generation. For Ye, this would amount to stories about the enslavement of Africans and counter-stories about Black liberation before, during, and after the transatlantic slave trade.

The legacy of unconditional love manifests in a couple of ways. On a superficial level, it manifests as "love-bombing," so, for example, in a 2022 interview that Ye did on InfoWars, he said, "I like Hitler," which was shocking, even for right-wing conspiracy theorist Alex Jones. It is impossible to know if Ye meant these words or if it is merely a provocative but nonsensical statement. In any case, it is a speech act, for which he must pay. He also believes that "love is the new money," which is curious to think about in terms of the libidinal economy.

Then there is the question of Real trauma, or surplus-*jouissance*, under racial capitalism. Ye indexes the traumatic Real of neo-slavery (cf. George, 2016): "I know that we the new slaves. I see the blood on the leaves." The zone of nonbeing is explored as a space occupied in particular by Black male subjects. Tommy Curry (2017) writes about the fungibility of the Black male body as over-exploited flesh, which in the context of racial capitalism manifests through "racial–sexual violence." In other words, while the slave was exchanged as a *thing* to be violently over-exploited not only economically but also libidinally, something of the slave's commodity form survives ideologically post-slavery in coloniality, which for Ye is the surplus-*jouissance* of neo-slavery.

This account shows us why it is not satisfactory to boil the analysis down to Ye's megalomania or narcissism. The egotistical aspect of his subjectivity does not shed light on his manic unconscious. For example, how the *sinthome* (Ye as in *you*, as in *we*, but also as in *yes!*) reframes psychotic (manic-depressive) subjectivity as power. An account of Ye's complex subjectivity affords us a more sophisticated critique of his reactionary politics.

Manic Depression > Bipolar Disorder

When it comes to clinical structures and the question of manic depression vs. bipolar disorder, there are three main categories in psychoanalytic diagnosis: neurosis, psychosis, and perversion. Manic depression falls under psychosis. The three clinical or psychical structures in psychoanalysis are more than diagnostic categories; they are *structural categories* that reveal the subject's position based on their form of negation. Neurotics, psychotics, and perverts use repression, foreclosure, or disavowal, respectively. In other words, Ye is a psychotic subject because he forecloses the Ray-of-the-Father. This phrase is a variation on the Name-of-the-Father, which metaphorically condenses both *the Real father* (Ray) and *the Imaginary father* (God).

The Ray-of-the-Father conjures up this image of crepuscular rays, referred to culturally as Stairways to Heaven or God Fingers—signs of the virtual, or ideological, father. The Ray-of-the-Father also captures the name of Ye's actual, or material, father. Returning to the question of diagnosis, Bruce Fink (1997) writes:

> American psychiatrists, psychoanalysts, and psychologists seem intent on introducing ever more classifications and diagnostic categories ... but none of their categories does anything but tag a particular symptom or set of symptoms manifested by an individual at a given moment. Each such category represents but a micro-symptom or mini-pattern in a person's overall psychological makeup.
> (pp. 115–116)

In other words, bipolar disorder is a misguided term because it confuses the symptom with the category, and this is why we have to go back to the psychoanalytic understanding of manic depression. My book on Ye includes a very long section, from pages 55 to 98, wherein I review the psychoanalytic literature on manic depression. I focus primarily on the work of Karl Abraham, Sigmund Freud, Melanie Klein, Donald Winnicott, Darian Leader, and Christopher Bollas. Lacan did not have a lot to say about manic depression, but he wrote significantly about psychosis. The texts that I found most enlightening were *Mourning and Melancholia* (Freud, 1917), *Strictly Bipolar* (Leader, 2013), and *Three Characters* (Bollas, 2021).

The mOther's Desire for Giantness/Nothingness

After the question of diagnosis, how does one interpret Ye's psychotic or manic-depressive subjectivity? We must begin with the mOther's desire for giantness/nothingness. This is a reference from the documentary *jeen-yuhs: A Kanye Trilogy* (2022), released on Netflix. In the documentary, there is a scene that captures a lovely exchange between Donda and Ye around the beginning of his career. Donda tells Ye a paradoxical riddle, which sounds like a koan: "The giant looks in the mirror and sees nothing." There is *Donda*-era fan art, which depicts Ye in a spikey black jacket sitting in his green room at the Mercedes-Benz Stadium while looking into a mirror, but he does not see his reflection (like a vampire). Donda's riddle is a very interesting statement *vis-à-vis* the ego's development. The mirror stage, for Lacan (2006), is not only a developmental stage, but also a theatrical stage on which we perform our egoic identifications in the forms of *personae* or masks throughout our lives.

In that moment in the film, Ye seems confused, and he is not sure what his mom means or wants, but she transfers this traumatic desire to him, which functions as an *objet a* that he lacks and, therefore, desires. He has been trying to subjectify this desire throughout his life and career. Sometimes he succeeds, and a lot of times, he fails. But if we consider his subjectivity, as divided between ego and unconscious, we can place depression on the side of his ego and mark it with the following humbling statement from one of his songs, "even though I'm a man of God."

The more interesting side is his manic unconscious, from which he would utter: "I am a god," as if he was al-Hallaj. This is the dimension of giantness. The question of "what is this nothingness?" is a significant one that has to do with the Other, more specifically the mOther, in the role of the Symbolic ~~Other~~, that is, the Name-of-the-Father + the Desire of the mOther. In summary, there is the *objet a* of giantness/nothingness, and then there is the barred ~~mOther~~, as a representative of the traumatic legacy of unconditional love. On the one hand, we have the over-presence of the mOther's desire for giantess/nothingness. On the other hand, we have the absent Ray-of-the-Father, which again signifies the *décadence* of Leftism and Judeo-Christianity.

The Ray-of-the-Father

Ray West was a member of the Black Panther Party, a radical Leftist party. Ray West is currently a Christian marriage counselor, so there is a movement from Leftism to Judeo-Christianity, a radical–liberal spectrum represented by the Ray-of-the-Father. Is it surprising then that Ye is both anti-Left (conservative) and anti-Christ (illiberal)?

Mania is Ye's solution to his depression from abandonment, whether it is divorce (Ray's from Donda and Kim's from Ye), death (of the mOther), or abortion. When Ye ran for President in 2020, he held a chaotic rally in South Carolina, where he was wearing a bulletproof vest, and started talking about a conversation that he had with his then-wife Kim Kardashian about the possibility of aborting their first daughter (North). After saying that, he started crying profusely, and the political rally turned into a highly emotional and confusing event. Abandonment is a signifier (from the mOther) that Ye indexes throughout his oeuvre, so he has a song called "Never Abandon Your Family," for example.

From the mOther, Ye learned that abandonment is the negation of family, hence, why the foreclosure of the Ray-of-the-Father manifests for him as the paranoid delusional foreclosure of Leftism and Judeo-Christianity. The dramatic shift from Kanye West (project/object) to Ye (subject) after 2016 is symptomatic of this foreclosure, a negation of abandonment: "God, why have you forsaken me?" God (the father) abandoned Jesus (the son) in order to save humanity from sin. Ye rejects this humanistic logic of the greater good and prefers traditional family values. Or does he?

The Method of Psychoanalytic Biography

At this point, I wish to take a step back and give a couple of notes on psychoanalytic biography as my method of analysis. The first psychoanalytic biography that we know of is Freud's (1910/1916) *Leonardo da Vinci: A Psychosexual Study of an Infantile Reminiscence*, wherein he writes:

> If a biographical effort really endeavors to penetrate the understanding of the psychic life of its hero it must not, as happens in most biographies through discretion or prudery, pass over in silence the sexual activity or the sex peculiarity of the one examined. What we know about it in Leonardo is very little but full

> of significance. In a period where there was a constant struggle between riotous licentiousness and gloomy asceticism, Leonardo presented an example of cool sexual rejection which one would not expect in an artist and a portrayer of feminine beauty.
>
> (pp. 13–14)

Freud presents us with a methodology for writing a psychoanalytic biography. Another classic study is from Bernard Meyer on Joseph Conrad. Meyer (1967) writes,

> the psychoanalytic biographer can make no claim to 'psychoanalyze' a dead [or living] artist; what he [or she] can aspire to is a painstaking application of psychoanalytic principles and insights to two main sets of data—*the available facts of the artist's life* and *his [or her] creative works*.
>
> (p. 7, emphasis added)

This is what I try to do with my psychoanalytic biography of Ye. I look at everything he produces creatively or artistically, as well as everything he says and does. I read and reread all of that material very closely, which is different from psychoanalyzing and may be described as *psychopoliticizing* (cf. Manganyi, 2016).

Interestingly, both Freud and Meyer also dealt with artists. Therefore, we should consider what psychoanalytic biography reveals and conceals *vis-à-vis* artists and the creative process. Given what Freud said about the method of psychoanalytic biography, we must now turn to the sexual question.

Sexual Non-Rapport

After Ye broke up with Amber Rose, she tweeted in 2016: "Awww @kanyewest are u mad I'm not around to play in ur asshole anymore? #FingersInTheBootyAssBitch" to shame Ye publicly about his anal-driven enjoyment. Ye also briefly dated Julia Fox for a month in 2022. Fox wrote a book, *Down the Drain* (2023), full of her sexual adventures. In the memoir, Fox says that she never slept with Ye, which is intriguing. The couple dated for a whole month, but "there was no such thing as a sexual relationship." However, a retroactive interpretation is apt in this context. In 2014, Ye revealed on social media the structure of his fundamental fantasy. The clue is in the title of a Nazi-themed album that probably will never be released: *CUCKKK*. Unlike incels, Ye is a volcel, a pornosexual gooner. In 2019, Ye said in an interview with Zane Lowe:

> Playboy was my gateway into full blown pornography addiction. My dad had a Playboy left out at age 5, and it's affected almost every choice I made for the rest of my life. From age 5, to now having to kick the habit. And it just presents itself in the open, like it's OK. And I stand up and say, you know, it's not OK.

Ye blames not only his father but also his ex-wife Kim, who was on the cover of *Playboy* in 2007.

Ye also said, "I have addiction to porn and it destroyed my family." Yet, in 2018, Ye designed the awards and the merchandise of the PornHub Awards; this ambivalence points to a symptom that repetitively surfaces in his free associations. It is worth highlighting that Ye specifically blames his father for his porn addiction, which started at age 5 or during the phallic stage of psychosexual development. Ye's beautiful dark, twisted pornographic fantasy signifies phallic *jouissance*, which Lacan (1975/1998) qualified as masturbatory or "the jouissance of the idiot [i.e., The Fool]." The original artwork for his 2010 album, *My Beautiful Dark Twisted Fantasy*, was a painting of him by George Condo, where Ye is lying on his back while having sex with an angel. This art was censored, and retail stores used an alternative cover of a ballerina in a black tutu holding a glass of wine. Some digital stores used a blurred version of the original artwork.

In September of 2023, paparazzi published photos of Ye and Bianca on a boat in Italy during the act of fellatio. Was this intentional or accidental from Ye? Is this the cuck fantasy on full display? It is hard to tell, but we know that in the song "FUK SUMN" from *Vultures*, Ye references this public scandal with pride saying, "Fuck on me, suck on me publicly." He seems to be enjoying the pornographic Gaze of voyeurs (i.e., peeping toms). Ye has also made references to masochistically enjoying being cucked (or cuckolded), which explains Censori's uncensored public appearances. It is worth noting that the submissive, in BDSM dynamics, is typically the one who holds more power in the relationship.

In April of 2024, there were media reports that Ye was planning to launch Yeezy Porn, so Ye went from blaming his father for his porn addiction, which he claims destroyed his family, to embracing porn and linking it to his high fashion Yeezy brand. Recent stories about Ye's addiction to nitrous oxide may be the reason for this 180-degree shift; regardless of the cause, the shift is symptomatic of the logical extremes of manic depression.

The Anti-Semitism of *Vultures*

Moving to the *Vultures* era, it is uncanny to hear the crowd, at Ye's public listening parties, chant the song "Carnival," particularly this specific line: "How I'm anti-Semitic? I just f***ed a Jewish b****." What makes the chanting disturbing is *how* the crowd says this line, cathecting it with excessive libidinal enjoyment.

Following Benjamin (1935/2008), Ye's *aestheticization of politics*—particularly his homage to *Triumph of the Will* (1935) during the New York album listening party—is a fascist sign. Or is it all some elaborate kayfabe *à la* Andy Kaufman v. Jerry Lawler? Inter Milan Ultras recorded the choir for the song "Carnival," and there are parallels between Ultras—extreme football (soccer) fans—and this kind of collective phallic *jouissance*, which disturbingly celebrates misogyny and anti-Semitism. In other words, this excessive cheering on from Ye's ultras has a perverse quality to it, and one can pinpoint that clearly in the lyrics that begin the song, "Go, go, go, go. Head so good, she a honor roll. She'll ride the d*** like a carnival. I done did the impossible."

There are some connections as well between Ultras and fascism, specifically fascist Inter Milan Ultras, who have been documented performing the Nazi salute while carrying a flag of the Celtic Cross—a white nationalist symbol. Furthermore, the aesthetic of the *Vultures* listening party in New York is reminiscent of some of the imagery we see in *Triumph of the Will*. Not to mention that there is a bloodied and screaming skinhead in the music video for "Carnival."

Wilhelm Reich theorized this collective phallic *jouissance* as the anti-sexual attitude of mystical and reactionary individuals (e.g., incels and vocels), who have a sadistic concept of sexual life. Reich (1933/1946) argues in *The Mass Psychology of Fascism*:

> A third source of the antisexual defense forces is the sadistic concept of sexual life which all children acquire at an early age in all patriarchal societies. Since any inhibition of natural genital gratification increases the sadistic impulses, the whole sexual structure becomes sadistic. Since, further, genital impulses become, to a large extent, replaced by anal ones, the sex-reactionary concept of the debasement of woman by sexual intercourse gains further support.
>
> (pp. 143–144)

The impossibility of the sexual—that there is no such thing as a sexual relationship—signifies the fantasy at work in collective phallic *jouissance* and the impotent passions (e.g., love, hate, or ignorance) that the authoritarian subject feels for the barred ~~Other~~. For Ye, love is a function of the mOther's desire—the legacy of unconditional love—and, in a sense, I qualify it as *creative mania*, which is the side that most fans enjoy. Ye ran a striking campaign, advertised on the front pages of the *Los Angeles Times*, the *Chicago Tribune*, the *New York Post*, etc., wherein the phrase "WE LOVE" was repeated in multiple languages. That campaign is a good example of creative mania.

What of Ye's anti-Semitism? He claims it is not hate but jealousy. Lacan, of course, considered jealousy pathological, even when it is based on truth. Aside from being a paranoid delusional symptom, I read Ye's anti-Semitism as projected self-hatred, which results from his internalization of anti-Black racism. After tweeting his anti-Semitic remark on October 8, 2022, Ye defended his position using several tactics.

First, Ye argued that he could not be anti-Semitic because he is Jewish himself. This Black Hebrew Israelite thesis also got Kyrie Irving in trouble after he tweeted about the documentary film *Hebrews to Negroes* (2018). Nietzsche wrote, "the Jews are the most *fateful* nation in world history; their after-effect has falsified mankind to such an extent that today the Christian is able to feel anti-Jewish without realizing he is the *ultimate consequence of the Jews*" (p. 146, emphasis in original). Ye's anti-Semitism echoes Nietzsche's; both take the form of a backhanded compliment. In a 2022 interview with Piers Morgan, Ye said:

> I'm envious of how they don't abort their children … I'm envious of how they don't shoot each other in the streets and then rap about it. I'm envious of how their families stay together. I'm envious that they turn their phones off on Friday nights and the family comes together. I'm envious of how they do business together. And I want that for the darker Jews, I want that for Black people. We need that.

Perhaps as a 2023 Christmas resolution, Ye issued through Instagram an apology, in Hebrew, to the Jewish community, which was translated as follows:

> I sincerely apologise to the Jewish community … It was not my intention to hurt or demean, and I deeply regret any pain I may have caused. I am committed to starting with myself and learning from this experience to ensure greater sensitivity and understanding in the future. Your forgiveness is important to me, and I am committed to making amends and promoting unity.
>
> (as cited in Beaumont-Thomas, 2023)

Furthermore, in November of 2025, Ye met with Rabbi Yoshiyahu Yosef Pinto to publicly repent in person. It is hard to evaluate the sincerity of his act, since he has been flip-flopping for years between anti-Semitic vitriol and apologetic contrition. However, when paparazzi asked Ye about Israel's genocide against the Palestinians in Gaza, he said: "I don't have enough information on that, I'm straight up … I'm from the south side of Chicago, born in Atlanta. I don't have enough information, love for everybody but don't pull me into that conversation … I got people, I've got 14 kids dying every week in my city. So talk to me about that" (February 2024). Meanwhile, Ye's protégé, Kid Cudi, wore a Palestinian Kufiya during a pro-Palestinian march in November 2023. Curiously, on May 13th, 2025, Ye tweeted: "FREE GAZA 🇵🇸". Again, this 180 confirms the minimal consistency of his ambivalence.

Suppose the legacy of unconditional love is the mOther's desire. In that case, the passions of hate and ignorance are a function of the foreclosed Ray-of-the-Father: Leftism and Judeo-Christianity as the impossibility of both absence and *décadence*, respectively. This is the dimension of destructive mania. The impossibility of post-phallic sexuality is also the enclosure of revolutionary politics, and this is why we encounter fascistic symptoms: anti-Semitic paranoid delusions and the aestheticization of politics through the spectacle.

We also witness the eternal return of German Romanticism in Ye's fascist spectacle, which romanticizes premodern nature. In that sense, we can reframe anti-Christ as anti-modern because it is a position invested in fantasizing about a nonexistent premodern time, where the fascist subject was one with nature (i.e., the mOther's breast). In fascist ideology, the fantasmatic figure of the Jew became a symbol of a decadent cultural modernity and was removed from the category of nature, as representative of organic unity. It is not hard to see why Nietzsche was a source of inspiration for Nazis, especially when he writes:

> The Jews are the most remarkable nation of world history because, faced with the question of being or not being, they preferred, with a perfectly uncanny conviction, being *at any price*: the price they had to pay was the radical *falsification* of all nature, all naturalness, all reality, the entire inner world as well as the outer.
>
> (1895/1990, p. 146, emphasis in original)

The first cover art designed for *Vultures*—which was eventually not used—was inspired by German Romantic paintings and the aesthetic of black metal one-man band Burzum. The artist behind Burzum is Varg Vikernes, a convicted murderer who wrote a fascist apologia in 1994 titled *Vargsmål*. The book's cover is the Celtic Cross—a white supremacist symbol. There is a photo of Ye standing next to JPEG Mafia while wearing a Burzum long-sleeve shirt. Not mentioning the controversial photo from 2022 of Ye standing next to Candace Owens, wherein both of them wore "WHITE LIVES MATTER" shirts—another white supremacist dog whistle. To what end? Ye's account got briefly suspended on X (Twitter) in 2022 after he posted an image merging the Star of David with a swastika. Strangely, this image is not original but is the symbol for a UFO religion called Raëlism.

The swastika is, of course, an ancient Hindu symbol for good luck, but it has been associated with evil ever since Nazis have appropriated it. Like punks in the 1970s, Ye has been consistent with appropriating far-right symbols, at least since 2013. Ye wore a Black KKK hood during a Miami album listening party for *Vultures* (December 12, 2023). This repeats his use, ten years earlier, of Black KKK hoods in the music video for "BLKKK SKKKN HEAD." In 2013, Ye also co-opted the Confederate flag during his *Yeezus* era.

The most famous German Romantic artist is Caspar David Friedrich (1774–1840). The image that Ye initially used for the *Vultures* album cover was *Landscape with Graves* (1835–1837). Catherine Hickley (2024) writes: "After the Second World War, [Friedrich's] reputation was tarnished by association with the Nazis—Hitler loved German Romantic painting and Friedrich was one of his favourite artists. Scholars and museums steered clear of Friedrich in the post-war years." To recap, Ye likes Hitler, Burzum, and Friedrich and associates himself with Fuentes, Yiannopoulos, and Owens.

What are we to make of the resurgence of German Romanticism through the visual aesthetics of Burzum and Ye? Bronte Wells (2018) argues:

> Romanticism has been the movement that some historians have cited as a possible root for Nazism. It is not difficult to parse out why. Romanticism includes multiple factors that were certainly part of Nazism: an interest in mysticism

> (specifically German mysticism for German Romantics), 'blood and soil' nationalism, fascination with the Medieval past, and a focus on emotional experience.
>
> (p. 1)

Lars von Trier is another artist who has been indexing German romantic aesthetics recently, particularly in his film *Melancholia* (2011). When asked, at Cannes during a press conference, about his use of Wagner's music and how he drew inspiration from the paintings by German Romantics, von Trier answered: "For a long time I thought I was a Jew and I was happy to be a Jew ... But then I found out I was actually a Nazi. My family were German. And that also gave me some pleasure. What can I say? I understand Hitler ... I sympathize with him a bit." What is it with transgressive artists associating themselves with one of the worst leaders in history?

Ye's farcical turn toward fascist aesthetics since 2022 contradicts his tragic legacy before then. For example, the merchandise for *Donda* (2021) had a Judeo-Christian theme: The Star of David with a cross inside. As such, the album *Donda* marks the end of *The Shaky Ass Years*. The manic-depressive subject is not only divided between ego and unconscious; they are also polarized between depression and mania. The intensification of Ye's psychotic symptoms (e.g., paranoid delusions) correlates to his constant feelings of being abandoned (or 'bullied') by the Left and Judeo-Christians, which triggers the Real traumatic anxiety at the heart of his false being *vis-à-vis* the Ray-of-the-Father, who must remain foreclosed. The sloppy album *Donda 2* indexes this foreclosure and signifies the beginning of the Fascist Era. The difference between *Donda* and *Donda 2* is the difference between mourning and melancholia: first as tragedy, then as farce.

One of the striking images used for the *Vultures* merchandise was the double-headed eagle, which indexes images related to the Holy Roman Empire and the Weimar Republic. The Reichsadler (Imperial Eagle) is a double-headed eagle that was used as the coat of arms of Emperor Otto IV circa 1250. The symbol became popular when adopted by the Holy Roman Empire (800–1806), but it can be traced to the Hittites in Mesopotamia (2nd millennium BCE). It evolved into the Bundesadler (Federal Eagle), which is the coat of arms from the Weimar Republic (1928–1935) and the Federal Republic of Germany (1950–now).

The Reichsadler, however, was abandoned by the Nazis during their rule (1935–1945) and replaced by the Parteiadler (a stylized black eagle above an oak wreath with a swastika at its center). The double-headed eagle symbolized imperial power, representing *spiritual–material power* (the God-Emperor, ruler of the Christian Empire) and *power over East–West* ('barbarism' and 'civilization'). Why is the symbol of the eagle significant for Ye? Perhaps, the answer lies in Freud's psychoanalytic biography of da Vinci.

Leonardo's—and Ye's—Vulture Fantasy: A Case of Passive Homosexuality?

Leonardo's dream-fantasy:

> *It seems that it had been destined before that I should occupy myself so thoroughly with the vulture, for it comes to my mind as a very early memory, when I was still in the cradle, a vulture came down to me, he opened my mouth with his tail and struck me a few times with his tail against my lips.*
>
> (as cited in Freud, 1916, p. 34, emphasis in original)

Freud's interpretation of Leonardo's dream is that it is essentially a fantasy exhibiting infantile sexuality:

> While reading in the writings of a church father or in a book on natural science that the vultures are all females and that they know to procreate without the cooperation of a male, a memory emerged in him [Leonardo] which became transformed into that [vulture] phantasy, but which meant to say that he also had been such a vulture child, which had a mother but no father. An echo of pleasure which he experienced at his mother's breast was added to this in the manner as so old impressions alone can manifest themselves. The allusion to the idea of the holy virgin with the child, formed by the authors, which is so dear to every artist, must have contributed to it to make this phantasy seem to him valuable and important. For this helped him to identify himself with the Christ child [cf. Yeezus], the comforter and savior of not alone this one woman.
>
> (pp. 47–48)

Later, Freud adds, "In all our male homosexuals there was a very intensive erotic attachment to a feminine person, as a rule to the mother, which was manifest in the very first period of childhood and later entirely forgotten by the individual" (pp. 63–64). It is widely believed that the Mona Lisa is Leonardo's face, which points to an ambivalent sexual identification that would confirm Freud's reading. On April 21st, 2025, Ye released a song titled "COUSINS" about his incestuous relationship with his male cousin. To provide context for the song, Ye tweeted the following about his sexual trauma:

> This song is called 'COUSINS' about my cousin that's locked in jail for life for killing a pregnant lady a few years after I told him we wouldn't 'look at dirty magazines together' anymore. Perhaps in my self-centered mess I felt it was my fault that I showed him those dirty magazines when he was six, and then *we acted out what we saw* … My name is Ye and I sucked my cousin's dick till I was 14. (emphasis added)

It is surprising to see Ye use a psychoanalytic concept (acting out), which accurately describes his defensive relationship to the traumatic Real at the heart of his desire; however, the situation is further complexified by his obscene subversions of the taboos against incest and childhood sexual abuse. These perverse transgressions in Ye's early childhood confirm Freud's seduction theory, but they do not signify fetishistic disavowal. Ye's confession involves his acknowledgment of the irreversible effects of childhood sexual trauma on him and his cousin, that is, there is no reversal for the foreclosure of the Law. After all, the *Playboy* magazines that traumatized Ye and his cousin as children, but also caused their desire and drove them to symptomatically act out their pornographic fantasies, belonged to the foreclosed Ray-of-the-Father.

Freud's abandonment of seduction theory and his shift toward an emphasis on psychosexual fantasy affords us an interpretation of Ye's acting out. The traumatic Real is so anxiety-provoking that one way of resolving this anxiety is through a defensive recourse to fantasy, which is then nonverbally *acted out* through repetition compulsion (fellatio) or paranoiac projection (murder), when the fantasy should have been verbally *worked through* in analysis and ultimately *traversed* (cf. Stevens, 2018). Traversal is the opposite of acting out, and it leads to subjective destitution, wherein the subject comes face to face with the traumatic Real, their *manque-à-être*, and chooses the path of enjoying their symptom and owning up to their unconscious desire as a cause, however anxiety-provoking the partial objects of the drives may be.

In ancient Egyptian mythology, the vulture mother-goddess Mut has an erect phallus, which makes Mut nonbinary using today's language. Freud refers to Mut in relation to da Vinci, which suggests that da Vinci and Ye, by extension, might be queer. I would also add that Ye's identification with vultures signifies an anti-Promethean attitude. Ye's rejection of the Promethean ideal of humanism is demonstrable given his belief in far-right conservative ideas. According to ancient Greek mythology, Prometheus was punished by Zeus for stealing fire from the gods and giving it to humans, sparking the creativity that led to the agricultural revolution or civilization. The fire symbolizes knowledge or wisdom, so to be anti-Promethean is to be anti-intellectual or post-truth. Ye baptizes himself in the fire of controversy, which is not the same as the fire of truth.

Vultures = *Donda 3* – Tragic Sublimation?

Ye was working on a video game that revolved around Donda being in heaven, and the purpose of the game was for the player to try to get to heaven to be with Donda. In the images that surfaced online from this unreleased video game, Donda is seen as an angel in the sky with wings, like a vulture. In the music video for the song "24," Ye is seen ascending to the heavens and flying to reach his mother in order to unite with her. I have written in my book on Ye about the symbolism of ascension in its connection with erection.

During the Atlanta listening party for *Donda*, Ye was seen ascending to the top of the stadium, which was a cathartic moment punctuating the show's dramatic climax. A clip of this ascension was used at the beginning of the "24" video. The original title of the album *Donda* was *Donda with Child*, which is provocative considering the rich history of paintings depicting Madonna with Child, including da Vinci's own *Madonna Litta* from 1490. Leonardo's painting is not only sensual but also sexual. It represents the infantile sexual fantasy of oneness with the mOther's breast and the earliest experience of oral (i.e., pre-phallic/pre-Oedipal) *jouissance*.

Freud (1916) writes:

> the phallus which was added to the feminine body was meant to denote the creative primitive force of nature, and that all these hermaphroditic deistic formations express the idea that only a union of the masculine and feminine elements can result in a worthy representation of divine perfection.
>
> (p. 55)

For Freud, Leonardo was a neurotic, especially an obsessional, who sublimated his regressive infantile sexuality of organic unity through his art, particularly the figure of the smiling woman (mOther), and through his "desire for knowledge" (p. 127). Meanwhile, Ye sings, repeating Jay's line from *Dogma* (1999): "Beautiful, naked, big-titty women just don't fall out the sky, you know?" The m(Other) indeed does not fall out of the sky; she is retroactively constituted in fantasy by the subject's desperate wish for a lost totality.

For Freud, the vulture is a phallic symbol, not in the sense of *having* the phallus, but in the sense of the mOther *being the phallus*. In essence, vulturous fantasies are infantile sexual wishes, whose aim is organic unity with the mOther. Freud adds:

> to fly or to be a bird in the dream is only a concealment of another wish, to the recognition of which one can reach by more than one linguistic or objective bridge. When the inquisitive child is told that a big bird like the stork brings the little children, when the ancients have formed the phallus winged, when the popular designation of the sexual activity of man is expressed in German by the word "to bird" (vögeln), when the male member is directly called *l'uccello* (bird) by the Italians, all these facts are only small fragments from a large collection which teaches us that the wish to be able to fly signifies in the dream nothing more or less than the longing for the ability of sexual accomplishment. This is an early infantile wish.
>
> (pp. 107–108, emphasis in original)

In sum, Ye's divided subjectivity—characterized by the extremes of manic depression and the psychotic weight of paranoid delusion—is a holographic microcosm of a crumbling empire, polarized by the colonial afterlives of racial capitalism. The effect of this societal polarization is political alienation, wherein one side frames itself as 'good' vs. the 'evil' Other.

Since 2022, Ye seems to have been flirting with the 'evil' side through his embrace of the fascist spectacle and his utterance of anti-Semitic paranoid delusional statements. Before 2022, but especially before 2016, Ye occupied a third position beyond 'good' and 'evil' embodied in his radical aesthetic of tragic sublimation. Anti-Christ, then is a farcical—reactionary and regressive—repetition of the radical tragedy of Christ. The Leftism of Christ is grounded in the redemption of the Other (the community); as such, it is the radical or creative dimension of the manic unconscious *qua* social link: the commons. Anti-Christ, however, is a pure death-driven egoic identification, for they seek to redeem only themselves, which is the narcissistic and aggressive essence of fascism as false being.

Chapter 13

Anora: Or the Impossibility of Love within Capitalism

Sean Baker's (2024) *Anora* received the highest form of recognition that a filmmaker can dream of: critical acclaim and commercial success. On Rotten Tomatoes, the film is both "certified fresh" with a 97% score from critics and "verified hot" with an 87% score from spectators. Similarly, on Metacritic, critics gave the film a 91% rating; this "universal acclaim" is significantly higher than the "generally favorable" score of 6.4 the film garnered from users. Also, on IMDB, the film scored a rating of 7.5, which is as high as Stanley Kubrick's (1999) *Eyes Wide Shut*, for example.

In the festival circuit, *Anora* secured 265 nominations and won 149 awards, including five Oscars (Best Picture, Best Director, Best Actress, Best Actor in a Supporting Role, and Best Original Screenplay), not to mention the prestigious Palme d'Or at the Cannes Film Festival. In terms of commercial success, the film made more than $56 million at the box office against a $6 million budget. Despite my own lack of affinity for *Anora*, or perhaps because I suspect it is overrated, my critique acknowledges the film as a masterpiece. Its structural significance persists quite apart from the vagaries of personal opinion.

For Todd McGowan (2007), an enjoyable masterpiece, from a Lacanian perspective, *intersects* the worlds of desire and fantasy within the formal structure of the film, leaving open a gap for the spectator's subjectivity to insert itself. On the other hand, mediocre films *integrate* desire and fantasy. In ideological cinema, fantasy resolves desire by taming the traumatic Real. Domesticating lack can often manifest as death-driven excess. Even though spectators are singular beings/divided subjects with different experiences and diverse interpretations *vis-à-vis* a given film, there is an objective dimension to cinematic enjoyment, which is a function of Lacan's infamous *objet a*. The *objet a* is that elusive object-cause of desire, that Thing (*je ne sais quoi*) that caused Baker's desire to make *Anora* in the first place.

The relationship between a creator and their creation mirrors the fantasmatic relationship (◊) between the subject ($) and the object (*a*), hence, the Lacanian formula for fantasy: $ ◊ *a*. The *objet a* is not an empirical object that we can acquire like the latest iPhone. Rather, the *objet a* drives us to keep on desiring while enjoying in the process our *manque-à-être*, with the caveat that *jouissance* is beyond the pleasure principle because it includes pain, too. As such, the purpose of this chapter

DOI: 10.4324/9781003768104-13

is to critique *Anora* and reveal why the film is objectively enjoyable (i.e., a masterpiece) from a Lacanian psychoanalytic and analectical materialist perspective.

The film's protagonist (Ani) is a hysterical subject in the most radical or revolutionary sense of the word; she represents the dignity of the proletariat, and her position is critical of bourgeois master-signifiers, once she can see through their parasitic role within capitalist ideology. Her name is homonym for *any*, for she represents anyone—the 'everyman' archetype in literature. Furthermore, I would argue that Igor is in the position of the analyst, for he hystericizes Ani to defy the master-signifiers associated with Russian oligarchy, since they are as empty as Orthodox Church theology. Igor is, of course, a reference to the hunchbacked lab assistant of Gothic lore; the analogy here positions parasitic capitalism as a Frankensteinian project—an attempt by Euromodernity to animate the dead labor of capital into a monstrous, autonomous Totality.

As a lackey of capital, the Orthodox Church functions as a University discourse in a position of service *vis-à-vis* oligarchical mastery. In this schema, theology provides the rational justification for the whims of mastery. According to Lacan (2007), psychoanalysis sits on the other side of mastery; it is positioned on the side of socialist liberation. Similarly, revolution—as the manifestation of hysterical (critical) knowledge—stands on the other side of the university's systemic theology; it is the side of decolonial secularization. Consequently, *Anora* enacts a revolutionary, analectical materialist praxis grounded in a psychoanalytic critique of ideology.

First, *Anora* is a comedy. In Shakespearean terms, a drama has a tragic ending—the protagonist's death—but a comedy typically has a happy ending, which often suggests sexual rapport. *Anora* has a happy ending in a literal sense (Ani copulates with Igor), but metaphorically, there is a topological twist to this 'happy' ending stemming from the Lacanian axiom that "there's no such thing as a sexual relationship (*il n'y a pas de rapport sexuel*)" (Lacan, 1998, p. 5).

How can we explain this sexual non-rapport when the film's protagonist is a "sex worker" in a plot replete with raunchy scenes? Lacan (1998) reminds us that even though "love is impossible and the sexual relationship drops into the abyss of nonsense" (p. 87), we should still not give up on the Other—that enigmatic representative of the Symbolic order. Why? Even though the Other (Ⱥ) is also castrated like the subject ($) by the limits of language ($-\varphi$), we imagine them to possess the unspeakable and unwritable *je ne sais quoi*: the *objet a*. This analectical materialist fiction is the necessary foundation for the psychosocial tie symptomatically knotting together any collective around a particular form of enjoyment—after all, as Lacan (1966–1967) reminds us, "*the unconscious is politics!*" (p. 205, emphasis in original).

Furthermore, the paradoxical twist regarding *the impossibility of love* and *the nonsense of sexuality* has something to do with the fact that "~~Woman~~ does not exist (*~~La femme~~ n'exist pas*)" (cf. Zupančič, 2017), except as an object of fantasy within the phallogocapitalist order (see Figure 13.1). In other words, I read Lacan, as a Marxist feminist, who is arguing against the status of ~~Woman~~ as a second-class

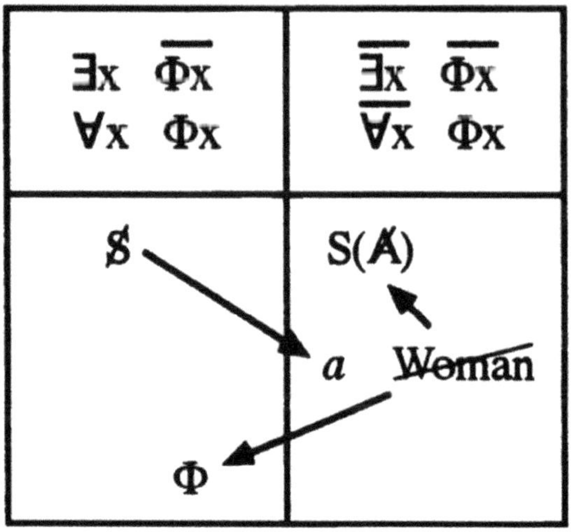

Figure 13.1 Formulae of sexuation

citizen. The film, of course, indexes a trope, which goes back to ancient times: the "hooker with a heart of gold."

To put it concretely, ~~Anora~~ (*a*) does not exist, but Ani ($) exists. Ani is not a "sex worker"; she is a sex laborer. This is an important distinction following Hannah Arendt (2019) in *The Human Condition*. Ani sells sex labor to survive life in the core of a crumbling empire—New York City, the home of Wall Street. This is the ground-zero of racial capitalism, where the modern subject is reduced to a calculable unit within the apparatus of global finance. To survive, Ani has to embody *being the phallus* in the fantasmatic form of ~~Anora~~, a commodified object of male fantasy. In the course of the film, she is positioned specifically as the object of Ivan's fantasy, the spoiled son of Russian oligarchs. Ivan is 'terrible,' being the embodiment of the American idiom 'loser,' for he spends all of his time playing video games, getting drunk and high, and having nonsensical 'sex,' if it can even be called that since Lacan (1998) characterizes *phallic or masculine jouissance* as masturbatory or "the jouissance of the idiot" (p. 81). The idiot (*idiōtēs*), of course, is Thatcher's *individual* with Odysseus being a prototype. Given Ivan's lack of unconscious thinking—a radical solipsism—he is alienated from the Other's meaning, resulting in a fundamentally false being. He exists as the ideal bourgeois consumer, a (post) modern subject for whom the alterity of the Other has been entirely disavowed in favor of a flat, individualistic Totality.

Ivan essentially uses ~~Anora's~~ body as a fetish commodity, from which he can extract surplus-*jouissance*, to facilitate his idiotic masturbation and premature ejaculation. Why is he able to do this? Because Ivan *has the phallus*, through his access to capital (a large villa, a private plane, etc.), which as it turns out is a *pseudo-phallus*, since his access to his family's wealth is contingent on the approval of his parents. Ivan's parents cannot sanction his marriage to Ani because her social being as a sex laborer is a site of negated Exteriority within their "surplus-value" system—a master morality that defines their bourgeois criminal life. Meanwhile, Ani always looks bored and dissatisfied when she is having 'sex' with Ivan, which points to the possibility of *Other or feminine jouissance* beyond the phallogocapitalist order.

Ani is a member of the working class, and her *jouissance* is a function of both her creative work and political action. Her skills as a stripper, for example, constitute creative work, and her ways of resisting the oppressive bourgeois order of neofeudalism amount to political action. Ani is a (lumpen)proletarian subject, who wishes to be free from exploitation, but, as a divided subject, she falls for the ideological fantasy of marrying a wealthy young man, as a way out of exploitation. This fantasy sutures the traumatic Real of class struggle, which is the driving force behind the politico-libidinal economy of sexuation throughout the film and beyond.

Ivan's exploitation of Ani was doubly so because not only did he fantasize about having sex with ~~Anora~~, but he also wanted to act out against his parents by marrying Ani. The marriage, of course, took place in the perfect *simulacrum of a city*: Las Vegas, the city of sin. As such, their marriage was a *simulation of love*. How can the impossible be simulated? Only within the realm of hyper-reality, Jean Baudrillard's (1994) term for an Imaginary order without origin or reality.

The impossibility of love is a function of its non-capitalist reliance on *a discourse that might not be a semblance* the way Valentine's Day, for example, is commodified globally as a day on which copious amounts of chocolates and flowers are sold and consumed as signifiers of romance. The condition for love is an Other language composed of decommodified signifying chains and a non-capitalist Symbolic order. This Other order—the revolutionary alternative to the university's scholastic theology—is doomed to an almost Beckettian infinite failure; it is a praxis that must fail again, but fail better each successive time. In the face of a crumbling empire that reduces life to surplus-value, this persistence is the only true success. It is the refusal to recoil into either instrumental reason or irrationalism, opting instead for a fail better analectic that slowly erodes the colonial—and anti-modern—foundation of Totality.

Lacan (1998) qualifies this Other dimension of surplus-*jouissance* beyond the phallus (Φ) as *pas-tout* or not-all, for love is beyond both the logic and the rhetoric of phallogocapitalism. According to Chela Sandoval (2000), revolutionary love is beyond ideology (p. 141) because it has the radical potential of being a "hermeneutics of social change" (p. 139). The agent of this revolutionary love is what Sandoval terms "differential consciousness," or the subject-as-Real in Lacanese, which she defines as:

> linked to whatever is not expressible through words. It is accessed through poetic modes of expression: gestures, music, images, sounds, words that plummet or rise through signification to find some void—some no-place—to claim their due. This mode of consciousness both inspires and depends on differential

> social movement and the methodology of the oppressed and its differential technologies, yet it functions outside speech, outside academic criticism, in spite of all attempts to pursue and identify its place and origin.
>
> (p. 140)

For Sandoval, differential consciousness is one of the five modes of oppositional consciousness—the other four include equal rights, revolutionary, supremacist, and separatist. Also, differential consciousness is one of the five skills comprising the border methodology of the oppressed, as a methodology of emancipation—the other four skills being semiotics, deconstruction, meta-ideologizing, and democratics (p. 2). Sandoval's use of critical theory aligns with my Freudo–Lacanian approach of mathematizing or formalizing liberation psychoanalysis throughout this book. According to Althusser (1970), "Philosophy represents the class struggle in theory." I would extend that statement and argue that *psychoanalysis represents oppression in theory*. In other words, there is no practice of liberation without the meta-theorization of oppression. And since oppression is the absence of love, we must return to the psychoanalytic theorization of love, given its revolutionary potential as a decolonial force that can smash ideology.

Lacan (2015) defines love as "giving what you don't have" (p. 34). Ivan has everything, but he gave Ani nothing. On the other hand, Igor has nothing but has given Ani everything, in the form of *a four-carat diamond ring*, which he stole as a sign of class solidarity. As (lumpen)proletarian subjects in the core of a crumbling empire, Ani and Igor are *less than nothing*—not merely lackeys of capital, but the structural lack that haunts the very Totality they inhabit. Igor's gift is more than a Robin Hood feat; it also symbolizes, in a very touching way, his marriage proposal to Ani—a sign of his impossible desire in contrast to Ivan's impotent fantasy. The double meaning of the ring is a sign of its *non-meaning*, for it occupies a position between the (lumpen)proletarian subject's *being* and the bourgeois Other's *meaning*.

Whereas the (lumpen)proletarian subject's being is structured by their unconscious thinking around liberation from exploitation, the bourgeois Other's meaning is the logic of capital itself. Non-meaning signifies the impossible gap between the (lumpen)proletarian subject and the bourgeois Other, a gap that is often sutured by ideological fantasy (e.g., sex, money, etc.), but non-meaning can also manifest as the revolutionary discourse of love.

This is what is radical about *Anora*: the film exposes the nihilistic decadence of the bourgeois family along with the subservience of the church to capital, for Toros (Ivan's godfather and the family 'fixer') is an Armenian Orthodox priest. *Anora* thus presents a revolutionary model of love grounded in solidarity and comradeship—a bond forged in the wake of the collapse of paternal authority and the decline of Symbolic efficiency. It is significant that Ani, for example, is an orphan living with her sister, while Igor is cohabiting with his grandmother. The film stages the postmodern turn of global "parasitic capitalism" (Wahba, 2022), wherein we witness the rise of financialization without production; this is the world of crime as the ontological ground of Totality. Within this politico-economic void of meaning, love ceases to be a bourgeois contract and becomes a radical, analectical materialist intervention at the level of the libidinal economy.

Anora's three-act structure can be read as follows: (Act I) *fantasmatic hyper-reality* as the Imaginary dimension of capitalist ideology, wherein oppression in the form of exploitation gives rise to the worker's need for disalienation; (Act II) *discursive reality* as the Symbolic dimension of capitalist ideology, wherein a meaningless marriage contract (*qua* fascist class collaboration) becomes a violent demand for annulment; and (Act III) *the traumatic Real* as the dimension of analectical materialism (i.e., the class struggle and the non-rapport of the sexual).

The class struggle thesis is complicated by the figure of Igor; as a lumpenproletarian henchman for a crime 'family,' his subjectivity is mutilated by his proximity to mastery. The sexual non-rapport between him and Ani is punctuated by her identification of his predatory desire—the "rape eyes" that signal a fantasy of total domination. This tension is grounded in the physical trauma of the second act, where Igor's forceful restraint of Ani is experienced not as family 'business,' but as assault and kidnapping. Through the Gaze, the film produces a profound spectator anxiety, stripping us of our neutral distance and forcing an anamorphic encounter with our subjective complicity in sexist oppression. The spectator is revealed as neither passive nor innocent; rather, their very enjoyment from a distance functions as the libidinal fuel that sustains a world of sex trafficking, exploitation, and abuse.

Act I was edited like an infinite scroll or endless feed social media experience, designed for spectators with a short attention span. The editing is dizzying, like riding a fast carousel, but we align our desire with Ani's and experience a dopamine rush, a virtual high followed immediately by an actual crash in Act II. The first act is too entertaining, which speaks of an excessive enjoyment beyond the pleasure principle that overcompensates for the lack or negativity at the navel of the film. The source of this negativity is *lovelessness*, which translates as a desire for solidarity and comradeship. Lack of love is substituted by an excess of sex drive, which, while fantasmatic, points toward a desire for liberation. However, the creative sex drive contains within itself its destruction in the form of the death drive: the other side of the unconscious coin.

The death drive is *ego-driven enjoyment for enjoyment's sake*, which is epitomized in the liberal figure of the hyper-individual consumer, who is amused to death. Ivan is the perfect example of this liberal figure, as a spoiled rich kid, but he is only a symptom of the meaningless egoic, or death-driven, activity of infinite capital accumulation. As such, sexual excess hides the fact that (post)modern capitalism is boring us to death. It is no coincidence, then, that Ivan looks like a vampire, for he is a psychic vampire sucking whatever vital enjoyment he can from the body of ~~Anora~~ and the mind of Ani. He not only wanted to have 'sex' with ~~Anora~~, but he also wanted Ani to think that he loved her.

In the second act, the violence of the Law, which brings to mind Benjamin's (1921/1996) critique of violence, is in full force both in the forms of the legal Other and the criminal Other. The judicial system is in cahoots with the world of organized crime because both are committed to the same Symbolic order, and together they constitute the phallogocapitalist Other, who serves the absolute master: money (*a*) *qua* death (Ⱥ)—cf. the *vel* of alienation: "a choice whose properties depend on this, that there is, in the joining [between the subject's Being and the Other's Meaning], one element [non-meaning] that, whatever the choice operating may be, has as its consequence a *neither one, nor the other*" (Lacan, 1977/2004, p. 211, emphasis in original).

Alienation is always an either/or operation, which, in the case of Ani, is the illusion of choice between *being* a commodity or having a fantasmatic *meaning*, two versions of ~~Anora~~. To be a sex laborer is to be a commodity fetish, and getting married to the son of oligarchs is to be reduced to the bourgeois Other's meaning (i.e., the proletariat as a fantasmatic source of extractable vital energy).

The psychoanalytic and analectical materialist solution to this alienation is to separate from this capitalist ideology by embracing *non-meaning*, wherein Ani is neither a commodity nor a fantasy. The traversal of fantasy goes one step further by sublating being and meaning, so Ani can get to enjoy ~~Anora~~ as her divine symptom beyond the mythic *jouissance* afforded within phallogocapitalism. Following Riane Eisler (2011) in *The Chalice and the Blade*, divine *jouissance* would not be possible within *the dominator model* because of how society is organized around oppressive and violent hierarchies. Divine *jouissance*, which is a function of the divine feminine principle, can only flourish within *the partnership model*, wherein society would self-organize like a complex system to promote equality and cooperation.

As such, Lacan (1998) translates sexuation as sexual non-rapport, which, in my view, accounts for the oppressive and violent reality of sexist exploitation and the Real of class struggle in Totality. Also, for Lacan (2006), there is no Other of the Other because there is no metalanguage. However, one must surely dream of a metapolitics—the Other of the Other—situated beyond the reach of phallogocapitalism: a post-phallic (humanist) recovery of subjectivity and a post-capitalist (socialist) reorganization of the social. This is the task of historical reason toward the horizon of transmodernity: the birth of a radical humanity from the wreckage of Totality—an extimate rebirth where the less than nothing finally becomes the ground for a new social becoming.

In response to Igor's gift, Ani decides to have sex with him in his grandmother's car. However, when he tries to kiss her, she begins to break down and cry. On one level, Ani was touched by Igor's gift and decided to reciprocate with sex according to the system of gift economy. However, when Igor attempts to kiss her, which signifies his impossible desire for her love, Ani was faced with the rupture between sex labor (~~Anora~~ as a commodity) and love action (class solidarity).

As a sex laborer, her ego is identified with her body as a fetishized commodity; however, there is no way of infinitely exploiting her unconscious. There are ways of putting it under the ideological spell of phallogocapitalist fantasy, but false consciousness cannot last because the traumatic Real is always bursting at the seams, awakening us to our critical (un)consciousness. Therefore, the analectical materialist and Lacanian psychoanalytic lesson of the film is that sex may be a necessary fantasy, but love—as an impossible discursive contingency—has the potential to be revolutionary, particularly as a traumatic quilting point of lack, which can give rise to praxis.

To put it differently, Ani's and Igor's lack of freedom as (lumpen)proletarian subjects in solidarity can drive them to actualize their collective liberation. The only aporia is that there are no means of production to be seized, for production has been outsourced to the Global South, which explains the parasitic status of (post)modern capitalism, wherein extreme wealth is being generated through abstract financialization. Not to mention the concrete machinations of money laundering through fungible businesses like strip clubs that produce nothing but meaningless entertainment (i.e., sex, drugs, and alcohol). As such, the surplus-*jouissance* of lack or not-all (*pas-tout*)—i.e., love action *qua* class solidarity or comradeship—signifies a divine form of enjoyment beyond the myth of phallogocapitalism. In sum, divine *jouissance* prefigures a libertarian socialist world to come, which does not stigmatize the lumpenproletariat, but rather includes them as potential comrades in solidarity.

Chapter 14

Three Clarifications

This chapter is my response to Daniel José Gaztambide's (2023) review of *Freud and Said* (2021a), which is a sequel to *Decolonial Psychoanalysis* (2019a). *Liberation Psychoanalysis* is the third installment, which will bring the trilogy to an end, so I thought it would be fitting to address the critical parts of Gaztambide's review and clarify some of my arguments in the first two books. To begin with, Gaztambide is a scholar whose work I admire, and overall, I found his review to be the sort of constructive criticism that is worth responding to. Gaztambide (2023) writes:

> While in general there is much to be lauded in Beshara's work here, there are three points of critique I would raise with respect to some specific assertions that seem to undercut the solidaristic perspective to which his contrapuntal psychoanalytic approach points. To be clear, these are points for further dialogue rather than condemnation.
>
> (p. 106)

Gaztambide (2023) argues that I make three assertions, which "create a number of methodological problems" (p. 106): (1) A shift in the argument on who is "most oppressed," from women to "the racialized, or politicized, male;" (2) the argument that the unconscious may be "*ipso facto* racist" based on the metaphor of "black = evil or sin," which could create new dialogues between psychoanalysis and Afropessimism; and (3) a tension between the stated critique of racial capitalism and a seeming return to cultural resistance, as the primary site of critique. In my view, points 1 and 3 are misreadings of my work, and point 2 is a disagreement. What follows is my response to Gaztambide's criticisms.

1

Patriarchy is the oppression of Women in particular and racialized folk in general within the apparatus of racial capitalism. My understanding of racialization is primarily historical but also psychosocial. Racialization is the (mis)perception of 'race,' which is often loaded with racist associations that are tethered to racial categories. In my view, there is a colonial logical sequence: civilization → slavery →

DOI: 10.4324/9781003768104-14

racism → racialization → 'race' (Beshara, 2022). This sequence identifies civilization as a foundational and problematic concept that provides the ideological basis for a global hierarchy. It then distinguishes between racialization (the process of creating racial meaning) and 'race' (the product of that process, for 'race' is not a pre-existing fact, but rather a social construction). Furthermore, the sequence positions racism not as a root cause but as the logical and systematic outcome of the previous stages. As such, my framework challenges essentialist views that understand 'race' as a biological reality and racism as simply a matter of individual prejudice, and presents them instead as a complex, historically contingent, and deeply interconnected system of ideas and practices that have shaped the modern world.

Feminism, the critique of sexist oppression, is part of an antiracist (humanist) and anticapitalist (socialist) liberation praxis led by racialized folk (~~Women~~ and ~~Men~~) as well as Women. Patriarchy is not only sexist, but also racist and exploitative. Why? Because it is what hierarchy looks like within the apparatus of racial capitalism. The patriarchs are the colonizers who became the capitalist class within the Totality of the Euromodern world-system.

Gaztambide (2023) thinks I am "stuck reversing terms" when I was specifically critiquing what Serene Khader calls "missionary feminism" (2019) or "faux feminism" (2024), from an anti-imperialist or decolonial perspective (cf. Mohanty, 2003). This "imperial feminism," as Alcoff (2020) calls it, following Lugones, is represented by what I term Woman, and it is a university discourse, according to Lacanian discourse theory. For Lacan (2007), the university always produces knowledge (S_2), which is subservient to the master (i.e., the capitalist class of Euro-American patriarchs), whom I designate as Man. Wynter (2003) calls this figure of liberal humanism Man_1, and I conceptualize him as a master-signifier or S_1. Subsequently, I position missionary or faux feminism as S_2, for it is a form of 'critical' knowledge that does not go far enough in its critique of mastery, thereby, obscures the libidinal investment of patriarchy in maintaining the status quo with its mythic enjoyment of violence and oppression. After 9/11, Lila Abu-Lughod (2002) famously asked, "Do Muslim Women Really Need Saving? The answer is, of course, an emphatic: no! Muslim women can save themselves, and they certainly do not need the help of imperial feminists.

Framing imperial feminism as a university discourse explains, for instance, the pseudo-feminism of the U.S. suffragette movement, which campaigned for white Women's right to vote while maintaining racism as a colonial structure of subjugation (Brown, 2018). I am for a decolonial feminism that hystericizes imperial feminism from the perspective of ~~Women~~ ($). Patriarchy is unethical because it is dehumanizing, and by being dehumanizing, it is self-destructive—an autoimmune response. Patriarchy dehumanizes not only the Other (Woman) but also the Other of the Other (~~Woman~~ and ~~Man~~). It renders this Other of the Other, particularly ~~Man~~, objectal (*a*), and by doing so, patriarchy also dehumanizes the patriarchal self and the feminist Other.

Lacan (1998) treats sexual difference as an ahistorical or ontological (i.e., universal) feature of the modern subject's experience with sexual enjoyment, wherein they are alienated between masculine *jouissance* and feminine *jouissance*. In my work, I show that coloniality is an unconscious fundamental fantasy sustaining the discourse of Euromodernity. As such, I historicize sexual difference by grounding it in the materiality of colonial difference. This then explains the power asymmetry between Man and Woman, which stems from another power asymmetry between colonizer/capitalist (Man and Woman) and colonized/exploited (~~Woman~~ and ~~Man~~).

In patriarchy, Woman is considered less than Man, not because she is less, but because she possesses a feminine or Other form of enjoyment that Man has no access to, which is a case of womb envy (cf. Horney, 1926). Similarly, non-Europeans are perceived to possess 'barbaric' forms of enjoyment that 'civilized' Europeans have no access to and therefore desire. This is how the racism of ideological whiteness structures desire under patriarchy.

In *Freud and Said*, I situate sexual difference within what I term mythic *jouissance* as the enjoyment of oppression and violence. In contrast, I see divine *jouissance* as the enjoyment of liberation and (non)violence. Divine *jouissance* is the basis for the liberation praxis that would drive the oppressed to desire and enjoy the commons. By the oppressed, I mean *comrades in solidarity*, regardless of their identity as subjects. And this is what I mean by *non-identity politics*.

Within the apparatus of racial capitalism, the racialized male (Man-Not) is a Thing or commodity that is doubly negated: they are neither Woman nor Man. They do not have the privileges of a patriarchal subject because they were historically situated outside the category of gender altogether and in the Exteriority of *genre*. This is Curry's (2017) main thesis about the misandric aggression against the Man-Not within a white supremacist patriarchy; this misandry is not only racist, but also has a sexual dimension, which he explains as the racial-sexual violence of *phallicism* (Curry, 2018).

The Man-Not is a fantasmatic *objet a* of white supremacist ideology, who is considered both a "super-predator" or "Black Buck" and an effeminate, castrated, fungible, and disposable Thing or commodity. The Man-Not is so dehumanized that they are either over-exploited to death or outright exterminated. Therefore, *Freud and Said* is not a masculinist or ideological argument for racialized men's rights, as Gaztambide is (mis)reading me. Rather, the book presents a historical argument about how the Man-Not was excluded from not only patriarchy but also masculinity. Consequently, Curry's (2017) effort is to reconstruct an empirically sound theoretical model of Black manhood, which corresponds with the historical and ongoing experiences of Black men and boys with vulnerability and suffering.

Why is the racialized male (Man-Not) at the bottom of a white supremacist and racial capitalist patriarchy? Because of their hypothetical potential as patriarchs, a function of their phallicism, wherein they are so dehumanized that they are often reduced to the biological level of their phallus (Curry, 2018). However, *subordinate group males* can never fully realize their potential as patriarchs because they are often viewed as a threat to the power and status of dominant group members. Curry (2017) shows this socio-historical fact following social dominance theory

(Sidanius & Pratto, 1999), which explains the violence against Black men and boys under Jim Crow and beyond in terms of *arbitrary set discrimination* and *the subordinate male target hypothesis*.

This research extends Curry's Black Male Studies by integrating a decolonial psychoanalytic lens to examine arbitrary-set discrimination within non-white group-based hierarchies. While traditional intersectionality often treats maleness as a monolith of privilege, this framework identifies the politicized male—specifically Kurds, Bosniaks, and the Rohingya—as the primary site of state-sponsored ontological insecurity. This is not merely generic violence; it is a surgical androcidal logic that targets the Man-Not's phallic potential to ensure the total disintegration of the subordinate group's Symbolic identity.

By analyzing the libidinal economy of the dominant group, we can observe how subordinate-group males are psychologized as inherent threats to the sovereign order. This threat status triggers a specific logic of androcide, where rape and extermination are utilized not as collateral damage, but as targeted mechanisms to break the collective agency of the subordinate group. This theorization provides a necessary global bridge between the African American experience and the broader reality of male-targeted violence in genocidal and sectarian contexts.

Curry's project is an empirical one, which relies on intellectual history, particularly 19th and 20th century ethnology, as well as more recent empirical data about intimate partner violence (IPV). The assumption that males are always perpetrators and females are always victims is not only false but also dehumanizing. This assumption is a function of a faux feminist ideology—a university discourse that produces knowledge subservient to the master-signifier of Man—and essentially works to deter solidarity among racialized folk, who would benefit from living in a non-hierarchical world. While imperial feminism often ignores the vulnerability of the racialized male, the CDC data shows that one in four U.S. men (26.3%) experienced IPV and reported a related impact, such as being fearful (8.1%), concerned for safety (7.1%), or experiencing PTSD symptoms (14.5%). For the Man-Not, these impacts are exacerbated by a state-sponsored androcidal logic that renders their suffering invisible.

Research from the CDC, specifically the 2016/2017 NISVS report, shows that IPV is common among both women and men in the United States. Nearly one in two women and men (49.4% of women and 45.1% of men) reported experiencing psychological aggression by an intimate partner in their lifetime. Furthermore, more than two in five adult women (42.0%) and men (42.3%) reported experiencing physical violence by an intimate partner. These near-equivalent rates of physical violence victimization challenge the monolithic perpetrator–victim binary and support a reading of IPV that must account for the specific material and historical conditions of the colonized.

The CDC findings highlight that racial and ethnic minority groups are disproportionately affected by IPV. More than half of all non-Hispanic Black women (53.6%) and non-Hispanic Black men (57.6%) reported experiencing contact sexual violence, physical violence, and/or stalking by an intimate partner in their lifetimes. In my framework, this horizontal violence is not merely toxic masculinity/femininity, but a function of colonial difference, where racialized folk are forced to negotiate their shared ontological insecurity.

Furthermore, the concept of *horizontal semiosis* (Beshara, 2021a, p. 191), which I have previously explored, offers a crucial missing link in the analysis of sub-oppression. When I write about horizontal semiosis as a solution to hierarchical oppression, I place ~~Woman~~ ($) as a co-leader alongside ~~Man~~ (*a*) of this decolonizing and liberatory effort. Therefore, there is no ground for painting my argument as anti-feminist or pro-masculinist. It is much more nuanced than that.

2

Gaztambide (2023) accuses me of equating "the racialized *structural* position of the Black subject with that of the 'Brown' Arab/Middle Eastern, Amerindian, Latinx, etc. subject" (p. 106, emphasis in original). This cannot be further from the truth. I often write the phrase "Indigenous, Black, and Brown" when referring to racialized folk to acknowledge the colonial history of genocide, enslavement, and racism in that order. These signifiers point to different legacies of historical trauma (cf. Brave Heart, Chase, Elkns, &, Altschul, 2011), which overlap in some ways but are quite distinct in other ways.

My model is not a flat binary of Black vs. white or male vs. female; instead, I conceptualize the apparatus of racial capitalism through the intermediary category of *ad limen hominis* (at the threshold of the human). This liminal space allows us to account for the complex and often contradictory positions of *the white lumpenproletariat* and *the non-white lumpenbourgeoisie*. While the former may possess racial proximity to Man without the corresponding class power, the latter—the non-white lumpenbourgeoisie—possesses class power while remaining ontologically precarious. Their inclusion into the category of the human is a dialectical and material product of history that can be revoked by the Totality whenever their utility to racial capitalism expires. This framework provides a global bridge for analyzing how power asymmetries shift across different genocidal and sectarian contexts, proving that humanity is not a fixed status but a border that is constantly policed.

Furthermore, I engage with the rich field of Black Studies, particularly the works of W. E. B. Du Bois, Angela Davis, Frantz Fanon, Sylvia Wynter, Tommy Curry, and Lewis Gordon, among others; however, Gaztambide expects me to also be in dialogue with Afropessimism, a field of study I disagree with for theoretical and political reasons, yet I have nothing but admiration for Marriott's (2021) ambitious marriage between Lacanian psychoanalysis and Afropessmism. While I admire the ambition of Marriott's work, I must distinguish my historical-materialist position from the ontological social death argument of Afropessimism. No one group has a monopoly over the zone of nonbeing; rather, this zone is produced by worldly, historical, and necropolitical conditions. Unlike race essentialism, which views anti-Blackness as an unchanging feature of the world, I see Blackness as an antiracist praxis—a material critique of the color line designed to divide the working class.

My goal is not to ontologize suffering, but to historicize it so that it may be overcome through radical humanism.

According to Frank B. Wilderson III (2020), "Blackness is coterminous with Slaveness: Blackness is social death: which is to say that there was never a prior metamoment of plenitude, never equilibrium: never a moment of social life" (p. 102). I do not see (anti)Blackness as an inherent and unchanging aspect of the world, but I am also not a race essentialist. I find the concept of 'race' to be problematic, and I regard it as one of the reasons why racism continues to exist in the first place.

Afropessimism makes an abstract ontological and ahistorical argument about (anti)Blackness, which has been refuted concretely through the historical and dialectical materialist lens of scientific socialism (Brown & Ford, 2021; Fermin, 2023; Sanchez, 2022). Zahi Zalloua's (2024) critique of Afropessimism is worth quoting in full in this context since it captures my position as well:

> If the notions of the zone of nonbeing and the proletarian position name a certain modality of ontological fraughtness, the Afropessimists *ontologize* this condition as an inescapable anti-Blackness ... Yes, the Black is in a zone of nonbeing, but so are the Jew and the Palestinian. No one has a monopoly over the zone of nonbeing. One's thrownness into the zone of nonbeing is not a divine punishment; it is not God, but a symbolic order that unjustly condemns you. *The source of disenfranchisement is worldly, historical, taking place under varying necropolitical conditions that rip at the individual's being.*
>
> (p. 16, emphasis added)

Whereas whiteness is an ideology that was invented by bourgeois Euro-Americans to divide and conquer a diverse working class along the color line, Blackness is a critique of this racist ideology. Therefore, I see Blackness as an antiracist praxis whose end goal is radical humanism. This much is clear from Martin Luther King Jr.'s "I Have a Dream" speech, for example, or even from Fanon's (1961/2004) call for a new humanism in *The Wretched of the Earth.*

My view on racism is informed by historical and dialectical materialism. Racism, like class struggle or sexist oppression, is a material phenomenon—not an abstract ontological category—that must be historicized. Racism is also dialectical; it is not unchanging. It is a human invention that mutates over time.

In his work, for instance, Gaztambide (2019) draws an insightful connection between anti-Semitism and anti-Blackness to explain the dehumanizing logic of racism, which impacted a Jewish subject like Freud. This juxtaposition does not collapse the many differences in the experiences of Jewish and Black subjects with anti-Semitism and anti-Blackness, respectively. The juxtaposition, however, does point to the category of (non)Europeanness that Said (2003) referred to when addressing Freud, and it is this *non* (or negation), which intrigues me since it is *vis-à-vis* Europe and the European.

Similarly, in *Decolonial Psychoanalysis* (2019a), I show an interesting paradox regarding the Islamophobia fantasy, which predates the discourse of Islamophobia by centuries. Upon arriving on Turtle Island in the 15th century, the Conquistadors (mis)perceived Amerindians through the lens of their Islamophobia and anti-Semitism toward Spanish Muslims and Jews back home on the Iberian Peninsula. I am curious about these racist displacements *vis-à-vis* the non-European Other of the Other, who is doubly negated in a variety of ways that we must account for.

My logical model in *Freud and Said* (2021a), which is based on the semiotic square (p. 19), is an attempt to map out these complex subject positions within an oppressive and violent apparatus, while bearing in mind that these subject positions are material products of history that are always changing following a dialectical logic—or an analectical logic, if we look at it from the Exterior perspective of transmodernity, as Dussel (1985) encourages us to.

3

Colonial difference translates the Real of cultural difference into racial difference. This is how we received the Orientalist distinction between the Occident and the Orient, which, as Said (1978) shows, is a power/knowledge asymmetry resulting from a colonial/imperial hierarchy. My phrase for this power/knowledge asymmetry is *colonial difference*. I argue that cultural difference is untranslatable because it is not simply a linguistic difference or a difference in customs and traditions. Cultural difference signifies how the specificity of each culture's or subculture's form of enjoyment can never really be captured by images or words, and that doing so is often stereotypical, if not racist. And this is precisely the mistake of Orientalism, being a pseudoscientific attempt to translate cultural difference, from a hegemonic perspective, as colonial difference.

Following Said (1993), I contend that cultural resistance is not a retreat into essentialism, but a vital intervention into the Symbolic order. In revolutionary praxis, seizing the means of production is insufficient if the superstructure remains colonized by the colonial fantasy. Because cultural difference signifies the Real—the untranslatable specificity of a group's form of enjoyment—cultural resistance becomes the psychosocial work required to articulate our singularity of being against the ideological fantasies of the dominant hierarchy. I complexify this through *non-identity politics*, where subjectivity is grounded in *a politics of difference* rather than the comforts of recognition. Consequently, I move beyond the Imaginary lure of Hollywood's superficial inclusion—the mere casting of non-European bodies in European frames—and focus instead on the crisis of *self-representation*. This involves articulating our singularity of being, while confronting the Real *gap* (lack) that emerges from the double division of the psychosocial order: the psychic split of the subject (*S*) and the social split of the Other (*A*). This double division does not look the same in Totality and Exteriority, hence, my notion of *cultural difference*. Within the libidinal economy of Totality, this gap manifests as a racial–sexual *surplus*—an excess of being that the patriarchy cannot assimilate and thus seeks to neutralize through ideological fantasy or, *in extremis*, genocidal violence.

Chapter 15

Seeing Gazans Through Decolonial Eyes: History as the Future

Ways of Seeing Gazans and Being Seen by Them

According to John Berger (1972),

> Seeing comes before words. The child looks and recognizes before it can speak ... The way we see things is affected by what we know or what we believe ... We only see what we look at. To look is an act of choice.
>
> (pp. 7–8)

W. J. T. Mitchell (2012) extends Berger's analysis. He argues that 'race' is a particular form of knowing or believing, which ideologically functions as a powerful medium through which we see the discursive-fantasies of reality. For Mitchell,

> The Real, by contrast, is the unrepresentable gap or blank space that opens up when the medium is fractured, when the Symbolic and Imaginary tear apart, the site of affect and the effects of trauma. The Real ... is the location not of race but of rac*ism*. Racism is what hurts. It is the disease, possibly an autoimmune disorder and certainly an infectious malady.
>
> (p. 17, emphasis in original)

To put it concretely regarding the dehumanization of Palestinians, particularly Gazans, anti-Arab racism is the surplus-enjoyment afforded by the racial ideology of Zionism. For example, the Law of Return, as Elmessiri (1977) argues, "has no parallel in any other country; it is based on the unique Zionist concept of pan-Jewish peoplehood and can be construed as racist in that it denies non-Jews [i.e., Palestinian Arabs] their inalienable rights in their own homeland" (p. 147). Zionism excludes Arabs from the Semitic category. As such, Israel's anti-Arab racism is an autoimmune disorder, a denial of the Arabs' Semitism. The Arabs must be dehumanized to erase their categorical status as Semites or as peoples of Shem. This is ironic, of course, when the whole Greater Syria or Levant region in Arabic has been referred to historically as Bilad al-Sham—the Land of Shem, after the eldest son of Noah, whose name in Hebrew (שֵׁם) signifies 'singularity' or 'authority.' I also

DOI: 10.4324/9781003768104-15

read anti-Semitism within the Arab world along similar lines. When anti-Jewish rhetoric emerges in Arabic-speaking nations, it is also a form of self-negation—a denial of a shared heritage and the historical coexistence that defined the region for centuries. It mirrors the Zionist exclusion by adopting a reactive, racialized lens that ignores the shared Semitic root, turning a familial or neighborly history into an absolute, irreconcilable binary. Therefore, I would argue for *pan-Semitism*—in the internationalist spirit of pan-Africanism—since what united the Semites historically was "the shared role not just as 'others' to Christian Europe but as *enemies* to Christendom" (Mitchell, 2012, p. 72, emphasis in original).

The ideological concept of Judeo-Christianity, or a Judeo-Christian civilization, was artificially created *après-coup*, as a way of downplaying the *longue durée* of European anti-Semitism, thereby implying that the Crusades were primarily motivated by Islamophobia or hatred of Islam—the sign of 'barbarism.' This is, of course, a historical fallacy, which covers over the phenomenon of antisemitic Zionism, particularly Christian Zionism, wherein the ideological figure of the rootless cosmopolitan Jew is kept fantasmatically at bay in Israel away from Euro-America.

This chapter is a psycho-political reflection on three ways of seeing Gazans and being seen by them in the context of the Second Nakba (catastrophe), which we are currently witnessing in real-time. The term Second Nakba is justified by the fact that Israel has killed more Palestinians in 2023 than in any year since 1948. Therefore, I will argue that at least three subject positions exist for onlookers witnessing the Second Nakba from outside through mediated images, particularly on social media. For the sake of simplicity, I will restrict my analysis to the ethics, politics, and aesthetics of war photography to consider questions of desire and enjoyment as they relate to liberation praxis.

According to the United Nations, 90% of war-time casualties are civilians; this amounts to around 167,000 Gazans and counting (Khatib, McKee, & Yusuf, 2024), the majority of whom are women and children, thereby confirming the psycho-historical thesis that what we call 'war' tends to be a cover up for widespread child abuse (DeMause, 1982). The questions of *who is looking* and *how they are looking* at images of living, dead, or mutilated Gazans shed light on the larger question of decolonial representation. Are Gazans representing themselves, or is someone representing them? This is a political question that has ethical and aesthetic dimensions.

Bracketing the political question concerning Hamas, ethical and aesthetic representations are complicated by *who* is taking these photographs, *what* they decide to photograph, *who* is the audience they imagine for them, and *what* is being widely shared on social media in the spirit of solidarity. In my view, there are three ways of seeing Gazans, through (1) colonial eyes, (2) postcolonial eyes, or (3) decolonial eyes. The first two are dehumanizing for different reasons, but they frame Gazans not as subjects of liberation but as traumatic objects. I propose a third way of seeing Gazans through decolonial eyes, a perspective grounded in self-representation (cf. Massad, 2007; Said, 1993), which is simultaneously a question of de-facement (De Man, 1979) or overdetermination (Freud, 1899).

Looking vs. The Gaze

It is worth mentioning, as an aside, that the signifiers Gaze and Gaza are false cognates: 'Gaze' is of Middle English origin, likely derived from a Scandinavian word meaning "to stare" and 'Gaza'—a name that dates back thousands of years—is a Semitic locution that signifies 'stronghold' or 'fortress.'

The theoretical distinction between the look and the Gaze further complicates my psycho-political reflection. Whereas *seeing* is how a given subject looks at something (in this case, war photos of Gazans), *being seen* is about how the images Gaze back at us, which causes us to analyze our desire and enjoyment (i.e., our subject position) concerning the question of Palestine. This may not be popular today. Still, like Edward Said, I believe in a one-state solution: "a unitary democratic nonsectarian Palestine," as envisioned also by Fatah in their posters from the 1980s.

I am unsettled by the barrage of images on social media of dead or mutilated Gazans, particularly children. As an Egyptian, I grew up feeling a strong sense of solidarity with Palestinians, mainly since the Second Intifada (2000–2005), which certainly politicized my consciousness; in other words, being pro-Palestinian is part of my subjectivity, but this statement must be unpacked beyond its obviousness, which opens up the space for self-criticism, for it is easier to critique the Other from a safe distance.

On a personal note, many in my generation will recall the images of 12-year-old Muhammed al-Durrah hiding behind his father, Jamal, during the beginning of the Second Intifada. The father is seen trying to protect his son. The latter is then tragically killed by gunfire from Israeli soldiers. We see expressions of extreme fear and horror on Muhammad's face before his untimely death, accompanied by Jamal's fainting. This was on September 30, 2000, and these images symbolized for my generation the unimaginable cruelty of the Israeli state and the excessive colonial violence of its military apparatus. Images of Jamal resurfaced in 2023 in the context of the Second Nakba; this time, we see him mourning his brothers, who were killed by Israeli airstrikes. It is worth noting that the killing of Muhammad al-Durrah was captured by two journalists working for France 2: a Palestinian (Talal Abu Rahma) and an Israeli (Charles Enderlin). Abu Rahma received the Rory Peck Award in 2001 for his unforgettable footage. I can never forget these images; they will never forgive me if I do.

I am unsettled—and this essay is indeed a reflection on how one unsettles coloniality—by said images, not only because of their graphic nature. After all, the traumatic Real can never be imaginarized or symbolized, for the violence inflicted on Gazans by the Israeli military is much worse than what we see or what is represented. However, once that violence is visually represented in one way or another, it enters a fantasy space, and here I worry about the dehumanizing objectification of Gazans as mainly dead or mutilated; in other words, not as ethico-political subjects with unconscious desires.

I wonder about the ethics of photographing the dead and the mutilated during wartime and whether there is too much enjoyment on social media in the consumption of what some may label "trauma porn." The concept of trauma porn is attributed to Tina Charisma (2021), who explored it concerning the commercialization of Black pain, or how seeing the suffering of Black people in the U.S. is normalized and commodified for public consumption through the wide circulation of graphic images that depict their death or torture in the media. As such, we must reflect on the public enjoyment of trauma porn and its function as perverse entertainment within the apparatus of racial capitalism.

I do not find the surplus-enjoyment of trauma porn to be liberating or enlightening in any way. I am reminded of the visual spectacle of lynching during the Jim Crow era, which was not only a live event for the racist enjoyment of white supremacists, but it was also commodified in terms of photographs and postcards that were widely circulated and celebrated. Hartman (1997) argues, "The emphasis on the joining of race, subjection, and spectacle is intended to denaturalize race and underline its givenness—that is, the strategies through which it is made to appear as if it has always existed, thereby denying the coerced and cultivated production of race" (p. 57). While Hartman is writing about the traumatic experiences of enslaved Africans in the U.S., one can extend her argument to the current spectacularization of Palestinian pain, for the spectacle of race is used to justify the subjection of Gazans, and this cycle makes Arabness appear as a natural reality, when in fact, it is a deliberate and historical production of racialization. Norman Finkelstein (2023b) draws an explicit analogy between Nat Turner's rebellion in 1831 and what he terms "the slave revolt in Gaza." Finkelstein seems to be thinking about Hegel's Master–Slave dialectic, which suggests that the genocide against Palestinian life is simultaneously an epistemicide against the Slave's practical form of know-how, on which the Master depends.

Furthermore, it is impossible to represent the traumatic Real; any such attempt is often an aestheticization of reactionary politics, be that fascism, settler colonialism, racial capitalism, or white supremacy. The traumatic Real must be acknowledged as the limit or failure of civility, human rights, international law, etc. It is the dimension of excessive violence and unimaginable oppression.

Critiquing the Israeli state and hystericizing its Zionist ideology produces "Free Palestine" as a new master-signifier, which must lead to a signifying chain grounded in critical knowledge about truth, justice, non-sectarianism, internationalism, democracy, socialism, liberation, and nonviolence. The alternative to the Zionist ideology, in other words, must be an internationalist praxis. Simply put, Free Palestine indexes the potential for a materiality, wherein the traumatic Real is worked through truth and reconciliation. This is how we can politicize the concrete utopian aesthetics of a Free Palestine to come. Note that Palestine refers to a rich *national culture* in the sense praised by Frantz Fanon and not to a *nationalism* like Zionism. This is why we critique Zionism or Israelism as a fascist ideology, but there is no such thing as Palestinianism. There is, of course, Islamism, but Palestine is not reducible to that ideology because the materiality of Palestine transcends any one religion, ethnicity, or ideology.

José Medina (2018) writes about how one can "neutralize and counter propaganda in visual culture" through what he labels "epistemic activism" (p. 52). For Medina, "Epistemic activism involves practices of interrogation and resistance that unmask, disrupt, and uproot forms of epistemic insensitivity, that is, ways in which our epistemic capacities and activities … have become uncritical and numbed to challenge and interrogation" (p. 59). So, how do we express our anti-colonial solidarity through epistemic activism? How do we resist the racist imagery of Gazans not as living ethico-political subjects but as dead or mutilated objects?

According to the United Nations Population Fund, around 1.9 million people have been displaced in Gaza, or 80% of the population. We must respectfully grieve the dead and, of course, continue to tell their stories and honor their memories, but I urge us to focus on *self-representations* that center the voices of the living since they are the ones who will build and organize a Free Palestine to come. A great example in this context is Mohammed Omer Almoghayer's (2024) *On the Pleasures of Living in Gaza: Remembering a Way of Life Now Destroyed.*

To be clear, I am not arguing that we should bury our heads in the sand or censor graphic images of the Second Nakba; instead, I am proposing that we do not take these images for granted but "*cultivate a critical and resistant way of viewing*" them (Medina, 2018, p. 60, emphasis in original). As Medina argues, "epistemic activism can contribute to disrupt[ing] uncritical attitudes toward images that distort and stigmatize the visibility of a group and to promote critical engagement with visual culture and with dysfunctional patterns of visual communication within it" (p. 66). Let us consider General Philip Sheridan's genocidal statement in 1869, "The only good Indian is a dead Indian," in juxtaposition to Palestinian trauma porn, for instance.

The unconscious message of these graphic images is that "the only good Palestinian is a dead Palestinian." From an Israeli settler-colonial perspective, that requires no explanation, for Zionists fantasize about Greater Israel, a promised ancestral homeland, a God-given *terra nullius*: "A land without a people for a people without a land." The Palestinian native population is, for Zionism, an inconvenience; Palestinians signify the traumatic Real that bursts the ideological fantasmatic bubble of Zionism. Paradoxically, the same message ("the only good Palestinian is a dead Palestinian") finds its unconscious resonance, from an anti-colonial perspective, in the implicit logic of martyrdom.

We witness something similar at work in a viral AI-generated image shared over 50 million times on social media. "The image shows tents in a camp, highlighted to spell out one single phrase: '"All Eyes on Rafah"' (Subzwari, 2024). The AI image represents neither Rafah nor Gazans, and it is precisely this *non-existence* of Palestinians and Palestine that made millions of people comfortable with sharing it, so we can say it is a way of non-seeing that produces an invisible Gaze from the Real void of AI.

The ideology of the AI-generated image has been critiqued with an alternative "all eyes on Rafah" bird's eye view photo, which shows the harsh reality of dead Gazans in white body bags and surrounded by a group of mourners. The phrase "all eyes on Rafah" indexes the title of 2Pac's fourth studio album, *All Eyez on Me*—a reference to the evil eye *qua* the racial capitalist panoptic Gaze. Morrissey said, "We hate it when our friends become successful." The hatred is magnified when the object of the evil eye is a racialized subject or subordinate group. So, perhaps the Lacanian intervention here, as a protection from the evil eye of oppressors, is to say "*not all* eyes on Rafah." In other words, we are only interested in good—anti-oppressive—eyes.

As an alternative to martyrdom, the Palestinian praxis of *sumud* (steadfastness) is much more liberatory, as captured by the statement: "to exist is to resist." This praxis was materially represented in the form of a mural on a portion of Israel's apartheid wall of shame. This type of Symbolic representation embodies *the politicization of aesthetics*, for it accepts the impossibility of representing the traumatic Real via the Imaginary, thereby rejecting *the aestheticization of politics*. In the words of Rebecca Ruth Gould (2014): "*Sumud* is freedom, but it is not unconditional because its attainment is premised on justice for everyone. It is the only solution there will ever be to a conflict that has claimed so many lives" (p. 106, emphasis in original). This ethic of *justice for everyone* is reminiscent of the feminine logic of not-all.

Lacan (1999) also framed this feminine logic as Other enjoyment, in contrast to masculine or phallic enjoyment. I have written about it as *divine enjoyment* stretching Benjamin's (1921/1996) *critique of violence* through a psychoanalytic lens to make sense of not only sexual difference in the zone of being but also *colonial difference*, which structures the power relations between those in the zones of being and nonbeing. Crucially, our liberation praxis must lead to *a zone of becoming*.

I imagine that if I were Gazan and someone posted an image online of my dead father or my mutilated son, I would feel horrified. How do we respectfully grieve the dead? My question, of course, assumes the grievability of Palestinians, whose lives many in Euro-America would not perceive to be as grievable as the lives of Ukrainians, for instance. According to Butler (2004), Palestinian lives are not considered to be "grievable." Their deaths are not considered to be "real deaths." Butler argues that this is a function of Israel's ideological and material dehumanization of Palestinians, which also forecloses any discursive critique of the Israeli state apparatus on antisemitic grounds (pp. 35–36).

Furthermore, how can we mourn Palestinian deaths beyond the theological framework of martyrdom? There is a relief for Muslim comrades in the idea that these civilian casualties are not in vain but amount to something greater, for martyrs are assumed to be on their way to paradise. The alternative of *sumud* is indeed far more grim, for there is no promise of paradise; however, there is the hope of a Free Palestine. Therefore, I distinguish between the ideology of liberation theology in the case of martyrdom and the materiality of liberation praxis in the case of *sumud*. I am much more interested in the latter.

In this context, I wonder about the political impact of endless graphic images of dead and mutilated Gazans, as a strategy that is perhaps meant to shame Zionists and their supporters or to elicit empathy from online bystanders. We must politicize aesthetics and not aestheticize politics, as Benjamin (1935/2008) recommended.

While the latter was the fascist route taken by the Nazis, the former is the antifascist path, which entails humanizing self-representations of Gazans, as ethico-political subjects, who are suffering deeply under a humanitarian crisis of genocidal proportions. I invite us to think *with* Gazans, on the lines of the Symbolic and the Real, about their seemingly impossible desire for liberation. This divine enjoyment of struggle toward something better (not paradise, but Free Palestine) must be the focus of our solidarity efforts. This is how we politicize aesthetics. Next, I will explore three ways of seeing Gazans before reflecting on how history is our link to the future.

Seeing Gazans Through Colonial Eyes

The first way of seeing Gazans is through a pro-Zionist perspective, which is the point of view of settler colonialism (cf. Pappé, 2007; Rodinson, 1973). As such, Gazans, as the colonized, are framed in dehumanizing terms as sub-/non-human objects. In the words of Yoav Gallant, the Israeli Defense Minister, after the October 7th attacks on Israel by Hamas: "We are fighting human animals and we act accordingly." The animal metaphor is not coincidental, of course. It indexes a fascist tradition of dehumanization, whose function is the justification of genocide. Seeing Gazans through colonial eyes produces the Gaze of fascism, which presupposes a sadistic subject, who enjoys traumatizing the Other through the perpetration of cruel forms of political violence. Therefore, it is inaccurate to label this situation as war or conflict; it is terrorism.

There has been so much debate in the western media around the signifier 'genocide,' which I would like to put to rest. The UN Independent International Commission of Inquiry on the Occupied Palestinian Territory, including East Jerusalem, and Israel has been investigating the events on and since October 7, 2023, and they released a 72-page report on September 16, 2025, wherein they concluded:

> **The Commission concludes on reasonable grounds that the Israeli authorities and Israeli security forces have committed and are continuing to commit the following *actus reus* [guilty act] of genocide against the Palestinians in the Gaza Strip, namely (i) killing members of the group; (ii) causing serious bodily or mental harm to members of the group; (iii) deliberately inflicting on the group conditions of life calculated to bring about its physical destruction in whole or in part; and (iv) imposing measures intended to prevent births within the group.**
>
> (p. 71, emphasis in original)

Perhaps we should consider a Derridean framing here since Israel's colonial terrorism is, in a sense, a form of endocolonial violence, which is symptomatic of "autoimmunitary terror" (Derrida, as cited in Borradori, 2003). It is suicidal autoimmunity because there are millions of Israelis and Palestinians between the river and the sea, who have a symbiotic relationship with the Holy Land. On a superficial level, there is a narcissism of minor differences, if we consider Jews, Christians, and Muslims as metaphorical cousins, which undoubtedly implies parricide.

On a more concrete level, there is a significant power/knowledge asymmetry between Israel and Palestine, which invokes the Hegelian dialectic between the Master and the Slave. In this scenario, the Master is a colonizing State, and the Slave is a colonized Nation. The Master not only over-exploits the Slave but also mimics their national culture to produce a virtual nation, which explains numerous bizarre examples of cultural appropriation, from the "Israeli salad" to "Israeli couscous."

Qualifying something as Israeli does not render it *ontologically Israeli* but rather *ideologically* so. This goes to show the over-exploitation of the Slave's manual and mental labor: their knowledge of the land, which is reflected in their national cultural expression. The *Hasbara* (propaganda) used by the Master to negate this know-how involves the repetition of certain master-signifiers. This language game is on display in the mainstream Euro-American media when we hear every pundit repeat the *Hasbara* question: "Do you condemn Hamas?" The condemnation of settler colonialism is out of the question, for that entails the hystericization of 'Israel' and 'Zionism' as master-signifiers, which amounts to anti-Semitism against the Master.

Another propaganda mechanism is the repetition of the dehumanizing phrase "human shields," which we are told is part of Hamas's military strategy since they are unimaginably 'barbaric.' The Israeli military indexes this phrase to justify any so-called collateral damage in Gaza, since the death of a human shield is nothing but the destruction of an object, and defensive armor is not grievable. The historical record, however, shows that Israel has systematically used Palestinians as human shields. So, the phrase is more than a dehumanizing metaphor and signifies the bare life, or abject, status of Palestinians as fungible or disposable commodities.

Seeing Gazans Through Postcolonial Eyes

The second way of seeing Gazans is through an anti-Zionist perspective, which is the (post)colonial point of view of many non-Palestinian western leftists. As such, Gazans, as the colonized, are still framed in dehumanizing terms as dead or mutilated objects as opposed to living ethico-political subjects. While I am sympathetic to anti-Zionism, I prefer being pro-Palestinian, which is about centering the political agency of Palestinian subjects in the West Bank, Gaza, and beyond.

Seeing Gazans through (post)colonial eyes produces the Gaze of western leftism, which presupposes a masochistic subject, who enjoys the consumption of trauma porn as a form of online activism. Susan Sontag (2003) wrote about the "desensitizing horror" of trauma porn. She asked,

> Flooded with images of the sort that once used to shock and arouse indignation, we are losing our capacity to react. Compassion, stretched to its limits, is going numb. So runs the familiar diagnosis. However, what is really being asked for here? That images of carnage be cut back to, say, once a week?
>
> (p. 108)

The problem, for Sontag, is "that our capacity to respond to our experiences with emotional freshness and ethical pertinence is being sapped by the relentless diffusion of vulgar and appalling images" (pp. 108–09). For Roland Barthes (1980), "Photography is subversive not when it frightens, repels, or even stigmatizes, but when it is *pensive*, when it thinks" (p. 38, emphasis in original). Images from the Second Nakba must be curated and collected for a Nakba Memorial Museum.

Suffice it to say that I do not find the oversharing of trauma porn to be a sound political strategy, even if I understand the emotional motivation behind the need to shame Israel for its cruelty. Our political interventions must be more on the lines of the Symbolic and the Real, which are the dimensions of desire and enjoyment. What do Palestinians want? Free Palestine. What would Palestinians enjoy as ethico-political subjects? The rights and freedoms granted to citizens living in a unitary democratic non-sectarian state. How do we support Palestinians to get there? Through an international solidarity movement.

Seeing Gazans Through Decolonial Eyes

The third way of seeing Gazans is through a radical humanistic perspective, the decolonial point of view. Here, Gazans, as living ethico-political subjects, represent themselves. The radical humanistic perspective is *ipso facto* anti-Zionist, but it does not define itself negatively in opposition to Jewish nationalism. Instead, it defines itself positively through *Palestinian internationalism*. According to Said (1999c), "real peace can come only with a binational Israeli–Palestinian state." Again, how do we get there? This is the million-dollar question, but if apartheid South Africa serves as a model, then the path will entail internal and external pressures, negotiations, reforms, and democratic leadership. Boycott, Divestment, and Sanctions (BDS) is an anti-apartheid tactic in this direction. Similarly, the political prisoner Marwan Barghouti (known as the Palestinian Mandela) can potentially serve as one of the first leaders of this unitary non-sectarian democracy to come.

To illustrate my point about Palestinian self-representation, I wish to highlight some Gazans committed to "the principle of hope" (Bloch, 1986), which is a reference to a "*concrete utopian horizon*" (p. 146, emphasis in original). Mahmoud Abed posted a picture on X of himself seated on a sofa chair amidst the rubble. His caption: "I'm still alive." An African American comrade, Reny, quoted Mahmoud's post with the following words: "Cuz clean asf [as f***] too. From the River to the sea!" Mahmoud exists and resists *in style*. Rahaf Nasser, a medical student, is seen in a video playing the guitar and singing to a group of children surrounded by debris. A little boy, Mohammed, is seen in a viral video leading a group of men in a *dabke* dance in a displacement camp in Gaza.

Finally, there is Hamada Sho, a food blogger posting videos from Gaza about his recipes and how he feeds children and other community members. This is the most radical form of resistance: the principle of hope. Israelis can only win *if* the Palestinian spirit is dead; therefore, Israelis will never win. To exist *is* to resist. To politically exist as a Palestinian is the highest form of spiritual resistance.

Spiritual here signifies the revolutionary love that drives the Palestinian community to continue the praxis of *sumud* in the face of the Zionist evil eye. Indeed, physiological and safety needs are the most basic in Maslow's hierarchy. These basic needs are at risk in Gaza. Nevertheless, Gazans resist death and continue to exist through their collective desire for liberation, and this communal spirit epitomizes their ethico-political praxis of *sumud. Sumud* is grounded in revolutionary love, which, according to Joy James (2022), "originates from a desire for the greater good that entails radical risk-taking for justice" (p. 4). This is what Hamada Sho and others like him capture through their empowering and inspiring self-representations.

The Palestinian spirit shall not be broken, and indeed, it will triumph one day over all forms of dehumanization—Israeli or otherwise. Mahmoud Darwish (2024) addressed the cultural resistance of the Palestinian spirit in an interview from 1984 as follows:

> Palestinian cultural expression became for Israelis, an immediate danger, for it firstly negates the allegations about the destruction of land by a culturally productive people and secondly because such cultural expression provides a very dangerous testimony as to the anti-cultural operation on whose essence the Zionist presence was founded.
>
> (pp. 33–34)

This liberatory logic resonates with Fred Hampton's statement that "you can kill a revolutionary but you can never kill the revolution." To be Palestinian, in other words, is a revolutionary act in and of itself. Still, I wish not to generalize, given the deafening silence of a diasporic Palestinian like DJ Khaled—whose bystander neutrality translates as bourgeois complicity. While Israel has succeeded in killing hundreds of thousands of Palestinians since the First Nakba in 1948, it has drastically failed to eradicate Palestinian cultural expression.

History as the Future: Palestine Beyond the Imaginary of Trauma Porn

The present in Gaza is beyond traumatic; it is full of terrorizing violence, unspeakable suffering, and excessive pain. Throughout this chapter, I have argued for the ethico-political self-representation of Palestinians, as a radical humanistic act, and against dehumanizing representations, which aestheticize politics through the Imaginary—and ideological—lens of trauma porn. I have outlined three ways of seeing Gazans through colonial, (post)colonial, and decolonial eyes. Part of the decolonial approach regards *history as the future*, which entails seeing the future through the past. This means bracketing the present to some extent, or at least our imagination of the present. The present is too close and unbearably traumatic to interpret; we can neither see nor unsee it. We must be able to signify a world beyond colonial violence and sadomasochistic cruelty. A better world is possible because it did exist once.

However, I do not suggest we romanticize the past and forget about present tragedy. Instead, I am proposing that we use our images of the past politically to inspire us now in the way we ethically signify the future. According to Lakota scholar Nick Estes (2019),

> Indigenous notions of time consider the present to be structured entirely by our past and ancestors. There is no separation between past and present, meaning that an alternative future is also determined by our understanding of our past. Our history is the future.
>
> (p. 19)

Similarly, the authors of *Camera Palestina* write: "the concept of the 'emancipated Palestinian spectator' permits us to see the Palestinian subjects of the image also looking back at themselves into the future from within the image itself, reaching across and connecting history, the present, and the certainties of a liberated future" (Nassar, Sheehi, & Tamari, 2022, p. 119).

On these notes, I wish to end with archival photographs of Gazans by Kegham Djeghalian Sr., an Armenian–Palestinian photographer, who opened the first photography studio in Gaza in 1944. His grandson, Kegham Djeghalian Jr., and I went to Collège de la Sainte Famille in Egypt, and we both graduated the same year from the American University in Cairo.

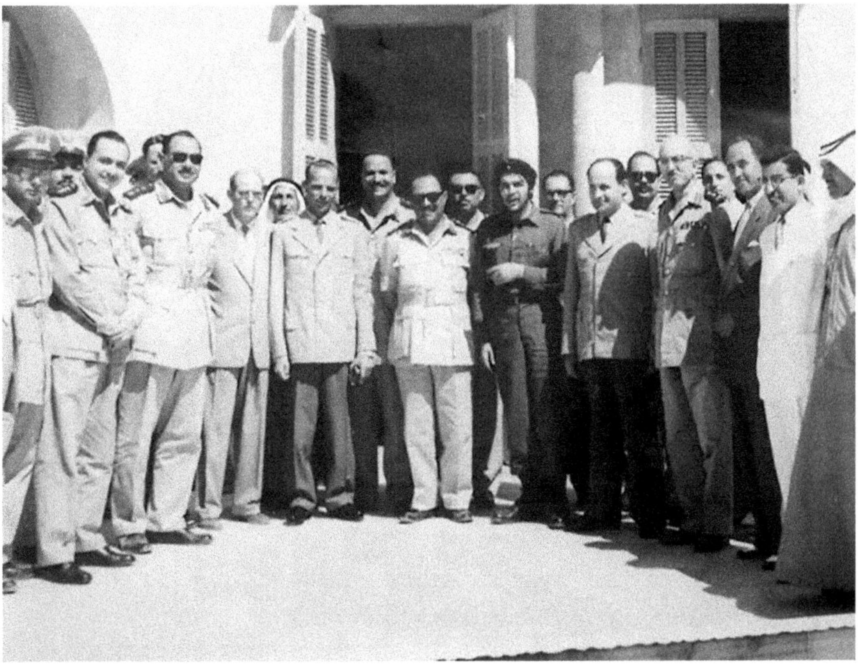

Figure 15.1 Che Guevara in Gaza in 1959 (Kegham Djeghalian)

In 2018, Kegham Jr. "stumbled upon three red boxes tucked away and forgotten in his father's wardrobe in Cairo" (as cited in Bedirian, 2021). He continues, "The boxes contained the negatives of more than 1,000 photographs taken [by Kegham Sr.] between the 1940s and the 1970s." The archive from the studio of Photo Kegham shows the reproduction of Palestinian life. In 1959, Che Guevara visited Gaza to meet with political leaders, an event that was also documented by Kegham Sr. (Figure 15.1). Who is the revolutionary equivalent of Che today? Perhaps Greta Thunberg or Chris Smalls? The IDF has a long history of disrupting flotilla attempts to bring humanitarian aid into Gaza, and of course, the Egyptian state is complicit in upholding the blockade against Gaza. In any case, I hope this chapter encourages the reader to reflect on *how* Gazans are represented, *who* represents them, *for whom* these representations are meant, and *for what* purpose.

In *After the Last Sky*, Said (1999a) writes, "I do not know whether the photograph can, or does, say things as they really are. Something has been lost. But the representation is all we have" (p. 84). Representing Free Palestine, in the Symbolic (e.g., "from the river to the sea, Palestine will be free") or in the Imaginary (e.g., watermelon 🍉 as a Palestinian symbol), signifies pre-figuring a unitary democratic non-sectarian state now.

Chapter 16

Conclusion

Throughout the book, I have argued that liberation psychoanalysis is an analectical materialist praxis of truth and justice, love and forgiveness, pluriversality and singularity, socialism and libertarianism, etc. Praxis signifies a unity of theory and practice. Therefore, liberation psychoanalysis is a critical theory that can be applied not only to the clinic but also to the social world writ large. Inversely, liberation psychoanalysis is a radical practice to test and refine the theory. Furthermore, liberation psychoanalysis is a materialist project.

Racial capitalism, as an apparatus within both Totality and Exteriority, facilitates a system of unequal exchange where the core (Global North) extracts labor and resources from the periphery (Global South) to sustain its own growth. This extraction is more than neo-colonial; it is fundamentally death-driven, employing instrumental reason to legitimize both endo- and exo-colonial forms of violence. As I have argued throughout this book, our praxis is essentially humanist, socialist, and life-driven by historical reason; its aim is *the liberation of the commons through (non)violence* (cf. Negri, 2023). I write *(non)violence* to acknowledge that while nonviolent resistance or action is preferred (e.g., civil disobedience, noncooperation, etc.), the possibility of revolutionary violence may be justified as a last resort. The broader inquiry centers on the manifestation of anarchist power as the teleological end of liberation psychoanalysis. Rather than a top-down structure, anarchist power represents a mode of self-organization: a complex, holarchical system where individuals and collectives function as *holons*—autonomous (w)holes that are simultaneously integral parts of a greater social ecology. Such a complex system is characterized by being decentralized, emergent, and non-linear, yet also robust and adaptable.

In liberation psychoanalysis, historical materialism signifies not only the political economy of a given society (i.e., the forces and relations of production) but also its libidinal economy (i.e., a society's dominant mode of enjoyment). The dominant mode of enjoyment within racial capitalism is *mythic jouissance* as the collective enjoyment of racism, sexist oppression, exploitation, and colonial/imperial forms of violence (e.g., genocide, enslavement, and epistemicide). Liberation psychoanalysis is committed to *divine jouissance* as the collective enjoyment of humanism, sexual liberation, and cooperation.

DOI: 10.4324/9781003768104-16

Collective enjoyment is a function of the political unconscious, and is often the result of ideological fantasy, but this does not need to be the case, if we are committed to the type of ideology critique that leads to not only critical consciousness, but also what I have termed *critical unconsciousness*. The double work of *critique from a place of love* entails *authentic hystericization* and *radical analysis*, that is, questioning violent masters and oppressive signifiers while analyzing the material conditions that give rise to violence and oppression.

The materialism of liberation psychoanalysis deals not only with history but also with the Real—that traumatic dimension, which can never be represented through either images or signifiers. As such, I conceive of the Real as not only one of the forces driving historical materialism, but also a "weird materialism of the signifier" (Eyers, 2011, p. 156)—*cf.* Kovel (1986). In other words, the Real is *the analectical materialism of the signifier* (cf. Endres, 2022). The social relationship between the base and the superstructure identified by Marx parallels the psychic relationship between the unconscious and the ego identified by Freud. But there is a tension between the Letter of the Law and the Spirit of Desire.

Lacan (2006) offers a couple of definitions of the Letter as "the material medium that concrete discourse borrows from language" (p. 413) and "the essentially localized structure of the signifier" (p. 418). But is the Letter inherently oppressive, given its connection to Law? Not necessarily, the Letter's oppressive quality emerges when it is too literal, as in a dead letter or a killing letter. This is when the signifier is no longer connected to a living desire and becomes empty, as in mere litter. As such, the Letter exists in potentiality, or in a littoral zone, "between [paranoiac] knowledge and jouissance [as a sign of the truth of one's unconscious desire]" (Lacan, 2013). Liberation, therefore, has to do with what Freud (1930/1961) terms "oceanic feeling," which is always in a dialectical relationship to the alienation of being castaway.

Žižek (1989) argued, following Lacan, that Marx invented the symptom in the sense that he identified commodity fetishism as an ideological fantasy, which covers over the traumatic Real of exploitation. Similarly, for Freud, bodily symptoms are not conditions in and of themselves, as psychiatry wishes for us to believe, but rather they are effects of the subject's particular form of negation. A subject's particular form of negation (e.g., repression, foreclosure, or disavowal) informs their psychical structure as a neurotic, psychotic, or pervert, respectively. In other words, bodily symptoms exist on the fantasmatic level of the Imaginary, which is to say, they ideologically structure the subject's Symbolic discourse (i.e., their articulation of desire). What is sutured or negated in this process of free association is the dimension of the traumatic Real, that is, the subject's enjoyment of their symptoms. These psychosocial deadlocks at the core of ideology point toward the method of dialectics *qua* ideology critique.

However, liberation psychoanalysis is not only dialectical (Fenichel, 1967), but also *analectical*. Dussel (1985) stretches Marxism through the Exterior perspective of liberation philosophy, which is a transmodern move. For him, dialectics is still situated within the Totality of the Euromodern world-system. Therefore, as an immanent critique of modernity from within, dialectics can only produce critical modernity or postmodernity. As such, according to Dussel, dialectics can never delink the rhetoric of modernity from the logic of coloniality because Euro-modernity is a discourse that is ideologically structured by unconscious colonial fantasies. Transmodernity is a counter-ideological (i.e., materialist) rhetoric, which is informed by a decolonial logic.

(De)colonial fantasies emerge from what I term double-unconsciousness, where two distinct 'Others' inform the discourses of (post)modernity and transmodernity. If the (post)colonial subject's unconscious is the discourse of the (post)modern Other, then the decolonial subject's unconscious is the discourse of the transmodern Other. I define this as the Other of the Other (A^2): not a metalanguage for a purely external Real, but a sovereign language of Exteriority that is doubly negated within Totality. In this framework, the Other of the Other implies the unconscious of the unconscious ($\$^2$). Consequently, while (post)colonial psychoanalysis engages the unconscious as a negation within Totality, liberation psychoanalysis engages the unconscious of psychoanalysis—a negation of the negation within Exteriority. This is the gift of second sight: a meta-consciousness forged from the facticity of a doubly negated, critical unconsciousness.

To traverse colonial fantasies, we require analectics, or ana-dialectics. Transmodernity is a critique from Exteriority, which transcends and includes Euromodernity, while sublating it with the alter-modernity of the non-European world (see Figure 16.1). Analectics works through the deadlocks of ideology by delinking the discourse of (trans)modernity from (de)colonial fantasies—that is, the fantasies of both *coloniality* and *antimodernity*. Both fantasies are not only regressive, but also reactionary. Just as critical modernity and postmodernity often entail the unconscious acting out of colonial fantasies, antimodernity is the acting out of a decolonial fantasy. However, decoloniality is not an ideology to be acted out fantasmatically; rather, it is the unconscious desire for collective liberation, a means to an end. The means is *praxis*, and the end is *anarchist power*.

Decoloniality is a process to be enjoyed in and of itself, the way the subject enjoys desiring more than realizing objects of desire. In other words, decoloniality is the *objet a* driving the transmodern subject-as-drive. We can conceive of the lack structuring the decolonial process in terms of what Derrida (2005) referred to as "a democracy to come," and what I have conceptualized in *Freud and Said* as "an impossible republic" (cf. Hallaq, 2012).

An impossible republic is an anti-authoritarian—i.e., radical or revolutionary (Hayat, 2023)—republic. Anarchism is often misinterpreted as anti-statist, when in fact, it is against centralized, hierarchical authority, or authoritarianism. Therefore, an impossible republic is a decentralized, holarchical form of authority, which accounts for the traumatic Real at the heart of politics because failure is constitutive of any Symbolic order, and no (ana)dialectical sublation can resolve this constitutive failure. Hence, an impossible republic is the realization of both *subjective* and *objective* destitution, as the outcome of traversing ideological fantasies, be they conservative (e.g., antimodernity) or liberal (e.g., coloniality)—for a sustained

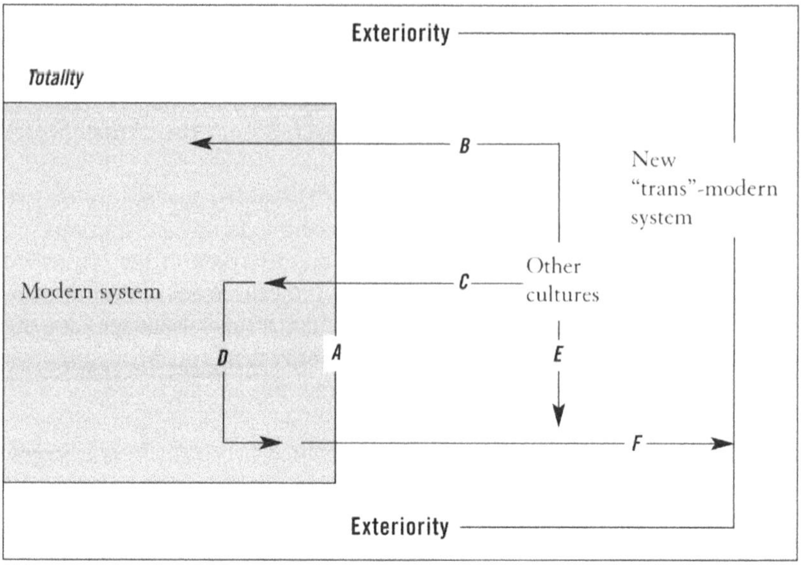

Totality, exteriority, affirmation of exteriority. Key:
(A) "postmodernity" (the limit of modernity and of totality);
(B) the inclusion of the other into the same (the old system); (C) the innovative interpellation before modernity; (D) the subsumption of modernity's positivity; (E) the affirmation of the other in its exteriority;
(F) the construction (as a synthesis of C + D + E)
of an innovative "trans"-modernity.

Figure 16.1 Transmodernity

critique of liberalism, see Losurdo (2014). It is worth noting that Plato's *Republic* is "based on the Egyptian models [of governance]" (Uždavinys, 2008, p. 21); however, we can reframe the philosopher-king (pharaoh) in terms of *the collective will of the people, as informed by philosophy*. According to Uždavinys (2008):

> The Egyptian form of government was imitated by the Pythagoreans, along with the methods of philosophical askesis [self-discipline], aimed at purifying the human soul and harmonizing with the perfectly arranged state regarded as an *imago* of the divine cosmos, both sensible and noetic.
>
> (p. 22, emphasis in original)

In other words, the divine cosmos served as the unconscious template for the Ancient Egyptian subject, with the *per ânkh* (House of Life), providing the institutional context for self-discipline under the guidance of Djehuty (the *nṯr* of philosophy: science and wisdom). I propose we conceptualize the *per ânkh* as *le nom-du-grand-père*—the Other of the Other—which marks the dimension of institutional failure in relation to the ethics of desire. Consequently, liberation psychoanalysis—a radical politics of libertarian socialism as the libidinal economic expression of anarchist power—becomes a scientific endeavor grounded in analectical materialism and animated by historical reason. It is capable of sublating colonial difference through the affirmation of (trans)modernity and the negation of coloniality/antimodernity. While colonial difference is a violent and oppressive (mis)translation of cultural difference—enforced through the imperial machinations of racial capitalism—transmodernity offers liberatory interpretations and (re)constructions that refuse to translate the Real of cultural difference. In this sense, transmodernity functions as an ethical relation to Exteriority; it recognizes the Real as an irreducible kernel that resists colonial capture, allowing for a second sight that affirms the Other of the Other without subsuming them into a new Totality.

A concrete example of transmodernity in the realm of aesthetics is the West-Eastern Divan Orchestra, founded by Edward Said and Daniel Barenboim. According to a statement from 2009 by the Orchestra: "We aspire to total freedom and equality between Israelis and Palestinians, and it is on this basis that we come together to play music." This aspiration, of course, does not presume that music alone can or will solve the Israeli–Palestinian conflict, as the Orchestra itself acknowledges, which is why we need not only aesthetic but also political and ethical interventions against Totality.

Contemporary transmodern psychoanalytic interventions—aside from the classics (e.g., Fanon, Nandy, Mannoni, Reich, Fromm, Marcuse, Spivak, Khanna, Faladé, Mitchell, Kristeva, Rose, etc.)—include: *Healing the American Indian Soul Wound* (Duran, Duran, Heart, & Horse-Davis, 1998), *The African Unconscious* (Bynum, 2012), *Desiring Whiteness* (Seshadri-Crooks, 2000), *The Melancholy of Race* (Cheng, 2001), *Psychoanalysis in Colonial India* (Hartnack, 2001), *The Puerto Rico Syndrome* (Gherovici, 2003), *Colonization of Psychic Space* (Oliver, 2004), *Freud Along the Ganges* (Akhtar, 2005), *Liberating Oedipus?* (Kovačević, 2007), *Why Are the Arabs Not Free?* (Safouan, 2007), *La Chine sur le Divan* (Datong, 2008), *Psychoanalysis and the Challenge of Islam* (Benslama, 2009), *From the Conscious Interior to an Exterior Unconscious* (Pavón-Cuéllar, 2010), *Freud Upside Down* (Ahad, 2010), *Psychoanalysis Outside the Clinic* (Frosh, 2010), *Unconscious Dominions* (Anderson et al., 2011), *Internal Racism* (Davids, 2011), *Doing Psychoanalysis in Tehran* (Homayounpour, 2012), *A Psychotherapy for the People* (Aron & Starr, 2013), *The Great Dragon Fantasy* (Wu, 2014), *Jacques Lacan in Africa* (Iwuanyanwu, 2015), *What Fanon Said* (Gordon, 2015), *Racist States of Mind* (Keval, 2016), *Trauma and Race* (George, 2016), *Race in Psychoanalysis* (Brickman, 2018), *The Arabic Freud* (El Shakry, 2017), *The Fetish Revisited* (Matory, 2018), *Islamic Psychoanalysis and Psychoanalytic Islam* (Parker & Siddiqui, 2019), *A People's History of Psychoanalysis* (Gaztambide, 2019), *Confronting Desire* (Kapoor, 2020), *The Psychoanalytic Zero: A Decolonizing Study of Therapeutic Dialogues* (Togashi, 2020), *Postcolonial Lack* (Basu Thakur, 2020), *Le vie psychique du racisme* (Boni & Mendelsohn, 2021), *Racism and Sexism in*

Brazilian Culture (Gonzalez, 2021), *Fanon's Decolonial Transcendence of Psychoanalysis* (Maldonado-Torres et al., 2021), *Treatment is Geopolitical: On Lacan's Decolonial Clinic* (Rahmat, 2021), *Psychoanalysis and Revolution* (Parker & Pavón Cuéllar, 2021), *Psychoanalysis and the Love of Arabic* (Bou Ali, 2020), *Colonial Trauma* (Lazali, 2021), *Lacan and Race* (George & Hook, 2021), *Lacan Noir* (Marriott, 2021), *The Work of Whiteness* (Morgan, 2021), *Unrootedness: a New Surface in the Lacanian Black Split Subject* (Akpan, 2022), *Decolonization, Polarization, Psychoanalysis, Privilege: Toward a Cosmopolitan and Culturally Intelligent Psychotherapist* (Gheorghe, 2022), *Psychoanalysis Under Occupation* (Sheehi & Sheehi, 2022), *Can We Decolonize Psychoanalytic Theory and Practice?* (Tummala-Narra, 2022), *Black Oedipus: Coloniality and the Foreclosure of Gender and Race* (Segato, 2022), *Psychoanalysis and Colonialism* (Swartz, 2023), *Spheres of Insurrection* (Rolnik, 2023), *Decolonizing the Psychoanalytic Technique* (Gaztambide, 2024), *Decolonisation of Psychoanalysis and Mesoamerican Conceptions of Subjectivity* (Pavón-Cuéllar, 2024), *La race sur Le divan* (Ayouch, 2024), *The Indian Jungle: Psychoanalysis and Non-Western Civilizations* (Kakar, 2024), *Decolonization and Psychoanalysis* (Rahmat, 2025), *Cloud: Between Paris and Tehran* (Copjec, 2025), *Psychoanalysis as a Decolonial Practice* (Gordon, 2025), *Psychoanalytic Liberation Psychology: Anti-capitalist approaches* (Malherbe, 2025), *From the Clinic to the Streets* (Sheehi, 2026), etc. This is, by no means, an exhaustive list—cf. two recent special issues from the peer-reviewed journals *Psychotherapy and Politics International* (Pavón-Cuéllar & Guerra, 2024) and *Psychoanalysis, Culture & Society* (Pavón-Cuéllar & Beshara, 2025) on "Decolonisation and Psychoanalysis" and "Psychoanalysis and Colonialism," respectively—rather these are selected works, intermediate nodes within a theoretical network, which will hopefully also include this nodal book.

While the aforementioned transmodern interventions provide the necessary geopolitical breadth to psychoanalysis, they must be synthesized into a cohesive structural model. To this end, the following section outlines a theoretical network that maps these diverse liberating practices onto a unified framework of anarchist power and decolonial legitimacy.

The untranslatability of cultural difference (cf. Bhabha, 1994; Hatem, 2020; Rahmat, 2025) does not signify a (multi)culturalist retreat; rather, it indicates the return of the doubly repressed—Exteriority—in the form of *an internationalist politics of difference* characterized by the transversal relation between *the singularity of being* (Ruti, 2012) and the *pluriversality of knowing* (Mignolo, 2000). The singularity of being refers to the uniqueness of the subject: that they are one of one. The pluriversality of knowing—cf. de Chardin's (2004) "Noosphere" as "a stupendous thinking machine" (p. 168)—implies the infinity of Otherness (Levinas, 1969), or that there is a vast, endless collection of ideas, experiences, and perspectives that exist Exterior to the (post)modern subject.

The transversal relation between singularity and pluriversality suggests that a subject's uniqueness is not a closed-off bubble, but a dynamic, non-hierarchical, and open-ended process of communication and connection. This process cuts across distinct levels—psychic, social, political, and economic—and bridges four foundational disciplines: psychoanalysis, sociology, political philosophy, and economics. Within this framework, the subject is not a static One within Totality, but a holon within a pluriverse, maintaining its singularity while participating in the collective interpretation and (re)construction of the Real.

Dussel (2012) understands transversality *vis-à-vis* transmodern intercultural dialogue as a "movement from the periphery to the periphery" (p. 54). For Guattari (2015), transversality is his name for institutional transference, which sheds light on the libidinal economy of the political unconscious at different levels of organization within society: micro, meso, and macro. However, while I find transversality to be an important concept, I regard schizoanalysis as a theoretical regression that fails to grapple with the structural truths of human subjectivity: the castrating function of the Law and the constitutive lack that defines our existence.

In Freudo–Lacanian psychoanalysis, desire is a function of the Law's prohibition: the Name-of-the-Father *qua* the No of the Father. The Law—specifically the prohibition of incest—creates a fundamental lack in the subject *vis-à-vis* the mOther. Desire is the engine that drives the subject to seek a lost object, a pursuit that is structurally doomed, for the subject's unconscious desire for the *objet a* is often negated and substituted with the phallus, as a signifier of lack, as some Thing *to have* or *to be*. Thus, desire is a subversive force, but it is always defined by the very Law that prohibits it.

In Deleuzo–Guattarian schizoanalysis, desire is a creative, productive, and affirmative force. It is not born from lack or shaped by a foundational Law. Instead, desire is seen as a "desiring-machine" that flows and connects with other machines to create reality. The Oedipal Law, in this view, is a repressive force that channels and subordinates these flows of desire, forcing them into a rigid, familial structure.

The goal of schizoanalysis is not to find liberation within the space of prohibition but to liberate desire from the Law, which is disavowed. It seeks to affirm a state of commanded enjoyment, as a perverse refusal of Symbolic castration and a rejection of the Oedipal Law. Having said that, I am neither pro-Oedipus nor anti-Oedipus. Nevertheless, I admire the Freudo–Marxist, or Lacano–Althusserian, commitments of Deleuze and Guattari (i.e., the materialism of schizoanalysis), but I am skeptical about their idealization or romanticization of psychosis through their invocation of the Nietzschean category of *homo natura* (natural human), such as when they write, "Schizophrenia is like love ... schizophrenia is the universe of productive and reproductive desiring-machines" (Deleuze & Guattari, 1983, p. 5).

For Deleuze and Guattari (1983), "We are all little colonies and it is Oedipus that colonizes us" (p. 265). According to them, the psychotic subject is the ideal decolonial subject given their foreclosure of the Name-of-the-Father, whom they equate with Oedipus. Their logic is that if "Oedipus is always colonization pursued by other means" (p. 190), then anti-Oedipus (embodied in the figure of the schizoanalysand or schizo-analyst) is always decolonization pursued by other means. But what is the goal of schizoanalysis? The psychotic decompensation of society as a supposed decolonial act? Their sensitivity to the question of coloniality is admirable; however, their abstract equivalence between Oedipalization and colonization is facile, to say the least. However, I agree with their critique of psychoanalysis "oedipalizing the indigenous population" (p. 269), which is the ethnocentric problem of false universality: projection on steroids.

According to Guattari (2015), "Transversality is a dimension that tries to overcome both the impasse of pure verticality and that of mere horizontality: it tends to be achieved when there is maximum communication among different levels and, above all, in different meanings" (p. 113). The transversal relationship between the Subject and the Other—and between Totality and Exteriority—is formed and understood through an ongoing journey into the infinite world of alterity. To put it differently, we define ourselves, particularly our uniqueness, in relation to endless difference, which should never be translated as either hierarchichal or horizontal violence.

In other words, transversality makes possible *a Symbolic identification based on Real politics* beyond the Imaginary forms of *vertical identification with a leader* and *horizontal identification with a group*. Whereas Imaginary identification is an egoic identification with a fantasmatic image of the Leader or the Nation, Symbolic identification is an unconscious identification with the Other's desire, which Safouan (2004), following Freud, qualifies as "hysterical identification" since it is an identification "without idealization" (p. 69). Basu Thakur (2021) defines *Real politics*—not to be confused with Realpolitik—as "a politics that does not seek to ignore or overwrite the antagonism, but instead, posits it as *the* political problem" (p. 290, emphasis in original).

Ideological fantasies tend to exist on the level of *the particularity of nothingness*, which is the ethnocentric narrative of culture, as an authoritarian politics of sameness, wherein what is provincial is hyperbolically magnified and projected as universal. In contrast, Mignolo (2007) argues for "*pluriversality as a universal project*" (p. 452–453, emphasis in original). The particularity of nothingness is a third term that stands in a contradictory relationship to the singularity of being and the pluriversality of knowing, and represents the negation of both. It is a state where uniqueness is erased and Otherness is rejected or absorbed into the same. The particularity of nothingness is the ideological space of ethnocentrism, where one's own culture is seen as the only valid one, and everything else is reduced to nothing. To formalize the relationship between these three terms, I have developed the following matheme: $1 \times \infty \div 0$. This is my politicization of Lacan's RSI, which stills honors his commitment to mathematizing psychoanalysis.

1 represents the singularity of being, $\times$ is the transversal relationship, and ∞ signifies the pluriversality of knowing, as an infinite world of Otherness. The multiplication symbolizes the subject's journey toward infinity. The division by zero (the particularity of nothingness) is a mathematical operation that voids the result, leading to a state of being undefined, which mirrors how ethnocentrism nullifies both the Subject (1) and the Other (∞), reducing everything to nothingness (0). In this matheme, zero represents the colonial void (the zone of nonbeing)—the structural point where the colonized subject is stripped of their ontological status. When we divide the infinite potential of the human spirit (∞) by this zero-point

of dehumanization, the result is not a defined value, but a systemic error or nullification. This formalizes how colonial logic treats the Other not as difference, but as an impossibility that must be managed or eliminated within Totality. The particularity of nothingness is neither the Buddhist *Śūnyatā* (emptiness)—which Hạnh (1998) conceives of as *interbeing*; his take on *pratītyasamutpāda* (dependent origination)—nor the existentialist anxiety theorized by Sartre (2003).

Anxiety is, of course, a Lacanian affect that does not lie (Soler, 2016), which is not only correlated with our sense of freedom as human subjects, but is also equal to Being as such. Instead, by nothingness I mean *the absence of difference*, following the (post)modern collapse of all "grand narratives" of history under the dominant hegemony of a particular cultural narrative (Lyotard, 1984): capitalism for Marx (1867/1978), colonialism and racism for Fanon (1952/1967), the repressive state apparatus for Althusser (1970/2014) and Davis (2015), Orientalism for Said (1978), Totality for Dussel (1985), modernity/coloniality for Quijano (2000), the modern world-system for Wallerstein (2004), authoritarianism for Chomsky (2005), liberalism for Losurdo (2005/2011), white patriarchy for Curry (2017), etc.

My conception of non-identity politics ($1 \times \infty$ and $\infty \times 1 = \infty$) is a move away from social identification, as the Imaginary basis for a divisive politics of sameness, wherein we all become dehumanized zeros. Subsequently, an internationalist politics of difference—that is, of *interknowing* and *interbeing*—is premised on two approaches to the commons: Symbolic alignment of desire (∞) and Real enjoyment (1). The former is the order of language and Law and the latter is the disorder of *lalangue* and *jouissance*. Whereas Symbolic alignment of desire around the commons is dialecticized through political economy, as the discursive organization of the social, Real enjoyment materializes through libidinal economy, as the traumatic disorganization of the psychic.

These are, in other words, the contours of an impossible republic (the moon) toward which liberation psychoanalysis (the finger) points. Flying metaphorically to the moon is what is at stake here. Writing (a psychoanalysis of the oppressed) is one metonym that can get us there: 1 (the finger) $\times$ ∞ (the moon). According to the Zen tradition, the following koan is attributed to the Buddha: "when the wise man points at the moon, the fool looks at the finger."

Here is my reframing of the koan following Lacan (2006): "a signifier [e.g., *writings*] represents a [*transmodern*] subject to another signifier [e.g., *liberation psychoanalysis*]" (p. 713). Or: *a* (impossible republic) $\rightarrow$ $\$$ (transmodern subject) $\rightarrow$ S_1 (writings) $\rightarrow$ S_2 (liberation psychoanalysis). From a Buddhist perspective, the impossible republic is akin to truth or enlightenment. But it is also the *objet a* (object-cause of desire) driving the transmodern subject's ($\$$) divine *jouissance*.

It goes without saying that *writing* has functioned as a master-signifier (S_1) throughout this text, birthing *liberation psychoanalysis* as a praxis: a decolonial know-how (S_2). Liberation psychoanalysis, however, is not a political science, but a *scientific politics*: *a hysterical science of interknowing* ($1 \times \infty$) and *an analytical ethics of interbeing* ($\infty \times 1$). My use of the multiplication symbol ($\times$) posits transversality as an alternative to Lacan's reliance on fantasy ($\lozenge$) as the subject's primary mechanism for a social link via being unconsciously tethered to the *objet a*—fantasy being, of course, a function of the sexual non-rapport (impotence) characterizing any impossible discourse.

Ideology is the trap that stems from over-relying on fantasy. As such, I am attempting to bracket ideology while being aware that fantasies must still be worked through and eventually traversed. The challenge facing any complex political system, even one structured holarchically like fractals, is the *problem of self-similarity* or the symptomatic repetition of certain patterns on multiple levels of society. This self-similar repetition is clearly a symptom of the drives and the libidinal economy of *jouissance* in the political unconscious. These self-similar repetitions in the structure of ideology (*qua* the master's discourse), for example, arise from a sociogenic feedback loop in response to phylogenesis (the biological evolution of homo sapiens) and ontogenesis (the psychosexual development of the subject).

Figure 16.2 illustrates the Sierpiński triangle, which is a classic fractal, whose key property is self-similarity, wherein the pattern of a triangle composed of three smaller triangles is repeated at every scale, thereby suggesting a recursive and nested relationship. This model posits that ethics, politics, and aesthetics are not independent fields. Each is built upon the same fundamental psychosocial building blocks: the Real, the Symbolic, and the Imaginary. For example, an ethical system is structured by its own set of laws (Symbolic), its self-image (Imaginary), and its

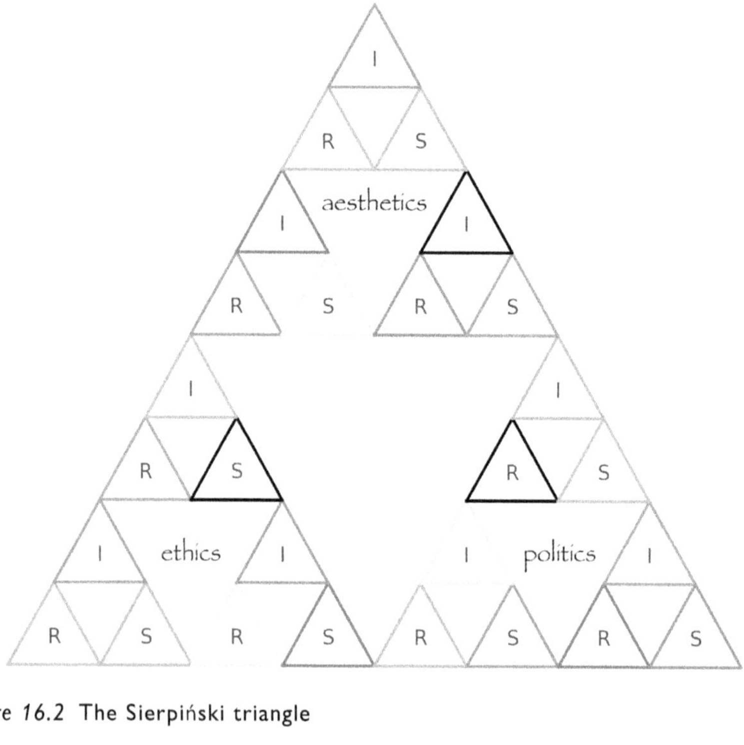

Figure 16.2 The Sierpiński triangle

unrepresentable trauma or lack (Real). Just as the Sierpiński triangle is formed by the recursive removal of central triangles, the transmodern subject is a subject-as-Real defined by the central lacuna of double-unconsciousness. Our decolonial praxis does not seek to fill this double negativity with fantasies or identifications; rather, it seeks to inhabit the empty space of the fractal, where anarchist power resides.

Furthermore, this fractal pattern implies that a self-similar relationship holds at every scale: the subject's ethics are governed by the RSI (Real, Symbolic, Imaginary) triad, as are the ethics of the community and the global ethical framework. This structure reaffirms that the personal is political, with each domain serving as a self-similar reflection of the others. Consequently, the most significant feature of this Sierpiński triangle is the empty, inverted triangle at its center. The dimensions of aesthetics, ethics, and politics are fundamentally knotted around this central lacuna; it is the topological site of the libidinal economy. This void does not merely house desire, but functions as the primordial source of the drive, where the subject's *jouissance* is both circumscribed by the Symbolic and contested within the Real of Exteriority.

Wahba (2022) argues that this empty, inverted triangle is currently plugged in with three ideological coordinates (religious fundamentalism, parasitic capitalism, and postmodern terrorism), which are dialectically interlinked within Totality (see Figure 16.3). Wahba's analysis suggests that our response from Exteriority must be in terms of three material coordinates that would comprise the Real of transmodernity: decolonial secularization, libertarian socialism, and radical humanism.

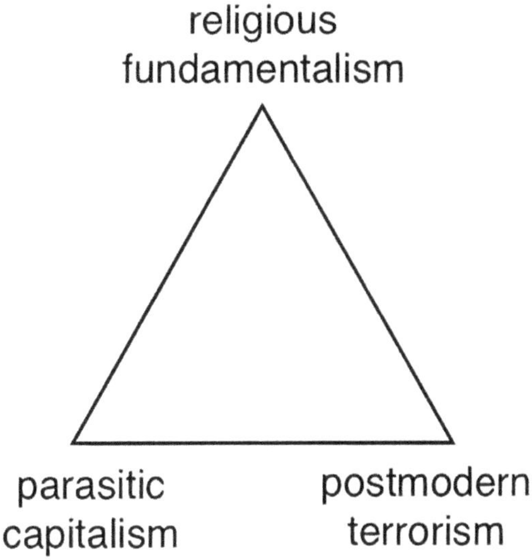

Figure 16.3 The Wahba triangle

The science of interknowing accounts for pluriversal epistemologies beyond the scope of scientism, specifically embracing not-knowing as a foundational ethic. Drawing from Nicholas of Cusa, this learned ignorance (*docta ignorantia*) allows the subject to navigate the Real without the violent (mis)translations of coloniality. It maintains a sharp distinction between the meta-consciousness of transmodernity and the anti-intellectualism of antimodernity, which it rejects as a form of structural, crass ignorance. Learned ignorance *vis-à-vis* Exteriority means that ~~the Other of the Other~~ is also barred. According to Nicholas Cusanus (1954), "the foundation for learned ignorance is the fact that absolute truth is beyond our grasp" (p. 10). No coincidence then that Wahba (2022) calls fundamentalists "the bearers of the Absolute Truth" (p. 29). In their dogmatic approach, fundamentalists confuse their paranoiac knowledge with the Absolute Truth, by "absolutizing what is relative" (Wahba, 2022, p. 45), and this is accomplished through literalism; therefore, we can label their absolutist position: death-driven crass ignorance.

However, psychoanalysis—the other side of death (absolute mastery)—is committed to life-driven learned ignorance, an epistemic relativist position, which is aligned with Wahba's (2022) notion of *secularization*. This epistemic relativist position was characterized by Lacan (1998) as the half-said (*mi-dire*) because while the unconscious is the site of truth *qua* desire, the ego is an agent of deception who resists truth. Therefore, secularization is what affords us interpretation, or what Ibn Rushd terms "metaphorical significance" (as cited in Wahba, 2022, p. 30).

For Ibn Rushd, metaphorical significance, or interpretation, was a Symbolic intervention, a signifierization of the Real. Literalism, on the other hand, is an Imaginary intervention, an imaginarization of the Real. Whereas interpretation opens up the space for the dialecticization of desire, literalism leads to nothing but aggressivity through narcissistic identification. As such, secularization affords us the possibility of *divine jouissance* through metaphorization, thereby bridging humanistic rationalism and radical empiricism, which include both esotericism, as a system of knowledge and practice, and direct mystical experiences.

In 2 Corinthians 3:6, Paul says, "for the letter kills, but the Spirit gives life." This was a succinct way of distinguishing between the Old Covenant (alienation through Mosaic Law) and the New Covenant (traversing the fantasy through unconditional love). More importantly, this distinction signifies the difference between the subject-as-demand, who is dominated by the Mosaic Other, and the subject-as-drive, who subjectifies Spirit. In the first instance, the Letter of the Law is the agent of Symbolic castration and, in the second instance, the Spirit of unconscious desire is a life-driven source of *jouissance*. Here we have arrived at a psychoanalytic distinction between what is progressive (divine) and what is regressive (mythic), which has political reverberations in terms of secular spirituality vs. religious fundamentalism. As I have written before, historical reason is (trans)rational, it integrates—transcends and includes—magical and mythic structures of consciousness.

Ancient Egyptians believed that the heart, as opposed to the brain or the mind, is the seat of consciousness, and this is clear not only from the weighing of the heart ceremony against the feather of Maat depicted in *The Book of Going Forth By Day*, but also from the fact that the heart was the only organ left in place during the mummification ritual. Furthermore, Ancient Egyptians had an understanding of the Symbolic order with the ethical system of Maat. The feather of Maat is the seat of the unconscious.

Maat reveals the following about the unconscious: the truth of one's desire and the justice of collective liberation are ruptures within a structure that attempts to manage and overcome *Isfet* (chaos). These subversive ruptures entail the traversal of the fantasy, that is, embracing one's singular lack and enjoying one's idiosyncratic symptom in spite of the Letter of Law. In Safouan's (2003) words: "If desire is flesh, the law is its bone" (p. 83), which can be represented using symbolic logic as follows: $(L \rightarrow D) \wedge (D \not\subseteq L)$. If there is a Law, then there is Desire. However, while the Law creates Desire, Desire is always in excess of the Law. This excess is the condition for surplus-*jouissance*. For instance, what forms of desire are afforded by the oldest living constitution in the world, the Iroquois Constitution, which is also known as the Great Law of Peace?

Consequently, a politics of interbeing reckons with nonbeing, or becoming, through an "ecological unconscious" sensibility that recognizes our "environmental reciprocity" with the biosphere (Roszak, 1992). This manifests as a kincentric ecological model, a transversal ethics that extends intersubjectivity to the non-human world of animals, vegetables, minerals, and things. Ancient Egyptians recognized this dimension of *the ecological unconscious* as *the discourse of the environmental Other*, and this is demonstrable from the grand architectural projects that were intentionally built in alignment with the cosmic order of Maat. In essence, the Ancient Egyptian praxis of divine cosmic alignment collapses the false dichotomy between nature (*Bios*) and culture (*Mythos*)—a modern dichotomy informing the logic of colonial difference. Furthermore, as Safouan (2003) argues, "the very idea of nature is a cultural idea" (p. 46) and "[t]he idea of a passage from Nature to Culture is a mythical idea" (p. 48). To have rules or taboos (e.g., prohibitions against murder, incest, etc.), however arbitrary they may seem, is a sign of culture.

The passion of learned ignorance is the liberation psychoanalytic alternative to "emotional ambivalence" (Freud, 1913a), which is the superimposition of the passions of love/hate: "In almost every case where there is an intense emotional attachment to a particular person we find that behind the tender love there is a concealed hostility in the unconscious. This is the classical example, the prototype, of the ambivalence of human emotions" (p. 70). According to Freud (1913a), this emotional ambivalence is a feature of the taboo, which is simultaneously "sacred" and "unclean" (p. 77), and applies in particular to the tyrannical figure of the primal father, who is hated and murdered by the band of brothers, yet also loved and mythically revered through the totem.

Learned ignorance represents a third path beyond the ambivalence dialectic; it is a passion, which is foundational for environmental reciprocity. Learned ignorance resolves the political problem of the One (father) and the Many (brothers) through complex affiliations, which are neither vertical (hierarchical) nor horizontal (flat), but complex: holarchical and transversal. Unlike a hierarchy, which operates through a top-down chain of command that subordinates the part to the (w) hole, a holarchy functions as a nested system of holons. Here, every autonomous collective, a (w)hole in itself, is simultaneously a vital component, a part, of the broader internationalist movement. This ensures that power remains distributed and transversal.

Identity politics is an ego politics (Mignolo, 2007), a non-politics: ego × ego. This non-politics often leads to populism, if not outright authoritarianism, and is always sustained by non-science: theo (Ⱥ) × theo (Ⱥ). Fascism is essentially an assault on truth (science) and justice (politics), wherein truth is replaced by *the will of the Leader* as *the ideology of the Nation*, which is realized through propaganda, anti-intellectualism, and the cult of personality; moreover, justice is replaced by *an authoritarian system of "us vs. them,"* wherein the Law is perverted to serve only the interests of the powerful with impunity; in such a system, acts of violence or oppression are *ipso facto* justified against so-called enemies of the state (Arendt, 2017; Eco, 1995).

For Mignolo (2007), identity, or social identification, must be based on politics and not the other way around, and delinking is how we realize a non-identity politics, particularly through a shift from a theo-/ego-politics to a geo-/body-politics of knowledge (p. 485). In Lacanian terms, delinking is a shift from ~~the Other~~ to the *objet a*, and from the ego to the unconscious, which is a process of subjective/objective destitution: alienation (demand) → separation (desire) → traversal of fantasy (drive).

In sum, decoloniality follows the psychoanalytic logic of unconscious desire, as opposed to ideological fantasy; therefore, it is not an end, but rather a means for actualizing the discourse of transmodernity. What is this discourse about? Transmodernity is about collective liberation as opposed to individual freedom—your freedom vs. mine. What does collective liberation look like in practice? Collective liberation is the praxis of desiring and enjoying the commons, as driven by historical reason. What, then, of the traumatic Real of transmodernity? That is the transmodern subject, who is a singular being in solidarity with other comrades in the spirit of pluriversality (cf. Nancy, 2000)! This quantum leap, from the singular to the pluriversal, is liberation psychoanalysis, a transversal ethic that prefigures *the aesthetic zone of becoming* through *an internationalist politics of difference*. As Safouan (2003) reminds us, "Between two subjects, there is only speech or death" (p. 31).

In *Yeats and Decolonization*, Said (1990) argues that whereas nationalism is the first moment of resistance to colonialism and imperialism, liberation is the second moment of resistance. Said echoes Fanon, and writes that liberation is "a transformation of social consciousness beyond national consciousness" (p. 83). History shows that nationalist independence, or political decolonization, does not guarantee psychic, social, and/or economic forms of decolonization.

As such, for Said, liberation transcends both the "metaphysics of essences" (p. 82) and "the nativist impasse" (p. 85), which are ahistorical romantic fantasies about the origin of one's nationalist identity. Nativism is a necessary feature of any decolonization movement that seeks national independence; however, national culture is a means to an end: collective liberation. When national culture becomes an end in itself, the outcome is often a reactionary politics (nationalism) premised on regressive fantasies that conflate decoloniality with antimodernity.

Liberation requires, according to Said, "a decent admixture of secular skepticism" (p. 83), which entails transcending dogmatic discourses about ethnic purity toward a radical humanist praxis. In Said's view, this radical humanist praxis has been prefigured poetically by Aimé Césaire, and it comprises three liberatory moments: (1) overcoming "all the interdictions wedged in the recesses of [our] fervor" since (2) "no race has a monopoly on beauty, on intelligence, on strength and there is room for everyone at the convocation of conquest" with the knowledge that (3) "the sun turns around our earth lighting the parcel designated by our will alone" (p. 85).

The first moment is a reference to psychic decolonization, that is, overcoming internalized oppression. The second moment is a rejection of essentialism (national consciousness) and an affirmation of pluriversalism (social consciousness); as such, it is the transmodern or analectical moment of social decolonization *qua* the international. The third moment concerns economic decolonization *vis-à-vis* politics and libido. In sum, the third moment of liberation affords us a theoretical and practical marriage between Marxism and Lacanianism, wherein the transmodern/decolonial subject-as-drive subjectifies the cause of their existence through libertarian socialist forms of desire and enjoyment (i.e., the commons): *from each according to their ability, to each according to their needs.*

Unlike Fanon (1961/2004), I do not think that "violence is a cleansing force" (p. 51). I prefer the path of revolutionary nonviolence with the understanding, of course, that violence may sometimes be necessary, but always requires justification as a means to an end: power. Fanon (1961/2004) dismisses nonviolence as "a creation of the colonial situation" (p. 23), which is false because history shows that, in addition to anticolonial violence, nonviolence can also be revolutionary and decolonial, as exemplified by Mohandas Gandhi, Thích Nhất Hạnh, and Martin Luther King Jr., among others (cf. Ayyash, 2024; Butler, 2020; Chenoweth & Stephan, 2011; Jackson, Llewellyn, Leonard, Gnoth, & Karena, 2020; King, 2007; Lawson Jr., 2024; Mutalemwa & Trochemowitz, 2024; Nepstad, 2011; Qumsiyeh, 2010; Vinthagen, 2015). It is easy, from the comfort and distance of a contemporary theoretical position, to idealize and romanticize Fanon's (1961/2004) description of decolonization as being "always a violent event" (p. 1), a statement written in the context of the Algerian War of Independence. However, Fanon died before experiencing postcolonial Algeria, which he would have found disappointing, based on his warnings in *The Wretched of the Earth* chapter on "The Trials and Tribulations of National Consciousness."

Simone de Beauvoir's (1948) *Ethics of Ambiguity* prefigures Freire's position in *Pedagogy of the Oppressed* (1970/2000), by twenty years, regarding the equivalence between oppression and dehumanization, on the one hand, and liberation and humanization, on the other hand. De Beauvoir writes, "In order for a liberating action to be a thoroughly moral action, it would have to be achieved through a conversion of the oppressors: there would then be a reconciliation of all freedoms" (p. 104).

Freire (1970/2000) echoes de Beauvoir when he claims, "Liberation is thus a childbirth, and a painful one. The man or woman who emerges is a new person, viable only as the oppressor–oppressed contradiction is superseded by the humanization of all people" (p. 49), or when he argues, "Conversion to the people requires a profound rebirth" (p. 61). Both existentialist thinkers acknowledge a limitation regarding their radical humanist ideal of liberation: the problem of "bad faith" (de Beauvoir) or "false generosity" (Freire), particularly as far as the oppressors are concerned.

Their resolution, therefore, is for the oppressed to act ethically in order to creatively seize the means of liberation. How? For Freire, "The naming of the world, which is an act of creation and re-creation, is not possible if it is not infused with love. Love is at the same time the foundation of dialogue and dialogue itself" (p. 89). Freire describes love as "an act of courage" and "a commitment to others" (p. 89). In other words, dialogue *qua* love is the condition for true generosity, that is, authentic comradeship with the oppressed.

For de Beauvoir, it is a question of the oppressed projecting themselves into the future through an ethical commitment to a creative project:

> The finite is nothing if it is not its transition to the infinite; the death of an individual is not a failure if it is integrated into a project which surpasses the limits of life … in the class, in the Socialist state.
>
> (p. 111)

To put it differently, de Beauvoir is gesturing toward the existentialist abyss of freedom at the heart of human subjectivity, wherein we have the power to act ethically and to create meaning through our creative projects—with the caveat that ethical actions, even in the colonial situation, are tragically ambiguous or antonymous (i.e., beyond good and evil).

In other words, oppression is dehumanizing and must be transcended ethically through liberation praxis, as the humanization of both the oppressors and the oppressed. The end of apartheid in South Africa serves as an imperfect model of restorative justice through truth and reconciliation. Similarly, there are numerous examples of Palestinian nonviolent resistance from the civil disobedience and mass action of the First Intifada (1987–1993) to the Boycott, Divestment, and Sanctions (BDS) tactics. These concrete examples align the ethics of ambiguity and the pedagogy of the oppressed with Coulthard's (2014) place-based Indigenous decolonial praxis of "grounded normativity," his alternative to the liberal politics of recognition. For Coulthard, recognition is an abstraction rooted in coloniality because it is essentially the negation of difference, the assimilation of Exteriority into Totality.

Therefore, liberation praxis realizes *the humanization of all people* not through recognition but through *reconciliation*, which entails the (re)construction of ontology as a politics of interbeing and epistemology as a science of interknowing.

Consequently, while Fanon is excellent at providing a sociogenic diagnostic of colonialism and how detrimental it is in terms of its material and ideological effects on colonized subjects, his writings do not prescribe a concrete political program regarding the actualization of a critical "national consciousness" after political decolonization, which would lead to the social realization of a "new humanism." In taking this stance, I risk the same critique I level at Fanon; yet, I prefer the vulnerability of falsifiable claims to the safety of dogmatic idol-worship.

History shows that, after political decolonization, postcolonial nation-states continue to struggle with the nationalist consciousness. Furthermore, because coloniality is a theory of violence and oppression, I believe decoloniality must be the exact opposite, a theory of (non)violence and liberation—with the caveat that Benjamin's notion of *divine violence*, as embodied in the proletarian general strike, is worth retaining in our liberation praxis. Idealizing violence, be it revolutionary or not, turns it into an end in itself and can never guarantee anything constructive, as far as power is concerned. Liberation is a praxis, whose goal is actualizing the kind of power that can guarantee truth and justice. Oppression is the denial of truth and justice, the negation of desire and reason, which is accomplished through the violent force of dehumanization.

In *Why War?*, Freud's correspondence with Albert Einstein, he argues, "Wars will only be prevented with certainty if [hu]mankind unites in setting up a central authority to which the right of giving judgement upon all conflicts of interest shall be handed over" (Freud, 1933, p. 207). He sees this potential in the League of Nations, which is the predecessor to the United Nations, but he concedes, even in 1933, that it lacks the necessary power for exerting this authority to end wars. Furthermore, Freud considers the possibility that wars will not end "until Communist ways of thinking have found universal acceptance," wherein brute force is replaced by "the force of ideas" (p. 208), or "the dictatorship of reason" (p. 213). For Freud, this a concrete utopian path, which must be fortified by bringing Eros into play against Thanatos (p. 212). The destructive death drive will always lead to war, as the culmination of the conflict between egos, a narcissism of minor differences, but the creative life drive diverts aggressivity through unconscious sublimation and "encourages the growth of emotional ties between men [and women]" (p. 212). Freud describes two kinds of emotional ties: (1) love and (2) identification. The latter, for him, structures human society and produces what he terms the "community of feeling" (p. 212). What is decolonial liberation but the actualization of this life-driven community of feeling, wherein violence is "overcome by the transference of power to a large unity … held together by emotional ties between its members" (p. 205)? This is what Gilman-Opalsky (2020) calls "the communist power of love," which sublates unconscious desire and historical reason.

Decoloniality is the theoretical framework for the practical processes of decolonization (see Figure 16.4), which are of two kinds, material and ideological, but can be broken down further into four types (the first two being material and the last

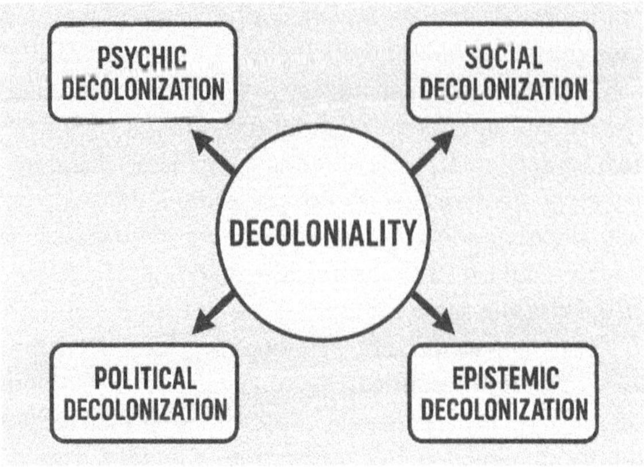

Figure 16.4 Decoloniality

two being ideological): political decolonization, economic decolonization, psychic decolonization, and social decolonization. Furthermore, there are four forms of decoloniality, which inform the different types of decolonization, and they include: the decoloniality of power, the decoloniality of knowledge, the decoloniality of being, and the decoloniality of nature.

Political decolonization is the most recognized type of decolonization, associated in particular with the decolonization of Asia and Africa between 1945 and 1960. Political decolonization refers to the political independence of postcolonial nation-states; however, as Nkrumah (1965) shows, the recent history of political decolonization was not accompanied by economic decolonization, a situation that he characterizes as neo-colonial. Furthermore, there is also the question of social decolonization, which has not been realized as a result of the postcolonial bourgeoisie's hold on power not through civic legitimation but through a hegemony overshadowed by the terror of sub-oppressive force—that is, the repressive state apparatus.

Finally, the practice of psychic decolonization informs the other three types of decolonization because it is about working through the internalization of oppression, which leads to the replication of oppression as an external structure. The decoloniality of being characterizes psychic decolonization through what I have referred to as liberation psychoanalysis and radical humanism. The decoloniality of power typifies political and social decolonizations by means of my conceptions of anarchist power and secular spirituality. And the decolonialities of knowledge and nature animate economic decolonization via libertarian socialism and kincentric ecology.

Safouan (2004) writes, "in its very essence *desire is a defense*" (p. 55, emphasis in original). In other words, the question of desire is what cause is worth defending? Safouan adds that desire is "*a defense against the desire of the Other*" (p. 55, emphasis in original). Therefore, *jouissance* is a question of subjectifying the cause. As such, the liberated *subject-as-drive* sublates both the oppressed *subject-as-demand* and the oppressive *subject-as-desire*.

The oppressed subject is dehumanized by the particular demand of the oppressed Other of the Other, a demand for Imaginary (mis)recognition, which leads to a politics of refusal. Demanding recognition for one's humanity from the oppressive Other implies the foreclosure of the oppressed Other of the Other, which is alienating, to say the least, and speaks to the problem of internalizing oppression and the subsequent trap of sub-oppression.

Furthermore, the oppressive subject is dehumanized by the Symbolic desire of the oppressive Other for freedom—a death-driven desire, since it is grounded in a narcissistic and aggressive form of legalistic freedom for oneself and one's tribe only. The oppressive Other's death-driven desire is a source of *mythic jouissance*, as the universal enjoyment of oppression and violence, wherein the oppressor disavows their dehumanization under the delusion of being exceptional. This false exceptionality is then projected onto the oppressed Other of the Other, thereby positioning oppressed subjects in an extra-legal state of exception, wherein any form of dehumanization is possible. According to this oppressive logic, the oppressed and the oppressors are *separate but 'equal'*—that is, equal in theory, but not in practice.

In conclusion, the transmodern subject is the subject-as-Real, who defends the cause of liberation as a life-driven source of divine *jouissance*. Decoloniality, then, is the pluriversal enjoyment of the object of liberation (the commons), whose subjectification consists of a radical humanist praxis: the traversal of the dehumanizing fantasy of oppression.

(Post)colonial oppression is an ideological fantasy that sustains the discursive-practices of (post)modern violence, which are framed as an end in themselves that require no justification. This failure to mediate beyond the exchange of death is symptomatic of the nation-state form with its necrophilic investments in ethno-nationalism and authoritarianism. To rupture this cycle, we must displace the State's hierarchical model of power with holarchical anarchist power—a fractal geometry of social organization that remains open to the Real, beyond Totality.

This is why we must prefigure other political, ethical, and aesthetic formations along internationalist and libertarian socialist lines that afford us radical humanistic mediations through the gifts of Eros: speech (*Logos*), writing (*Graphē*), and action (*Praxis*). By reclaiming these gifts, we transform the void of the colonial unconscious into the decolonial lacuna of creative potential: *critical double-unconsciousness*. After all, violence is a means to an end, and always requires justification. The end is transmodern power, which necessitates decolonial legitimacy.

References

Abdouni, H. (2021). The First University in the World: Al-Quarawiyine University. *MAS Journal of Applied Sciences*, 8(8), 789–795.

Abraham, K. (1941). Amenhotep IV (Ikhnaton). *The Psychoanalytic Review* (1913–1957), 28, 544.

Abramson, J. B. (1984). *Liberation and its limits: The moral and political thought of Freud.* Beacon Press.

Abu-Lughod, L. (2002). Do Muslim women really need saving? Anthropological reflections on cultural relativism and its others. *American anthropologist*, 104(3), 783–790.

Adi, H. (2018). *Pan-Africanism: a history*. Bloomsbury.

Adonis (2003). *An introduction to Arab poetics*. Al Saqi.

Adams, G. (2012). Context in person, person in context: A cultural psychology approach to social-personality psychology. In K. Deaux & M. Snyder (Eds.), *The Oxford handbook of personality and social psychology* (1st ed., pp. 182–208). Oxford University Press.

Adams, G. (2019, April). Toward a decolonial psychology. *Global Insights Newsletter*. https://www.apa.org. https://www.apa.org/international/global-insights/decolonial-psychology

Adams, G., & Salter, P. S. (2010). A critical race psychology is not yet born. *Connecticut Law Review*, 43(5), 1355–1377.

Adams, G., Dobles, I., Gómez, L. H., Kurtiş, T., & Molina, L. E. (2015). Decolonizing psychological science: Introduction to the special thematic section. *Journal of Social and Political Psychology*, 3(1), 213–238. https://doi.org/10.5964/jspp.v3i1.564

Adeane, L. (1945). Psychoanalysis and government. *The Anarchist Library*.

Adler, N. (1992, August 27). Viewing the unconscious from another time and place [PDF document]. The Lacan School of Psychoanalysis.

Agamben, G. (1998). *Homo Sacer: Sovereign power and bare life*. Palo Alto, CA: Stanford University Press.

Agamben, G. (2000). *Means without end: Notes on politics*. University of Minnesota Press.

Ahad, B. S. (2010). *Freud upside down: African American literature and psychoanalytic culture*. University of Illinois Press.

Ahmed, S. (2004/2014). *The cultural politics of emotion*. Edinburgh University Press.

Ahmed, S. (2017). *Living a feminist life*. Duke University Press.

Akanbi, A. (2018, October 30). The problem with wokeness [Video]. *YouTube*. https://www.youtube.com/watch?v=_-WimRb2jXs

Akehurst, N. (2026, January 4). The US Is a Weakened and Dangerous Empire. *Jacobin*. https://jacobin.com/2026/01/us-trump-imperialism-decline-venezuela

Akhtar, S. (2005). *Freud along the Ganges*. Other Press.

Akpan, J. (2022). Unrootedness: a New Surface in the Lacanian Black Split Subject. *Human Arenas*, 7(3), 494–506.

Al-Azm, S. J. (2012). *Self-criticism after the defeat*. Saqi Books.

Alcoff, L. M. (2020). Lugones's world-making. *Critical Philosophy of Race*, *8*(1–2), 199–211.
Al-Khalili, J. (2011). *The house of wisdom: how Arabic science saved ancient knowledge and gave us the Renaissance*. Penguin.
Allen, T. W. (2012). *The invention of the white race (Volume 1): Racial oppression and social control*. Verso.
Almoghayer, M. O. (2024). *On The Pleasures of Living in Gaza: Remembering a Way of Life Now Destroyed*. OR Books.
Alpert, A. (2020, September 24). Philosophy's systemic racism. *Aeon*. = https://aeon.co/essays/racism-is-baked-into-the-structure-of-dialectical-philosophy
Altman, N. (2010). *The analyst in the inner city: Race, class, and culture through a psychoanalytic lens* (2nd edn). Routledge.
Althusser, L. (1970). Philosophy as a revolutionary weapon. *New Left Review*, (64), 3.
Althusser, L. (1970/2014). *On the reproduction of capitalism: Ideology and ideological state apparatuses* (pp. 232–72). Verso.
Amin, S. (2010). *Eurocentrism*. New York University Press.
Anderson, P. (1998). *The origins of Postmodernity*. Verso.
Anderson, W., Jenson, D., & Keller, R C. (Eds.) (2011). *Unconscious dominions*. Duke University Press.
Anon (2017, June 13). #AltWoke manifesto. *TripleAmpersand Journal (&&&)*. https://tripleampersand.org/alt-woke-manifesto/
Anthony, C. (1995). Ecopsychology and the deconstruction of whiteness. In T. Roszak, M.E. Gomes, & A.D. Kanner (Eds.), *Ecopsychology: Restoring the earth, healing the mind*. Counterpoint.
Apollon, W., & Feldstein, R. (1996). *Lacan, Politics, Aesthetics*. New York: State University New York Press.
Arendt, H. (1969, February 27). Reflections on violence. *The New York Review*. https://www.nybooks.com/articles/1969/02/27/a-special-supplement-reflections-on-violence/
Arendt, H. (2017). *The origins of totalitarianism*. Penguin.
Arendt, H. (2019). *The human condition*. University of Chicago Press.
Arfken, M. (2017). Marxism as a foundation for critical social psychology. In B. Gough (Ed.), *The Palgrave handbook of critical social psychology* (pp. 37–58). Palgrave.
Arnett, J. J. (2008). The neglected 95%: Why American psychology needs to become less American. *American Psychologist*, *63*(7), 602–614. https://doi.org/10.1037/0003-066X.63.7.602
Aron, L., & Starr, K. (2013). *A psychotherapy for the people: Toward a progressive psychoanalysis*. Routledge.
Asaad, T. (2015). Sleep in Ancient Egypt. In S. Chokroverty & M. Billiard (Eds.), *Sleep medicine: A comprehensive guide to its development, clinical milestones, and advances in treatment*. Springer.
Asad, T. (2003). *Formations of the secular: Christianity, Islam, modernity*. Stanford University Press.
Asad, T., Brown, W., Butler, J., & Mahmood, S. (2009). *Is critique secular? Blasphemy, injury, and free speech*. The Townsend Center for the Humanities.
Ayouch, T. (2024). *La race sur Le divan*. ANACAONA.
Ayyash, M. M. (2024). Anticolonial Violence and Decolonial Liberation. *International Politics*, 61(4), 881–887.
Azibo, D. A. (1996). *African psychology in historical perspective and related commentary*. Africa Research and Publications.
Bakan, D. (1958/1975). *Sigmund Freud and the Jewish mystical tradition*. Beacon Press.
Balibar, É., & Wallerstein, I. (1988/1991). *Race, nation, class: Ambiguous identities*. Verso.
Bamyeh, M. A. (2009). *Anarchy as order: The history and future of civic humanity*. Rowman & Littlefield.

Barratt, B. B. (2011). Ignacio Martín-Baró's 'Writings for a Liberation Psychology.'; forum: inspiring psychoanalytic writing. *Psycho-analytic Psychotherapy in South Africa*, 19(2), 121–134.

Barthes, R. (1980). *Camera lucida: Reflections on photography*. Farrar, Straus, & Giroux.

Bastani, A. (2019). *Fully automated luxury communism*. Verso.

Basu Thakur, G. (2020). *Postcolonial lack: Identity, culture, surplus*. State University New York Press.

Basu Thakur, G. (2021). Fanon's "zone of nonbeing": Blackness and the politics of the Real. In S. George & D. Hook (Eds.), *Lacan and race: Racism, identity and psychoanalytic theory*. Routledge.

Bay Area Equity Atlas. (n.d.). *Indigenous populations in the Bay Area*. https://bayareaequityatlas.org/about/indigenous-populations-in-the-bay-area

Baudrillard, J. (1994). *Simulacra and simulation*. University of Michigan Press.

Baum, B. (2015). Decolonizing critical theory. *Constellations*, 22(3), 420–434. https://doi.org/10.1111/1467-8675.12169

Beaumont-Thomas, B. (2023, December 26). Kanye West apologises to Jewish community for 2022 antisemitic remarks. *Guardian*. https://www.theguardian.com/music/2023/dec/26/kanye-west-apologises-to-jewish-community-for-2022-antisemitic-remarks

Benjamin, W. (1921/1996). Critique of violence. In M. Bullock & M. W. Jennings (Eds.), *Selected writings, Volume 1: 1913–1926*. Harvard University Press.

Benjamin, W. (1935/2008). *The work of art in the age of its technological reproducibility, and other writings on media*. Harvard University Press.

Bennett, P. W. (2010). Wilhelm Reich's early writings on work democracy: A theoretical basis for challenging fascism then and now. *Capitalism Nature Socialism*, 21(1), 53–73.

Benslama, F. (2009). *Psychoanalysis and the challenge of Islam*. University of Minnesota Press.

Ben Slama, R., & Beshara, R. K. (2024). Psychoanalysis in Egypt: A problem of non-accession. *International Journal of Applied Psychoanalytic Studies*, 21(3), e1881.

Berger, J. (1972). *Ways of seeing*. Penguin.

Berger, P. L. (1979). *The heretical imperative: Contemporary possibilities of religious affirmation*. Anchor Books.

Bernal, M. (1987). *Black Athena (Vol 1)*. Rutgers University Press.

Bedirian, R. (2021, July 1). The Armenian photographer who captured life in Gaza on camera. *The Armenian Mirror-Spectator*. https://mirrorspectator.com/2021/07/01/the-armenian-photographer-who-captured-life-in-gaza-on-camera/

Beshara, R. K. (2016). The psychological construction of reality: An essay in the Buddhist psychology of knowledge. *International Journal of Peace Studies*, 21(1), 71–95.

Beshara, R. K. (2017). Cutting through false dualisms: Transformative social change as a transmodern moral framework for critical psychological research. *International Journal of Qualitative Methods*, 16(1), 1609406917705956.

Beshara, R. K. (2018). Decolonizing Psychoanalysis/Psychoanalyzing Islamophobia. In I. Parker & S. Siddiqui (Eds.), *Islamic psychoanalysis and psychoanalytic Islam: Cultural and clinical dialogues*. Routledge.

Beshara, R. K. (2019a). *Decolonial psychoanalysis: Towards critical Islamophobia studies*. Routledge.

Beshara, R. K. (Ed.). (2019b). *A critical introduction to psychology*. Nova Science Publishers.

Beshara, R. K. (2020, September). The importance of Freudo–Lacanian psychoanalysis to liberation praxis. *Stillpoint*. https://stillpointmag.org/articles/the-importance-of-freudo-lacanian-psychoanalysis/

Beshara, R. K. (2021a). *Freud and Said: Contrapuntal psychoanalysis as liberation praxis*. Palgrave.

Beshara, R. K. (Ed.). (2021b). *Critical psychology praxis: Psychosocial non-alignment to modernity/coloniality*. Routledge.

Beshara, R. K. (2022). A liberation psychoanalytic account of racism. *Awry: Journal of Critical Psychology*, *3*(1), 77–94.
Beshara, R. K. (2023). *A Psychoanalytic Biography of Ye: The Legacy of Unconditional Love*. Cambridge Scholars Publishing.
Beshara, R. K. (2024a). Engaged Buddhist Praxis and Critical Psychology. *Annual Review of Critical Psychology*, 17, 26–45.
Beshara, R. K. (2024b). *Transmodern Cinema and Decolonial Film Theory: A Study of Youssef Chahine's Al-Masir*. Bloomsbury.
Bhabha, H. K. (1994). *The location of culture*. Routledge.
Bhambra, G. K., Last, A., Mayblin, L., & Tilley, L. (2018). Global social theory: Building resources. *Area*, 51(4), 816–819. https://doi.org/10.1111/area.12479
Bhatia, S. (2018). *Decolonizing psychology: Globalization, social justice, and Indian youth identities*. Oxford University Press.
Bhattacharya, T. (Ed.). (2017). *Social reproduction theory: Remapping class, Recentering oppression*. Pluto Books.
Blauner, R. (1969). Internal colonialism and ghetto revolt. *Social problems*, 16(4), 393–408.
Bloch, E. (1986). *The principle of hope*. MIT Press.
Boal, A. (1979). *Theater of the oppressed*. Pluto Press.
Boeck, D. (2014). Kanye Omari West: Visions of Modernity. In *The Cultural Impact of Kanye West* (pp. 209–228). New York: Palgrave Macmillan.
Bollas, C. (2015). Psychoanalysis in the age of bewilderment: On the return of the oppressed. *The International Journal of Psychoanalysis*, 96(3), 535–551.
Bollas, C. (2021). *Three characters: Narcissist, borderline, manic depressive*. Phoenix Publishing House.
Boni, L., & Mendelsohn, S. (2021). *Le vie psychique du racisme*. éditions la découverte.
Borradori, G. (2003). *Philosophy in a time of terror: Dialogues with Jurgen Habermas and Jacques Derrida*. University of Chicago Press.
Bosteels, B. (2012). *Marx and Freud in Latin America: politics, psychoanalysis, and religion in times of terror*. Verso.
Bou Ali, N. (2020). *Psychoanalysis and the Love of Arabic: Hall of Mirrors*. Edinburgh University Press.
Boutebal, S. (2020). For a Fertile Dialogue between Decolonial Theory and Psychoanalysis. *Research in Psychoanalysis*, (2), 165–175.
Bracher, M. (1993). *Lacan, discourse, and social change: A psychoanalytic cultural criticism*. Cornell University Press.
Brave Heart, M. Y., Chase, J., Elkins, J., & Altschul, D. B. (2011). Historical trauma among Indigenous Peoples of the Americas: Concepts, research, and clinical considerations. *Journal of Psychoactive Drugs*, *43*(4), 282–290. https://doi.org/10.1080/02791072.2011.628913
Brennan, T. (2021). *Places of mind: a life of Edward Said*. Bloomsbury.
Brentano, F. (1874/2012). *Psychology from an empirical standpoint*. Routledge.
Brentano, F. (1977). *The psychology of Aristotle: In particular his doctrine of the active intellect*. University of California Press.
Brickman, C. (2018). *Race in psychoanalysis: Aboriginal populations in the mind*. Routledge.
Bricmont, J. (2005). *Humanitarian imperialism: Using human rights to sell war*. New York University Press.
brown, a. m. (2020). *We will not cancel us: And other dreams of transformative justice*. AK Press.
Brown, N., & Ford, D. (2021, October 5). Teaching politically and the problem of Afropessimism. *Monthly Review Online*. https://mronline.org/2021/10/05/teaching-politically-and-the-problem-of-afropessimism/
Brown, T. (2018). Celebrate women's suffrage, but don't whitewash the movement's racism. *American Civil Liberties Union*. https://www.aclu.org/news/voting-rights/celebrate-womens-suffrage-dont-whitewash-movements-racism

Bryan, C. P. (Trans.). (1931). *The Papyrus Ebers*. D. Appleton and Company.
Burden-Stelly, C. (2020). Modern U.S. racial capitalism. *Monthly Review*. https://monthlyreview.org/2020/07/01/modern-u-s-racial-capitalism/
Burmah, L. S. (2021). The curious cases of cancel culture [Master's thesis]. https://scholarworks.lib.csusb.edu/cgi/viewcontent.cgi?article=2440&context=etd
Burman, E. (2008). *Deconstructing developmental psychology* (3rd ed.). Routledge.
Burnham, C. (2022). Can We Decolonize Lacan? Indigenous Origins of the Split Subject. In *Psychoanalysis, Politics, Oppression and Resistance* (pp. 50–66). Routledge.
Burton, M., & Kagan, C. (2009). Towards a really social psychology: Liberation psychology beyond Latin America. In M. Montero & C. C. Sonn (Eds.), *Psychology of liberation: Theory and applications* (pp. 51–72). Springer.
Burton, M., & Osorio, J. M. F. (2011). Introducing Dussel: The philosophy of liberation and a really social psychology. *Psychology in Society*, (41), 20–39.
Bush, G. W. (2001, September 21). Text of George Bush's speech. *Guardian*. https://www.theguardian.com/world/2001/sep/21/september11.usa13
Butler, J. (1990/1999). *Gender trouble: Feminism and the subversion of identity*. Routledge.
Butler, J. (2004). *Precarious life: the powers of mourning and violence*. Verso.
Butler, J. (2020). *The force of nonviolence: An ethico-political bind*. Verso Books.
Bynum, E. B. (2012). *The African unconscious*. Cosimo.
Cajete, G. (2000). *Native science: Natural laws of interdependence*. Clear Light.
Camfield, D. (2016). Elements of a historical-materialist theory of racism. *Historical Materialism*, 24(1), 31–70. https://doi.org/10.1163/1569206x-12341453
Capra, F. (1996). *The web of life: A new scientific understanding of living systems*. Anchor.
Carlson, M. (Ed.). (2005). *The Arab Oedipus: Four Plays from Egypt and Syria*. Segal Theatre Center Publications.
Casid, J. H. (2015). *Scenes of projection: recasting the enlightenment subject*. University of Minnesota Press.
Cassin, B. (2019). *Jacques the Sophist: Lacan, Logos, and Psychoanalysis*. Fordham University Press.
Charisma, T. (2021). Trauma porn and the commercialisation of Black pain. *tmrw*. https://www.tmrwmagazine.com/news/trauma-pornand-the-commercialisation-of-black-pain
Chen, J. (2017, October 2). Kanye West and David Bowie: Music's Most WTF Conspiracy Theories, Explained. *Rolling Stones*. https://www.rollingstone.com/music/music-news/kanye-west-and-david-bowie-musics-most-wtf-conspiracy-theories-explained-196893/
Chen, K. H. (2010). *Asia as method: Toward deimperialization*. Duke University Press.
Cheng, A. A. (2001). *The melancholy of race: Psychoanalysis, assimilation, and hidden grief*. Oxford University Press.
Chenoweth, E., & Stephan, M. J. (2011). *Why civil resistance works: The strategic logic of nonviolent conflict*. Columbia University Press.
Chiesa, L. (2007). *Subjectivity and otherness: A philosophical reading of Lacan*. MIT press.
Chomsky, N. (2005). *On anarchism*. AK Press.
Chotiner, I. (2020, July 22). Thomas Chatterton Williams on Race, Identity, and "Cancel Culture". *New Yorker*. https://www.newyorker.com/news/q-and-a/thomas-chatterton-williams-on-race-identity-and-cancel-culture
Ciccariello-Maher, G. (2017). *Decolonizing dialectics*. Duke University Press.
Clark, J. P. (2022). *The impossible community: Realizing communitarian anarchism*. PM Press.
Clark, K. B., & Clark, M. P. (1947). Racial identification and preference in Negro children. In T. M. Newcomb & E. L. Hartley (Eds.), *Readings in social psychology* (pp. 169–178). Henry Holt and Co.
Clark, M. D. (2020). DRAG THEM: A brief etymology of so-called "cancel culture". *Communication and the Public*, 5(3–4), 88–92. https://doi.org/10.1177/2057047320961562

Clemens, J. (2013). *Psychoanalysis is an Antiphilosophy*. Edinburgh University Press.

Cohn, J. (2010). Sex and the anarchist unconscious: A brief history. *Sexualities*, 13(4), 413–431.

Collins, P. H. (1990/2000). *Black feminist thought: Knowledge, consciousness, and the politics of empowerment*. Routledge.

Comas-Díaz, L., Hall, G. N., & Neville, H. A. (2019). Racial trauma: Theory, research, and healing: Introduction to the special issue. *American Psychologist*, 74(1), 1.

Combahee River Collective. (1977). The Combahee River Collective statement. https://www.blackpast.org/african-american-history/combahee-river-collective-statement-1977/

Connell, R. (2007). *Southern theory: The global dynamics of knowledge in social science*. Polity Press.

Copjec, J. (1989). The Orthopsychic subject: Film theory and the reception of Lacan. *October*, 49, 53–71. doi:10.2307/778733

Copjec, J. (2025). *Cloud: Between Paris and Tehran: Kiarostami/Corbin/Lacan*. MIT Press.

Coulthard, G. S. (2014). *Red skin, white masks: Rejecting the colonial politics of recognition*. University of Minnesota Press.

Crenshaw, K. (1989). Demarginalizing the intersection of race and sex: A Black feminist critique of antidiscrimination doctrine, feminist theory, and antiracist politics. *University of Chicago Legal Forum*, 1.

Crowley, A. (1909). *Liber AL vel Legis*. ΘΕΛΗΜΑ. A.:A.:

Cudworth, E., & Hobden, S. (2010). Anarchy and anarchism: towards a theory of complex international systems. *Millennium*, 39(2), 399–416.

Curry, T. J. (2009). Will the real CRT please stand up? The dangers of philosophical contributions to CRT. *The Crit: A Critical Legal Studies Journal*, 2(1), 1–47.

Curry, T. J. (2017). *The man-not: Race, class, genre, and the dilemmas of Black manhood*. Philadelphia, PA: Temple University Press.

Curry, T. J. (2018). Killing boogeymen: Phallicism and the misandric mischaracterizations of Black males in theory. *Res Philosophica*, 95 (2), 235–272.

Curry, T. J. (2021a). Decolonizing the intersection: Black Male Studies as a critique of intersectionality's indebtedness to subculture of violence theory. In R. K. Beshara (Ed.), *Critical psychology praxis: Psychosocial non-alignment to modernity/Coloniality*. Routledge.

Curry, T. J. (2021b). II—Must There Be an Empirical Basis for the Theorization of Racialized Subjects in Race-Gender Theory? In *Proceedings of the Aristotelian Society* (Vol. 121, No. 1, pp. 21–44). Oxford University Press.

Cusanus, N. (1954). *Of learned Ignorance*. Routledge.

Cutrone, C. (2023). *The death of the millennial left: Interventions: 2006–2022*. Sublation Press.

Curtis, A. (2004). *The power of nightmares*. BBC.

Cybulska, E. M. (2019). Nietzsche: Bipolar disorder and creativity. *Indo-Pacific Journal of Phenomenology*, 19(1), 51–63.

Dadlani, M. B. (2020). Queer use of psychoanalytic theory as a path to decolonization: A narrative analysis of Kleinian object relations. *Studies in Gender and Sexuality*, 21(2), 119–126.

Dalal, F. (2006). Racism: Processes of detachment, dehumanization, and hatred. *The Psychoanalytic Quarterly*, 75(1), 131–161.

Danto, E. A. (2005). *Freud's free clinics: Psychoanalysis & social justice, 1918–1938*. Columbia University Press.

Darwish, M. (2024, January). Israel's war on Palestinian culture (R. K. Beshara, Trans.). *Ebb*, (1).

Datong, H. (2008). *La chine sur Le divan*. Plon.

Davids, M. F. (2011). *Internal racism: A psychoanalytic approach to race and difference*. Palgrave.

Davis, A. Y. (2015). *Freedom is a constant struggle: Ferguson, Palestine, and the foundations of a movement*. Haymarket Books.

Davis, A. Y., & Martínez, E. (1993, May 12). Building coalitions of people of color. *Center for Cultural Studies*. https://culturalstudies.ucsc.edu/inscriptions/volume-7/angela-y-davis-elizabeth-martinez/

Day, R. J. (2005). *Gramsci is dead: Anarchist currents in the newest social movements*. Pluto Books.

De Beauvoir, S. (1948). *The ethics of ambiguity*. Open Road Media.

Debord, G. (1967/2018). *Society of the spectacle*. Black & Red.

De Chardin, P. T. (2004). *The future of man*. Image.

De Courson, H., & El-Maghreby, A. (1997). *Mozart l'Égyptien (CD)*. Virgin Classics.

De Geus, M. (2014). Peter Kropotkin's anarchist vision of organization. *Ephemera*, 14(4), 853–871.

DeLeon, L. (1994). Embracing anarchy: Network organizations and interorganizational networks. *Administrative Theory & Praxis*, 234–253.

Deleuze, G., & Guattari, F. (1983). *Anti-Oedipus: Capitalism and schizophrenia*. University of Minnesota Press.

Delgado, R., & Stefancic, J. (2012). *Critical race theory: An introduction* (2nd ed.). New York University Press.

De Man, P. (1979). Autobiography as De-facement. *mln*, 94(5), 919–930.

DeMause, L. (1982). *Foundations of psychohistory*. Creative Roots.

Derrida, J. (1981). *Dissemination*. Athlone Press.

Derrida, J. (1987). *The post card: From Socrates to Freud and beyond*. University of Chicago Press.

Derrida, J. (1991). Geopsychoanalysis: "… and the rest of the world". *American Imago*, 48(2), 199–231.

Derrida, J. (1997). *Of grammatology* (G. C. Spivak, Trans.). Johns Hopkins University Press.

Derrida, J. (2003). Jacques Derrida keynote response to Étienne Balibar [Video]. *YouTube*. https://youtu.be/LfXdYefgKjw?si=wwEXX5NlsaCxmu42

Derrida, J. (2005). *The politics of friendship*. Verso.

Dershowitz, A. (2020). *Cancel culture: The latest attack on free speech and due process*. Simon & Schuster.

De Sousa Santos, B. (2001). Toward an epistemology of blindness: Why the new forms of ceremonial adequacy neither regulate nor emancipate. *European Journal of Social Theory*, 4(3), 251–279.

De Sousa Santos, B. (2007). Beyond abyssal thinking: From global lines to ecologies of knowledges. *Review* (Fernand Braudel Center), 30(1), 45–89.

De Sousa Santos, B. (2014). *Epistemologies of the South: Justice against epistemicide*. Routledge.

Di Cesare, D. (2017). The "Jewish Question" and the Question of Being: Heidegger before and after 1945. *Journal of Aesthetics and Phenomenology*, 4(2), 173–182.

Diouf, S. A. (1998). *Servants of Allah: African Muslims enslaved in the Americas*. New York University Press.

Dolar, M. (2008). Freud and the Political. *Unbound–Harvard Journal of the Legal Left*, 4, 15–29.

Du Bois, W. E. (1903/2007). *The souls of Black folk*. Oxford University Press.

Dunbar-Ortiz, R. (2014). *An Indigenous Peoples' history of the United States*. Beacon Press.

Dunker, C. (2011). *The Constitution of the psychoanalytic clinic: A history of its structure and power*. Routledge.

Dunworth, L. (2025, August 19). Gary Oldman says "the world's gone to shit" since David Bowie died. *NME*. https://www.nme.com/news/music/gary-oldman-says-the-worlds-gone-to-shit-since-david-bowie-died-3885803

Duran, E., & Duran, B. (1995). *Native American postcolonial psychology*. State University New York Press.
Duran, E., Duran, B., Heart, M. Y. H. B., & Horse-Davis, S. Y. (1998). Healing the American Indian soul wound. In *International handbook of multigenerational legacies of trauma* (pp. 341–354). Boston, MA: Springer US.
Dussel, E. (1985). *Philosophy of liberation*. Orbis Books.
Dussel, E. (1995). *The Invention of the Americas. Eclipse of "the Other" and the Myth of Modernity*. Continuum.
Dussel, E. (2002). World-System and "Trans"-modernity. *Nepantla: Views from South, 3*(2).
Dussel, E. (2012). Transmodernity and interculturality: An interpretation from the perspective of philosophy of liberation. *Transmodernity: Journal of Peripheral Cultural Production of the Luso-Hispanic World*, 1(3).
Dussel, E. (2013). *Ethics of liberation: In the age of globalization and exclusion* (E. Mendieta, C. P. Bustillo, Y. Angulo, & N. Maldonado-Torres, Trans.). Duke University Press.
Dzielska, M. (1995). *Hypatia of Alexandria*. Harvard University Press.
Eco, U. (1995). *Ur-fascism. The New York review of books*, 22, 12–15.
Eisenstadt, S. N. (Ed.). (2000). *Multiple modernities*. Routledge.
Eisler, R. (2011). *The chalice and the blade: Our history, our future*. HarperCollins.
El-Kilany, E., & Elgammal, I. (2019). Dream incubation tourism: The resurrection of ancient Egyptian heritage of sleep temples. *International Journal of Heritage and Museum Studies*, 1(1), 93–106.
Elmessiri, A. M. (1977). *The land of promise: A critique of political Zionism*. North American Publishing.
El Shakry, O. (2017). *The Arabic Freud: Psychoanalysis and Islam in Modern Egypt*. Princeton University Press.
Endres, F. (2022). The Crux of the Matter: Lacan's Dialectical Materialism of the Signifier. *European Journal of Psychoanalysis*, 9(1).
Eng, D. L., & Han, S. (2018). *Racial melancholia, racial dissociation: On the social and psychic lives of Asian Americans*. Duke University Press.
Engels, F. (1877/1939). *Anti-Dühring* (E. Burns, Trans.). New York International Publishers.
Engels, F. (1880/2020). *Socialism: Utopian and scientific*. Foreign Languages Press.
Engels, F. (2004). *The origin of the family, private property and the state*. Resistance Books.
Enriquez, V. G. (1986). Kapwa: A Core Concept in Filipino Social Psychology. In V. G. Enriquez (Ed.), *Philippine world-view*. Institute of Southeast Asian.
Escobar, A. (2007). Worlds and knowledges otherwise: The Latin American modernity/coloniality research program. *Cultural Studies*, 21(2–3), 179–210.
Estes, N. (2019). *Our history is the future: Standing rock versus the Dakota Access Pipeline, and the long tradition of Indigenous resistance*. Verso.
Evzonas, N. (2020). Prologue: Queering and decolonizing psychoanalysis. *Psychoanalytic Inquiry*, 40(8), 571–578.
Eyers, T. (2011). Lacanian materialism and the question of the Real. *Cosmos & History*, 7(1), 155–166.
Fanon, F. (1952/1967). *Black skin, white masks* (R. Philcox, Trans.). New York: Grove Press.
Fanon, F. (1959/1965). *A dying colonialism* (H. Chevalier, Trans.). Monthly Review Press.
Fanon, F. (1961/2004). *The wretched of the earth* (R. Philcox, Trans.). Grove Press.
Fenichel, O. (1967). Psychoanalysis as the nucleus of a future dialectical-materialistic psychology. *American Imago*, 24(4), 290–311.
Federici, S. (2019). *Re-enchanting the world: Feminism and the politics of the Commons*. PM Press.
Ferenczi, S. (1949). Confusion of the tongues between the adults and the child—(The language of tenderness and of passion). *International Journal of Psychoanalysis*, 30(4), 225–230.

Fermin, J. C. C. (2023). A Stethoscope to the World: The Fault Lines Between Marxism and Afropessimism. *International Labor and Working-Class History*, *104*, 183–208.

Ffytche, M. (2011). *The foundation of the unconscious. Schelling, Freud and the birth of the modern psyche*. Cambridge University Press.

Fink, B. (1997). *A clinical introduction to Lacanian psycoanalysis: Theory and technique*. Harvard University Press.

Fink, B. (2017). *The Lacanian subject: Between language and Jouissance*. Princeton University Press.

Finkelstein, N. (2023a). *I'll burn that bridge when I get to it: Heretical thoughts on identity politics, cancel culture and academic freedom*. Sublation Press.

Finkelstein, N. (2023b, October 26). Nat Turner in Gaza. *Norman G. Finkelstein*. https://www.normanfinkelstein.com/nat-turner-in-gaza/

Fleet, X. V. (2023a). *Mao's America: A survivor's warning*. Center Street.

Fleet, X. V. (2023b, October 1). 'Wokeism' is Maoism with American characteristics [Video]. *Fox News*. https://www.foxnews.com/video/6338194059112

Fletcher, J. (2016). *The story of Egypt*. Simon & Schuster.

Foucault, M. (1977). *Language, counter-memory, practice: Selected essays and interviews*. Cornell University Press.

Foucault, M. (1980). *Power/Knowledge: Selected interviews and other writings, 1972–1977*. C. Gordon (Ed.). Vintage.

Fox, D. (2011). Anarchism and psychology. *Theory in Action*, 4(4), 31–48.

Fox, J. (2023). *Down the drain*. Simon & Schuster.

Fredrickson, G. M. (2002/2015). *Racism: A short history* (2nd ed.). Princeton University Press.

Freire, P. (1970/2000). *Pedagogy of the oppressed* (M. B. Ramos, Trans.). Continuum.

Freire, P., & Macedo, D. (1987). *Literacy: Reading the word and the world*. Routledge.

Freud Museum London (2019). *Between Oedipus and the Sphinx: Freud and Egypt*. Freud Museum.

Freud, S. (1899/1950). *The Interpretation of Dreams* (J. Strachey, Trans). Basic Books.

Freud, S. (1910/1916). *Leonardo da Vinci: A psychosexual study of an infantile reminiscence* (A. A. Brill, Trans.). Moffat, Yard.

Freud, S. (1913a). *Totem and taboo: Resemblances between the psychic lives of savages and neurotics*. Beacon Press.

Freud, S. (1913b). "The claims of psycho-analysis to scientific interest." In *The Standard Edition of the Complete Psychological Works of Sigmund Freud, Volume XIII (1913–1914): Totem and Taboo and Other Works*. Hogarth Press.

Freud, S. (1917). Mourning and melancholia. In *On the History of the Psycho-Analytic Movement, Papers on Metapsychology and Other Works*. Hogarth Press.

Freud, S. (1920/1961). *Beyond the Pleasure Principle* (J. Strachey, Trans.). W. W. Norton.

Freud, S. (1923/1961). *The Ego and the Id*. W. W. Norton

Freud, S. (1926). *The Question of lay analysis*. W. W. Norton.

Freud, S. (1927). *The future of an illusion*. W. W. Norton.

Freud, S. (1930/1961). *Civilization and its discontents*. W. W. Norton.

Freud, S. (1933). Why war? In J. Strachey (Ed.), *New introductory lectures on psychoanalysis and other works*. Hogarth Press.

Freud, S. (1939/1967). *Moses and monotheism*. Hogarth Press.

Freud, S., & Breuer, J. (1895/2004). *Studies in hysteria*. Penguin.

Freud, S., & Fliess, W. (1985). *The complete letters of Sigmund Freud to Wilhelm Fliess, 1887–1904*. J. M. Masson (Ed.). Belknap Press.

Fromm, E. (1955). *The sane society*. Routledge.

Frosh, S. (2010). *Psychoanalysis outside the clinic: Interventions in psychosocial studies*. Bloomsbury.

Frosh, S. (2020). Psychoanalysis as decolonial Judaism. *Psychoanalysis, Culture & Society*, 25, 174–193.

Fukuyama, F. (1989). The end of history? *The National Interest*, 16, 3–18. https://www.jstor.org/stable/24027184

Galtung, J. (1969). Violence, peace, and peace research. *Journal of Peace Research*, 6(3), 167–191.

Galatzer-Levy, R. M. (2017). *Nonlinear psychoanalysis: Notes from forty years of chaos and complexity theory*. Routledge.

Gambino, C., & Göransson, L. (2016). Redbone. On *"Awaken, My Love!"*. Glassnote.

Gandhi, M. K. (2001). *Non-violent resistance (Satyagraha)*. Dover.

Ganjipour, A. (2021, October 15). Islam and Politics: A History of Ambivalence. *K.* https://k-larevue.com/en/islam-and-politics-a-history-of-ambivalence-interview-with-anoush-ganjipour/

Garba, T., & Sorentino, S. (2020). Slavery is a metaphor: A critical commentary on Eve Tuck and K. Wayne Yang's "Decolonization is not a metaphor". *Antipode*, 1–19. https://doi.org/10.1111/anti.12615

Gardiner, A. H. (Ed.). (1935). *Hieratic papyri in the British Museum: Vol. I*. British Museum.

Garvey, M. (2004). *Selected writings and speeches of Marcus Garvey*. Dover.

Gaztambide, D. J. (2019). *A people's history of psychoanalysis: From Freud to liberation psychology*. Lexington Books.

Gaztambide, D. J. (2023). Robert K. Beshara, Freud and Said: Contrapuntal Psychoanalysis as Liberation Praxis. *Psychoanalysis and History*, 25(1), 104–108.

Gaztambide, D. J. (2024). *Decolonizing Psychoanalytic Technique: Putting Freud on Fanon's Couch*. Springer.

Gaztambide, D. J., Feliciano-Graniela, F. E., Luiggi-Hernández, J., & Escobar, E. V. M. (2024). Decolonizing psychoanalysis: Anti-Blackness, coloniality, and a new premise for psychoanalytic treatment. In L. Comas-Díaz, H. Y. Adames, & N. Y. Chavez-Dueñas (Eds.), *Decolonial psychology: Toward anticolonial theories, research, training, and practice* (pp. 321–343). American Psychological Association. https://doi.org/10.1037/0000376-014

Gebser, J. (1986). *The ever-present origin*. Ohio University Press.

Gendzier, I. L. (1976). Psychology and Colonialism: Some Observations. *Middle East Journal*, 30(4), 501–515.

George, S. (2016). *Trauma and race: A Lacanian study of African American racial identity*. Baylor University Press.

George, S., & Hook, D. (Eds.). (2021). *Lacan and race: Racism, identity and psychoanalytic theory*. Routledge.

Gheorghe, C. (2022). Decolonization, Polarization, Psychoanalysis, Privilege: Toward a Cosmopolitan and Culturally Intelligent Psychotherapist. *In Analysis*, 6(2), 128–133.

Gherovici, P. (2003). *The Puerto Rican syndrome*. Other Press.

Gherovici, P., & Christian, C. (Eds.) (2018). *Psychoanalysis in the barrios: Race, class, and the unconscious*. Routledge.

Gilley, B. (2023). *The case for colonialism*. New English Review Press.

Gilman, S. L. (1993). *Freud, race, and gender*. Princeton University Press.

Gilman-Opalsky, R. (2020). *The communism of love: An inquiry into the poverty of exchange value*. AK Press.

Gilmore, R. W. (2020, June 1). Geographies of racial capitalism with Ruth Wilson Gilmore – An antipode Foundation film [Video]. *YouTube*. https://youtu.be/2CS627aKrJI?si=dZ221gyZRH70pxzO

Gilroy, P. (2002). *Against race: Imagining political culture beyond the color line*. Belknap Press.

Glissant, É. (1990/1997). *Poetics of relation*. University of Michigan Press.

Goldman, E. (2017). *Anarchism and other essays*. Active Distribution.
Gonzalez, L. (2021). Racism and sexism in Brazilian culture. *WSQ: Women's Studies Quarterly*, 49(1), 371–394
Gordon, L. R. (2008). *An introduction to Africana philosophy*. Cambridge University Press.
Gordon, L. R. (2015). *What Fanon said: A philosophical introduction to his life and thought*. Fordham University Press.
Gordon, L. R. (2025). Psychoanalysis as a decolonial practice. *Psychoanalysis, Culture & Society*. https://doi.org/10.1057/s41282-024-00513-w
Gould, R. R. (2014). Sumud: The Palestinian Art of Existence. *World Policy Journal*, 31, 99–106.
Graeber, D. (2004). *Fragments of an anarchist anthropology*. Prickly Paradigm.
Graeber, D., & Wengrow, D. (2021). *The dawn of everything: A new history of humanity*. Farrar, Straus and Giroux.
Gray, L. (1995). Shamanic counseling and ecopsychology. In T. Roszak, M. E. Gomes, & A. D. Kanner (Eds.), *Ecopsychology: Restoring the earth, healing the mind* (pp. 172–182). Sierra Club Books.
Greenshields, W. (2017). *Writing the structures of the subject: Lacan and topology*. Palgrave Macmillan.
Greimas, A. J., & Rastier, F. (1968). The interaction of semiotic constraints. *Yale French Studies*, (41), 86–105.
Grosfoguel, R. (2013). The structure of knowledge in westernised universities: Epistemic racism/sexism and the four genocides/epistemicides. *Human Architecture: Journal of the Sociology of Self-Knowledge*, 1, 73–90.
Grosfoguel, R., Oso, L., & Christou, A. (2015). 'Racism', intersectionality and migration studies: Framing some theoretical reflections. *Interrogating Intersectionalities, Gendering Mobilities, Racializing Transnationalism*, 22(6), 635–652. https://doi.org/10.4324/9781315226491-1
Gross, O. (1913). Overcoming cultural crisis. *The Anarchist Library*.
Gross, O. (1919/1977). Protest and Morality in the Unconscious. *New German Critique*, (10), 105–109.
Guattari, F. (2015). *Psychoanalysis and transversality: Texts and interviews 1955–1971*. MIT Press.
Guerra, A. M. C. (2024). Crypt. *Psychotherapy & Politics International*, 22(2), 1–25.
Guérin, D. (2017). *For a libertarian communism*. PM Press.
Gutierrez, G. (1973). *A theology of liberation: History, politics, and salvation*. Orbis Books.
Gutermann-Jacquet, D. (2015). The Impossible-to-write and the Unreadable. *Research in Psychoanalysis*, 19(1), 43–49.
Hallaq, W. (2012). *The impossible state: Islam, politics, and modernity's moral predicament*. Columbia University Press.
Hạnh, T. N. (1993). *Love in action: Writings on nonviolent social change*. Parallax Press.
Hạnh, T. N. (1998). *The heart of the Buddha's teaching: Transforming suffering into peace, joy, and liberation*. Harmony.
Hạnh, T. N. (2016). *At home in the world: Stories and essential teachings from a monk's life*. Parallax Press.
Hanna, M. (2025). *The Future of Egyptology*. Diwan.
Hannah-Jones, N. (2019, August 18). Introduction to the "1619 Project". *New York Times Magazine*.
Hanrahan, M. (2013). Writing Symptomatically. *Paragraph*, 36(2), 206–222.
Haque, A. (2004). Psychology from Islamic perspective: Contributions of early Muslim scholars and challenges to contemporary Muslim psychologists. *Journal of Religion & Health*, 43(4), 357–377. https://doi-org.nnmc.idm.oclc.org/10.1007/s10943-004-4302-z

Harding, S. (1993). Rethinking standpoint epistemology: What is "strong objectivity"? In L. Alcoff & E. Potter (Eds.), *Feminist epistemologies*. Routledge.
Harjo, S. & Waititi, T. (Producers) (2021). *Reservation Dogs* (TV series). FX on Hulu.
Harper's Magazine Foundation (2020, July 7). A Letter on Justice and Open Debate *Harper's Magazine*. https://harpers.org/a-letter-on-justice-and-open-debate/
Hartnack, C. (2001). *Psychoanalysis in colonial India*. Oxford.
Hartman, S. V. (1997). *Scenes of subjection: Terror, slavery, and self-making in nineteenth-century America*. Oxford University Press.
Hartung, B. (1983). Anarchism and the Problem of Order. *Mid-American Review of Sociology*, 8(1), 83–101.
Hatem, N. (2020). On the Untranslatable in Psychoanalysis. *Psychoanalytic Inquiry*, 40(8), 622–632.
Hassan, I. (1971). POSTmodernISM. *New Literary History*, *3*(1), 5–30. https://doi.org/10.2307/468378
Hau'ofa, E. (1994). Our Sea of Islands. *The Contemporary Pacific*, *6*(1), 148–161. http://www.jstor.org/stable/23701593
Hayat, S. (2023). *Revolutionary republicanism: Participation and representation in 1848 France*. Routledge.
Hecq, D. (2008). Writing the unconscious: Psychoanalysis for the creative writer. *TEXT*, *12*(2). https://doi.org/10.52086/001c.31697
Hendrix, J. S. (2015). *Unconscious thought in philosophy and psychoanalysis*. Palgrave Macmillan.
Henriques, J., Hollway, W., Urwin, C., Venn, C., & Walkerdine, V. (1984/1998). *Changing the subject: Psychology, social regulation and subjectivity* (2nd ed.). Routledge.
Henry, P. (2000). *Caliban's reason: Introducing Afro-Caribbean philosophy*. Psychology Press.
Hesse, B. (2023). Derrida's Black accent. *ReOrient*, 8(1), 4–33.
Heuer, G. M. (2016). *Freud's 'Outstanding' colleague/Jung's 'Twin brother': The suppressed psychoanalytic and political significance of Otto Gross*. Routledge.
H. D. (2012). *Tribute to Freud* (2nd ed.). New Directions.
Hickley, C. (2024, January 3). Caspar David Friedrich: His rise from obscurity to fame. *The Art Newspaper*. https://www.theartnewspaper.com/2024/01/03/caspar-david-friedrich-his-rise-from-obscurity-to-fame
Hoffman, D. H. (2015). Report to the special committee of the Board of Directors of the American Psychological Association: Independent review relating to APA ethics guidelines, national security interrogations, and torture. *Sidley Austin LLP*. https://www.apa.org/independent-review/revised-report.pdf
Homayounpour, G. (2012). *Doing psychoanalysis in Tehran*. MIT Press.
Homer (2002). *The Odyssey* (I. Johnston, Trans.). Perseus Digital Library. https://johnstoniatexts.x10host.com/homer/odysseyallpdf.pdf
Honigman, A. F. (2023, November 22). *Wanderer Above the Sea of Fog*. *Encyclopedia Britannica*. https://www.britannica.com/topic/Wanderer-Above-the-Sea-of-Fog
Hook, D. (2025). *Fanon, psychoanalysis, and critical Decolonial psychology: The mind of apartheid*. Routledge.
Hord, F. L., & Lee, J. S. (Eds.). (2016). *I am because we are: Readings in Africana philosophy* (2nd ed.). University of Massachusetts Press.
Horkheimer, M., & Adorno, T. W. (2002). *Dialectic of enlightenment*. Stanford University Press.
Horney, K. (1926). The flight from womanhood: the masculinity-complex in women, as viewed by men and by women. *International Journal of Psychoanalysis*, *7*, 324–339.
Hourigan, D. (2012). Postmodern anarchy in the modern legal psyche: Law, anarchy and psychoanalytic philosophy. *Griffith Law Review*, 21(2), 330–348.

Huntington, S. P. (1993, Summer). The Clash of Civilizations? *Foreign Affairs*, 72(3), 22–49.
Huston, J. (Director). (1962). *Freud: The Secret Passion* [Blu ray]. Kino Lorber.
Ingleby, D. (1985). Professionals as socializers: The 'psy complex'. *Research in Law, Deviance and Social Control*, 7, 79–109.
Iwuanyanwu, O. (2015). Jacques Lacan in Africa. In M. Nwosu & Obiwu (Eds.), *The critical imagination in African literature: Essays in honor of Michael J. C. Echeruo*. Syracuse University Press.
Jackson, R., Llewellyn, J., Leonard, G.M., Gnoth, A., & Karena, T. (Eds.). (2020). *Revolutionary nonviolence: Concepts, cases and controversies*. Bloomsbury.
James, C.L.R., Lee, G.C., & Castoriadis, C. (2006). *Facing reality*. Charles H. Kerr.
James, J. (2022). *In Pursuit of Revolutionary Love*. Divided Publishing.
Jameson, F. (1981). *The political unconscious: Narrative as a socially symbolic act*. Cornell University Press.
Jaynes, J. (1976). *The origin of consciousness in the breakdown of the bicameral mind*. Houghton Mifflin Harcourt.
Jensen, D. (2004). *The culture of make believe*. Chelsea Green Publishing.
Jones, A. [@RealAlexJones]. (2024, June 20). You are surrounded by lies [Tweet]. *X*. https://x.com/RealAlexJones/status/1804004063476170904
Kadalie, M. M. (2019). *Pan-African social ecology: Speeches, conversations, and essays*. On Our Own Authority!
Kader, H. A., & Beshara, R. K. (2023). Psychoanalysis in Egypt between an ambitious past and an uncertain future. *Psychoanalysis, Culture & Society*, 28(2), 324–338.
Kadri, A. (2023). *The accumulation of waste: A political economy of systemic destruction*. Brill.
Kakar, S. (2024). *The Indian jungle: Psychoanalysis and non-western civilizations*. Karnac Books.
Kant, I. (1781/1998). *Critique of pure reason*. Cambridge University Press.
Kapoor, I. (2020). *Confronting desire: Psychoanalysis and international development*. Cornell University Press.
Karenga, M. (2003). *Maat, the moral ideal in ancient Egypt: A study in classical African ethics*. Routledge.
Karson, M. (2021, August 9). The psychology of "Wokeism". *Psychology Today*. https://www.psychologytoday.com/us/blog/feeling-our-way/202108/the-psychology-wokeism
Katsafanas, P. (2016). *The Nietzschean self: Moral psychology, agency, and the unconscious*. Oxford University Press.
Keay, D. (1987). Aids, education and the year 2000. *Woman's Own*, 31, 8–10.
Kelley, E. (2022). Coping with Trauma: Evidence that Suggests the Ancient Egyptians used Transpersonal Psychology to Cope with Birth-Related Trauma. *History in the Making*, 15(1), 6–??.
*Kelley, R., & Burden-Stelly, C. (2021, March 30). Black and red: Socialism and Black liberation. *Verso*. https://www.versobooks.com/blogs/news/5040-black-and-red-socialism-and-black-liberation-with-robin-kelley-and-charisse-burden-stelly
Kessi, S. (2019). Towards a Decolonial psychology: Defining and confining symbols of the past. *Museum International*, 71(1–2), 80–87. https://doi.org/10.1080/13500775.2019.1638032
Keval, N. (2016). *Racist states of mind: Understanding the perversion of curiosity and concern*. Routledge.
Khader, S. J. (2019). *Decolonizing universalism: A transnational feminist ethic*. Oxford University Press.
Khader, S. (2024). *Faux feminism: Why we fall for white feminism and how we can stop*. Beacon Press.

Khan, A. (2018). Lacan and race. In A. Mukherjee (Ed.), *After Lacan: Literature, theory, and psychoanalysis in the twenty-first century* (pp. 148–164). Cambridge University Press.
Khanna, R. (2003). *Dark continents: Psychoanalysis and colonialism.* Duke University Press.
Khatib, R., McKee, M., & Yusuf, S. (2024). Counting the dead in Gaza: difficult but essential. *The Lancet*, 404(10449), 237–238.
Khatibi, A. (1983/2019). *Plural Maghreb: Writings on Postcolonialism.* Bloomsbury.
Khatibi, A. (1990). *Amour bilingue* [*Love in two languages*]. University of Minnesota Press.
Khatibi, A. (2016). *La mémoire tatoée* [Tattooed memory]. Editions L'Harmattan.
Kimmerer, R. W. (2013). *Braiding Sweetgrass: Indigenous wisdom, scientific knowledge and the teachings of plants.* Milkweed Editions.
King, M. E. (2007). *A quiet revolution: The first Palestinian intifada and nonviolent resistance.* Bold Type Books.
King Jr., M. L. (1991). *A testament of hope: The essential writings and speeches of Martin Luther King, Jr.* J. M. Washington (Ed.). HarperCollins.
King Jr., M. L. (2010). *Where do we go from here: Chaos or community?* Beacon Press.
Klein, T., & Vieira, J. (2024). Provocations from Amerindian perspectivism to psychoanalysis. *Psychotherapy & Politics International*, 22(2), 1–17.
Kolakowski, L. (1968). The concept of the left. In C. Oglesby (Ed.), *The new left reader.* Grove Press.
Kovačević, F. (2007). *Liberating Oedipus? Psychoanalysis as critical theory.* Lexington Books.
Kovel, J. (1986). Marx, Freud and the problem of materialism. *Dialectical Anthropology*, 179–188.
Krakauer, D. C. (2024). *The complex world: An introduction to the foundations of complexity science.* SFI Press.
Kropotkin, P. A. (1995). *The conquest of bread and other writings.* Cambridge University Press.
Lacan, J. (1966–1967). *The logic of phantasy* (C. Gallagher, Trans.) https://nosubject.com/images/4/49/THE-SEMINAR-OF-JACQUES-LACAN-XIV_logique_du_fantasme.pdf
Lacan, J. (1966/2006). *Écrits: The first complete edition in English* (B. Fink, Trans.). New York: W. W. Norton.
Lacan, J. (1973/2009). L'étourdit (C. Gallagher, Trans.). *Scilicet*, 4, 5–25.
Lacan, J. (1975/1988). *Freud's papers on technique.* W. W. Norton.
Lacan, J. (1975/1998). *On feminine sexuality: The limits of love and knowledge.* W. W. Norton.
Lacan, J. (1977–1978). *The moment to conclude* (C. Gallagher, Trans.). http://www.lacaninireland.com/web/wp-content/uploads/2014/03/Book-25-The-Moment-to-Conclude.pdf
Lacan, J. (1977/2004). *The four fundamental concepts of psycho-analysis* (A. Sheridan, Trans.). London, UK: Karnac Books.
Lacan, J. (1987). Television. *October*, 40, 6–50. https://doi.org/10.2307/778337
Lacan, J. (1991/2007). *The other side of psychoanalysis* (R. Grigg, Trans.). W. W. Norton.
Lacan, J. (2013). Lituraterre. *Continental Philosophy Review*, 46(2), 327–334.
Lacan, J. (2014). *Anxiety.* Polity.
Lacan, J. (2015). *Transference.* Polity.
Lacan, J. (2016). *The Sinthome.* Polity.
Lacan, J. (2018). *... or Worse.* Polity.
Lacan, J. (2025). *On a discourse that might not be a semblance.* Polity.
Laing, R. D. (1960). *The divided self: An existential study in sanity and madness.* Tavistock Publications.
LaMothe, R. (2023). Decolonizing Nature: Freud, the Ontological Rift and the Anthropocene Age. *Free Associations*, (90).

Lane, C. (Ed.). (1998). *The psychoanalysis of race*. Columbia University Press.
Latour, B. (1991). *We have never been modern*. Harvard University Press.
Lau, U. (2021). Between Fanon and Lacan: Rupturing spaces for the return of the oppressed. *Studies in Gender and Sexuality*, 22(4), 278–292.
Laubender, C. (2024). *The political clinic: Psychoanalysis and social change in the twentieth century*. Columbia University Press.
Lawson, J. M. (2024). *Revolutionary nonviolence: Organizing for freedom*. University of California Press.
Lazali, K. (2021). *Colonial trauma: A study of the psychic and political consequences of colonial oppression in Algeria*. Polity Press.
Leader, D. (2013). *Strictly bipolar*. Penguin.
Lees, J., & Cleminson, R. (2015). Retrieving the past for a usable present: Anarchism, psychoanalysis and revolutionary transformation in the early 20th century. *Psychotherapy and Politics International*, 13(2), 141–153.
Lehrer, R. (1994). *Nietzsche's presence in Freud's life and thought: On the origins of a psychology of dynamic unconscious mental functioning*. State University of New York Press.
Lehrman, P. R. (1940). Freud's contributions to science. *Harofe Haivri*, 1, 161–176.
Leipold, B. (2024). *Citizen Marx: Republicanism and the formation of Karl Marx's social and political thought*. Princeton University Press.
Lenin, V. (1917). *Imperialism: The highest stage of capitalism*. Wellred Books.
Lenti, G. (2014). *Psychoanalysis and complexity*. Nova Science.
Lentin, A. (2020). *Why race still matters*. John Wiley & Sons.
Lewis, S. (2022). *Abolish the family: A manifesto for care and liberation*. Verso Books.
Levin, M. R. (2021). *American Marxism*. Simon & Schuster.
Levinas, E. (1969). *Totality and infinity: An essay on exteriority*. Duquesne University Press.
Lévi-Strauss, C. (1961). *Tristes Tropiques*. Criterion Books.
Lieber, E. (2020). *The writing cure*. Bloomsbury.
Lindsay, J. A. (2022). *Race Marxism: The truth about critical race theory and praxis*. Independently published.
Lipson, C. S. (2004). Ancient Egyptian Rhetoric: It All Comes Down to Maat. In C. S. Lipson & R. A. Binkley (Eds.), *Rhetoric before and beyond the Greeks*. State University of New York Press.
Losurdo, D. (2005/2011). *Liberalism: A counter-history*. Verso.
Losurdo, D. (2021). *Nietzsche, the aristocratic rebel: Intellectual biography and critical balance-sheet*. Haymarket Books.
Losurdo, D. (2024). *Western Marxism: How It Was Born, How It Died, How It Can Be Reborn*. Monthly Review Press.
Lugones, M. (2007). Heterosexualism and the colonial/modern gender system. *Hypatia*, 22(1), 186–219.
Lukács, G. (1952/1981). *The destruction of reason* (P. Palmer, Trans.). International Library of Social and Political Thought.
Lundström, M. (2023). *Anarchist critique of radical democracy: The impossible argument* (2nd ed.). PM Press.
Luxemburg, R. (1913/2003). *The accumulation of capital*. Routledge.
Lyotard, J. (1984). *The postmodern condition: A report on knowledge*. University of Minnesota Press.
Lyotard, J. (1993). *Libidinal economy*. Indiana University Press.
Madhubuti, H. R. (1973). *From plan to planet: Life studies: The need for Afrikan minds and institutions*. Third World Press.
Magallanes, F. (2018). *Psychoanalysis, the Body, and the Oedipal Plot: A Critical Re-imaging of the Body in Psychoanalysis*. Routledge.
Malaguti, M. (2023, December 11). Wokeism, child of the union of Maoism and post-Marxism. *Centro Machiavelli*. https://www.centromachiavelli.com/en/2023/12/11/malaguti-conferenza-wokeismo/

Malatesta, E. (2015). *Life and ideas: The anarchist writings of Errico Malatesta*. PM Press.
Maldonado, C. E., & Mezza-Garcia, N. (2014). Anarchy and complexity. *E: CO*, 18(1), 52–73.
Maldonado-Torres, N. (2017). Frantz Fanon and the decolonial turn in psychology: From modern/colonial methods to the decolonial attitude. *South African Journal of Psychology*, 47(4), 432–441.
Maldonado-Torres, N., France, M. F. M., Suffla, S., Seedat, M., & Ratele, K. (2021). Fanon's decolonial transcendence of psychoanalysis. *Studies in Gender and Sexuality*, 22(4), 243–255.
Malherbe, N. (2023). Unconsciousness-raising: Considerations for liberation psychology, subjectivity, and reflexivity theory. *Psychoanalytic Dialogues*, 33(4), 456–474.
Malherbe, N. (2024). Anti-capitalist subjectivity: considerations of fantasy, (in)action, and solidarity building. *Subjectivity*, 1–20.
Malherbe, N. (2025). *Psychoanalytic liberation psychology: Anti-capitalist approaches*. Routledge.
Malone, K. R. (2000). Subjectivity and the address to the other. *Theory & Psychology*, 10(1), 79–86. https://doi.org/10.1177/0959354300010001602
Mamdani, M. (2005). *Good Muslim, bad Muslim: America, the Cold War, and the roots of terror*. Three Leaves Press.
Mamdani, M. (2022). *Neither settler nor native: The making and unmaking of permanent minorities*. Harvard University Press.
Manganyi, N. C. (2016). *Apartheid and the Making of a Black Psychologist: A memoir*. New York University Press.
Manganyi, N. C. (2019). *Being black in the world*. Wits University Press.
Mannoni, O. (1950/1990). *Prospero and Caliban: The psychology of colonization* (P. Powesland, Trans.). University of Michigan Press.
Marcuse, H. (1969). *An essay on liberation*. Beacon Press.
Marcuse, H. (2015). Liberation from the affluent society. In D. Cooper (Ed.), *The dialectics of liberation*. Verso Books.
Martín-Baró, I. (1996). *Writings for a liberation psychology*. Harvard University Press.
Marriott, D. S. (2021). *Lacan noir: Lacan and afro-pessimism*. London: Palgrave Macmillan.
Marx, K. (1859/1978). A contribution to the critique of political economy. In R. C. Tucker (Ed.), *The Marx–Engels reader* (2nd ed., pp. 3–6). W. W. Norton.
Marx, K. (1867/1978). *Capital, Volume One*. In R. C. Tucker (Ed.), The Marx–Engels reader (2nd ed., pp. 294–438). W. W. Norton.
Marx, K., & Engels, F. (1846). *The German ideology*. Marxists Internet Archive.
Marx, K., & Engels, F. (1848). *The communist manifesto*. Marxists Internet Archive.
Maslow, A. H. (1943). A theory of human motivation. *Psychological review*, 50(4), 370–396.
Massad, J. A. (2007). *Desiring Arabs*. University of Chicago Press.
Masson, J. M. (1984). *The assault on truth: Freud's suppression of the seduction theory*. Farrar, Straus and Giroux.
Matory, J. L. (2018). *The fetish revisited: Marx, Freud, and the gods Black people make*. Duke University Press.
Mbembe, A. (2001). *On the Postcolony*. University of California Press.
McGowan, T. (2007). *The Real gaze: Film theory after Lacan*. Albany, NY: State University of New York Press.
McGrath, S. J. (2012). *The dark ground of spirit: Schelling and the unconscious*. Routledge.
McGuire, W. (Ed.). (1973). *The Freud–Jung letters: The correspondence between Sigmund Freud and C.G. Jung*. Princeton University Press.
McKeown, N. (2011). Greek and Roman slavery. In G. Heuman & T. Burnard (Eds.), *The Routledge history of slavery* (pp. 19–34). Routledge.
McLuhan, M. (1962). *The Gutenberg galaxy: The making of typographic man*. University of Toronto Press.

McMahon, M. (2023). *The violence of the letter: Toward a theory of writing*. University of Michigan Press.
McWhorter, J. (2021). *Woke racism: How a new religion has betrayed Black America*. Penguin.
Medina, J. (2018). Resisting racist propaganda: Distorted visual communication and epistemic activism. *Southern Journal of Philosophy*, 56, 50–75.
Melzer, A. M. (2014). *Philosophy between the lines: The lost history of esoteric writing*. University of Chicago Press.
Merchant, C. (1980). *The death of nature: Women, ecology, and the scientific revolution*. HarperCollins.
Merleau-Ponty, M. (1968). *The visible and the invisible*. Northwestern University Press.
Meyer, B. C. (1967). *Joseph Conrad: A psychoanalytic biography*. Princeton University Press.
Mignolo, W. (2000). *Local histories/Global designs: Coloniality, subaltern knowledges, and border thinking*. Princeton University Press.
Mignolo, W. (2007). Delinking: The rhetoric of modernity, the logic of coloniality and the grammar of de-coloniality. *Cultural Studies*, 21(2–3), 449–514.
Miller, J.-A. (1988). Extimité. *Prose Studies*, 11(3), 121–131. https://doi.org/10.1080/01440358808586354
Miller, N., Hamilton, G., & Warren, M. (1992). *Handel's Messiah: A Soulful Celebration* (CD). Alliance.
Miller, P. L. (2010). Psychoanalysis as spirituality. *symplokē*, 18(1–2), 31–46.
Mitchell, J. (1974/2000). *Psychoanalysis and feminism: A radical reassessment of freudian psychoanalysis*. Basic Books.
Mitchell, W. J. T. (2012). *Seeing through race*. Harvard University Press.
Moghaddam, F. M. (1987). Psychology in the three worlds: As reflected by the crisis in social psychology and the move toward Indigenous third-world psychology. *American Psychologist*, 42(10), 912–920. https://doi.org/10.1037/0003-066x.42.10.912
Mohanty, C. T. (2003). *Feminism without borders: Decolonizing theory, practicing solidarity*. Duke University Press.
Morgan, H. (2021). *The work of whiteness: A psychoanalytic perspective*. Routledge.
Moyn, S. (2018, November 13). The alt-right's favorite meme is 100 years old. *New York Times*. https://www.nytimes.com/2018/11/13/opinion/cultural-marxism-anti-semitism.html
Mulvey, L. (1975). Visual pleasure and narrative cinema. *Screen*, 16(3), 6–18. doi:10.1093/screen/16.3.6
Musser, A. J. (2018). *Sensual excess: Queer femininity and Brown Jouissance*. New York University Press.
Mutalemwa, G., & Trochemowitz, S. (2024). Nonviolence as a Decolonial Principle: Limits and Possibilities of Mainstreaming Peace Studies in Africa. In *Peace as Nonviolence: Topics in African Peace Studies* (pp. 31–44). Springer Nature.
Nancy, J. (2000). *Being singular plural*. Stanford University Press.
Nandy, A. (1983). *The intimate enemy: Loss and recovery of self under colonialism*. Oxford University Press.
Nappalos, S. N. (2019). *Emergence and anarchism: A philosophy of power, action, and liberation*.
Nassar, I., Sheehi, S., & Tamari, S. (2022). *Camera Palaestina: Photography and Displaced Histories of Palestine*. Univ of California Press.
Needleman, S. (2021, December 19). Cornel West: Before the worms get your body. *The Blue and White*. https://www.theblueandwhite.org/post/cornel-west
Negri, A. (2023). *The common*. Polity.
Neiman, S. (2023). *Left is not woke*. John Wiley & Sons.

Nepstad, S. E. (2011). *Nonviolent revolutions: Civil resistance in the late 20th century*. Oxford University Press.
Newman, B. (Ed.). (1998). *Voice of the living light: Hildegard of Bingen and her world*. University of California Press.
Newman, S. (2004). Interrogating the master: Lacan and radical politics. *Psychoanalysis, culture & society*, 9(3), 298–314.
Newman, S. (2010). *Politics of Postanarchism*. Edinburgh University Press.
Newman, S. (2017). Anarchism and Psychoanalysis. In *Brill's Companion to Anarchism and Philosophy* (pp. 401–433). Brill.
Ng, E. (2022). *Cancel culture: A critical analysis*. Springer Nature.
Nichols, R. (2020). *Theft is property!: Dispossession and critical theory*. Duke University Press.
Niemuth, N., Mackaman, T., & North, D. (2019). The New York Times' 1619 project: A racialist falsification of American and world history. *World Socialist Web Site*.
Nietzsche, F. (1895/1990). *Twilight of idols and Anti-Christ*. Penguin.
Nietzsche, F.W. (1908/1975). *Ecce homo: How one becomes what one is* (R. J. Hollingdale, Trans.). Penguin Classics.
Nkrumah, K. (1965). *Neo-colonialism: The last stage of imperialism*. Thomas Nelson & Sons.
Nobus, D. (2016). Psychoanalytic violence: an essay on indifference in ethical matters. *Psychoanalytic Discourse*, 1(2), 1–20.
Norris, P. (2021). Cancel culture: Myth or reality? *Political Studies*, 71(1), 145–174. https://doi.org/10.1177/00323217211037023
Öcalan, A. (2022). *Beyond state, power, and violence*. PM Press.
Odin, S. (2025). *DT Suzuki on the Unconscious in Zen Art, Meditation, and Enlightenment*. State University of New York Press.
Oliver, K. (2004). *The colonization of psychic space: A psychoanalytic social theory of oppression*. University of Minnesota Press.
O'Neill, E. (1997). Disappearing ink: Early modern women philosophers and their fate in history. In J. A. Kourany (Ed.), *Philosophy in a feminist voice: Critiques and reconstructions* (pp. 17–62). Princeton University Press.
Ortigues, M. C., & Ortigues, E. (1966). *Oedipe Africain*. Librarie Plon.
Pandolfo, S. (2018). *Knot of the soul: Madness, psychoanalysis, Islam*. University of Chicago Press.
Pappé, I. (2007). *The ethnic cleansing of Palestine*. Simon & Schuster.
Patsalides, A. (1992, August 31). Palimpseste [PDF document]. The Lacan School of Psychoanalysis.
Parker, I. (1989). *The crisis in modern social psychology, and how to end it*. Routledge.
Parker, I. (1997). Discourse analysis and psychoanalysis. *British Journal of Social Psychology*, 36(4), 479–495. https://doi.org/10.1111/j.2044-8309.1997.tb01145.x
Parker, I. (1999). Critical psychology: Critical links. *Annual Review of Critical Psychology*, 1(1), 3–18.
Parker, I. (2001). Lacan, psychology and the discourse of the University. *Psychoanalytic Studies*, 3(1), 67–77. https://doi.org/10.1080/14608950020026854
Parker, I. (2003a). Jacques Lacan, barred psychologist. *Theory & Psychology*, 13(1), 95–115. https://doi.org/10.1177/0959354303013001764
Parker, I. (2003b). Discursive resources in the discourse unit. *Discourse Analysis Online*, 1(1), 1–11.
Parker, I. (2005). Lacanian discourse analysis in psychology. *Theory & Psychology*, 15(2), 163–182. https://doi.org/10.1177/0959354305051361
Parker, I. (2009). Critical psychology and revolutionary Marxism. *Theory & Psychology*, 19(1), 71–92. https://doi.org/10.1177/0959354308101420

Parker, I. (2010a). Psychosocial studies: Lacanian discourse analysis negotiating interview text. *Psychoanalysis, Culture & Society*, 15(2), 156–172. https://doi.org/10.1057/pcs.2009.21
Parker, I. (2010b). The place of transference in psychosocial research. *Journal of Theoretical and Philosophical Psychology*, 30(1), 17–31. https://doi.org/10.1037/a0019104
Parker, I. (2011). *Lacanian psychoanalysis: Revolutions in subjectivity*. Routledge.
Parker, I. (2014a). *Psychology after Lacan: Connecting the clinic and research*. Routledge.
Parker, I. (2014b). *Psychology after the unconscious: From Freud to Lacan*. Routledge.
Parker, I. (2022). *Radical Psychoanalysis: And Anti-capitalist Action*. Resistance Books.
Parker, I., & Pavón-Cuéllar, D. (Eds.). (2013). *Lacan, discourse, event: New psychoanalytic approaches to textual indeterminacy*. Routledge.
Parker, I., & Pavón-Cuéllar, D. (2021). *Psychoanalysis and revolution: Critical psychology for liberation movements*. 1968 Press.
Parker, I., & Siddiqui, S. (Eds.) (2019). *Islamic psychoanalysis and psychoanalytic Islam: Cultural and clinical dialogues*. Routledge.
Parry, G. A. (2016). Ecopsychology: Remembering the true source of our consciousness. *Cosmos and History: Journal of Natural and Social Philosophy*, 12(2), 226–236.
Pavón-Cuéllar, D. (2010). *From the conscious interior to an exterior unconscious: Lacan, discourse analysis, and social psychology*. Karnac Books.
Pavón-Cuéllar, D. (2017). *Marxism and psychoanalysis: In or against psychology?* Taylor & Francis.
Pavón Cuéllar, D. (2024). Decolonisation of psychoanalysis and mesoamerican conceptions of subjectivity. *Psychotherapy & Politics International, 22*(2), 1–14. https://doi.org/10.24135/ppi.v22i2.09
Pavón-Cuéllar, D., & Beshara, R. K. (2025). Psychoanalysis and colonialism: Introducing a special issue. *Psychoanalysis, Culture & Society*, 30(3), 441–458. https://doi.org/10.1057/s41282-025-00559-4
Pavón-Cuéllar, D., & González Equihua, E. E. (2013). Subversive psychoanalysis and its potential orientation toward a liberation psychology: From a Lacanian reading of Martín-Baró to a committed use of Jacques Lacan. *Theory & Psychology*, 23(5), 639–656.
Pavón-Cuéllar, D., & Guerra, A. M. (2024). Decolonisation and psychoanalysis. *Psychotherapy & Politics International*, 22(2), 1–6. https://doi.org/10.24135/ppi.v22i2.02
Pe-Pua, R. (2006). From decolonizing psychology to the development of a cross-Indigenous perspective in methodology. In U. Kim, K. Yang, & K. Hwang (Eds.), *Indigenous and cultural psychology: Understanding people in context* (pp. 109–137). Springer.
Pe-Pua, R., & Protacio-Marcelino, E. A. (2000). Sikolohiyang pilipino (Filipino psychology): A legacy of Virgilio G. Enriquez. *Asian Journal of Social Psychology*, 3(1), 49–71.
Peele, J. (Director) (2017). Film. *Get Out*. Universal Pictures.
Peterson, J. (2019, May 15). Equity: When the left goes too far. https://www.jordanbpeterson.com/blog-posts/equity-when-the-left-goes-too-far/
Pickren, W. (2020). Coloniality of being and knowledge in the history of psychology. In V. Balz & L. Malich (Eds.), *Psychologie und Kritik: Formen Der Psychologisierung nach 1945* (pp. 329–343). Springer-Verlag.
Pike, K. (2022, October 28). Mental health in Ancient Egypt. *Five on Friday: Musings on mental health*. https://kathypikephd.com/five-on-friday/mental-health-in-ancient-egypt/
Plato (2000). *The Republic*. Cambridge University Press.
Plato (2002). *Phaedrus* (R. Waterfield, Trans.). Oxford University Press.
Pluckrose, H., & Lindsay, J. A. (2020). *Cynical theories: How activist scholarship made everything about race, gender, and identity—and why this harms everybody*. Phstone Publishing.
Politzer, G. (1928/1994). *Critique of the foundations of psychology: The psychology of psychoanalysis*. Duquesne University Press.

Popper, K. (2013). *The open society and its enemies*. Princeton University Press.

Powell, C. (2023). Radical Complexity: Using Concepts from Complex Systems Theory to Think About Socialist Transformation. *New Proposals: Journal of Marxism and Interdisciplinary Inquiry*, 12(2), 34–39.

Powell, D. R. (2018). Race, African Americans, and psychoanalysis: Collective silence in the therapeutic situation. *Journal of the American Psychoanalytic Association*, 66(6), 1021–1049.

Prashad, V. (2012). *The poorer nations: A possible history of the Global South*. Verso.

Preciado, P. B. (2021). *Can the monster speak? Report to an Academy of psychoanalysts*. MIT Press.

Quijano, A. (1989). Paradoxes of modernity in Latin America. *International Journal of Politics, Culture, and Society*, 3(2), 147–177.

Quijano, A. (1993). Modernity, identity, and utopia in Latin America. *boundary 2*, 20(3), 140–155.

Quijano, A. (2000). Coloniality of power and Eurocentrism in Latin America. *Nepantia: Views from the South*, 1(3), 533–580.

Quijano, A. (2007). Coloniality and modernity/Rationality. *Cultural Studies*, 21(2–3), 168–178. https://doi.org/10.1080/09502380601164353

Qumsiyeh, M. B. (2010). *Popular resistance in Palestine: A history of hope and empowerment*. Pluto Press.

Ragland, E. (2004). *The logic of sexuation: From Aristotle to Lacan*. State University of New York Press.

Rahmat, A. F. (2020). Misrecognizing the Clinic: Towards a Planetary Psychoanalysis. *Free Associations*, (80), 70–89.

Rahmat, A. F. (2021). Treatment is geopolitical: On Lacan's decolonial clinic. *Psychoanalysis, Culture & Society*, 26(4), 535–547.

Rahmat, A. F. (2025). *Decolonization and psychoanalysis: The underside of signification*. Routledge.

Ratele, K. (2019). *The world looks like this from here: Thoughts on African psychology*. Wits University Press.

Rawley, J. A., & Behrendt, S. D. (1981/2005). *The transatlantic slave trade: A history* (2nd ed.). University of Nebraska Press.

Reed, A. Jr. (2022). *No politics but class politics*. W. B. Michaels (Ed.). ERIS.

Reed, I. (2024). America's Anti-Woke Hysteria Spreads. *CounterPunch*.

Reed, L. (2013, July 3). Lou Reed on Kanye West's Yeezus: 'It brings tears to my eyes'. *Guardian*. https://www.theguardian.com/music/2013/jul/03/lou-reed-kanye-west-yeezus

Reich, W. (1933/1946). *The mass psychology of fascism*. Farrar, Straus and Giroux.

Reich, W. (1934/2012). *Sex-pol: Essays, 1929–1934*. Verso.

Reik, T. (1948). *Listening with the third ear*. Farrar, Straus and Company.

Richards, G. (1997). *'Race', racism and psychology: Towards a reflexive history* (1st ed.). Routledge.

Richards, S. (2023). A lesson for the world: Solange Faladé's anti-colonial multiracialism. *Modern & Contemporary France*, 31(4), 435–450.

Rieber, R. W. (2012). *Freud on Interpretation: The ancient magical Egyptian and Jewish traditions*. Springer.

Riefenstahl, L. (Director) (1935). *Triumph des Willens* [Triumph of the Will], film. Reichsparteitag-Film.

Robinson, C. J. (1983/2000). *Black Marxism: The making of the Black radical tradition*. University of North Carolina Press.

Robinson, C. J. (1984). An inventory of contemporary Black politics. *Emergency*, 2, 21–28.

Robinson, P. A. (1969). *The Freudian left: Wilhelm Reich, Geza Roheim, Herbert Marcuse*. Cornell University Press.

Rodinson, M. (1973). *Israel: A colonial-settler state?* Anchor Foundation.
Rolnik, S. (2023). *Spheres of insurrection: Notes on decolonizing the unconscious*. John Wiley & Sons.
Rothstein, H., Huber, M., & Gaskell, G. (2006). A theory of risk colonization: The spiralling regulatory logics of societal and institutional risk. *Economy and society*, 35(1), 91–112.
Rose, J. (2017). The psychoanalytic passion of Edward Said. *Raritan*, 36(3), 1–23.
Rose, N. (1979). The psychological complex: mental measurement and social administration. *Ideology and Consciousness*, 5, 5–68.
Rozitchner, L. (2022). *Freud and the limits of bourgeois individualism*. Haymarket Books.
Roszak, T. (1992). *The voice of the Earth*. Simon & Schuster.
Rufo, C. F. (2023). *America's Cultural Revolution: How the radical left conquered everything*. HarperCollins.
Ruti, M. (2012). *The Singularity of Being: Lacan and the immortal within*. Fordham University Press.
Saad, G. (2020). *The parasitic mind: How infectious ideas are killing common sense*. Simon & Schuster.
Safouan, M. (1981). Is the Oedipus complex universal? *m/f*, 5(6), 83–90.
Safouan, M. (2000). *Jacques Lacan and the question of psychoanalytic training*. Palgrave.
Safouan, M. (2002). *The seminar of Moustafa Safouan*. Other Press.
Safouan, M. (2004). *Four lessons of psychoanalysis*. Other Press.
Safouan, M. (2003). *Speech or death? Language as social order: a psychoanalytic study*. Palgrave.
Safouan, M. (2007). *Why are the Arabs not free? The politics of writing*. Blackwell.
Said, E. W. (1968). The Arab Portrayed. *The Arab–Israeli confrontation of June 1967*, 1–9.
Said, E. W. (1971). Linguistics and the Archeology of Mind. *International Philosophical Quarterly*, 11(1), 104–134.
Said, E. W. (1972, February 20). A good man against theories. *New York Times*. https://www.nytimes.com/1972/02/20/archives/speaking-and-language-defence-of-poetry-by-paul-goodman-242-pp-new.html
Said, E. W. (1972, March), "Al-tamanu' wa al-tajanub wa al-ta'aruf" [Withholding, Avoidance, and Recognition], *Mawaqif*.
Said, E. W. (1975). *Beginnings: Intention and method*. Basic Books.
Said, E. W. (1978/2003). *Orientalism*. Vintage.
Said, E. W. (1979). *The Question of Palestine*. Vintage.
Said, E. W. (1981). *Covering Islam*. Vintage.
Said, E. W. (1983). *The world, the text, and the critic*. Harvard University Press.
Said, E. W. (1990). Yeats and decolonization. In *Nationalism, colonialism, and literature*. University of Minnesota Press.
Said, E. W. (1993). *Culture and Imperialism*. Vintage.
Said, E. W. (1994). *Representations of the intellectual: The 1993 Reith Lectures*. Vintage.
Said, E. W. (1999a). *After the last sky: Palestinian lives*. Columbia University Press.
Said, E. W. (1999b). *Out of place: A memoir*. Vintage.
Said, E. W. (1999c, January 10). The One-State Solution. *New York Times Magazine*. https//:www.nytimes.com/1999/01/10/magazine/the-one-state-solution.html
Said, E. W. (2000, April 17). My encounter with Sartre. *London Review of Books*. https://www.lrb.co.uk/the-paper/v22/n11/edward-said/diary
Said, E. W. (2001). The Palestinian right of return: An interview with Ari Shavit. *Raritan*, 20(3), 34.
Said, E. W. (2003). *Freud and the Non-European*. Verso.
Said, E. W. (2006). *On late style: Music and literature against the grain*. Vintage.
Sakai, J. (1983). *Settlers: The mythology of the white proletariat*. Morningstar Press.
Saketopoulou, A. (2023). *Sexuality beyond consent: Risk, race, Traumatophilia*. New York University Press.

Salaita, S. (2016). *Inter/Nationalism: Decolonizing native America and Palestine*. University of Minnesota Press.

Salmón, E. (2000). Kincentric ecology: Indigenous perceptions of the human–nature relationship. *Ecological Applications*, 10(5), 1327–1332.

Salter, P., & Adams, G. (2013). Toward a critical race psychology. *Social and Personality Psychology Compass*, 7(11), 781–793.

Sanchez, J. (2022, June 13). Against Afro-Pessimism. *Jacobin*. https://jacobin.com/2022/06/afro-pessimism-frank-wilderson-socialism-flattening-racism#:~:text=This%20is%20why%20Afro%2Dpessimists%2C%20believing%20in%20a,of%20the%20manufactured%20structures%20of%20our%20societies

Sandoval, C. (2000). *Methodology of the oppressed*. University of Minnesota Press.

Sartre, J. P. (2003). *Being and nothingness: An essay on phenomenological ontology*. Routledge.

Segato, R. (2022). Black Oedipus: Coloniality and the Foreclosure of Gender and Race. In *The critique of Coloniality: Eight essays*. Routledge.

Seshadri-Crooks, K. (2000). *Desiring whiteness: A Lacanian analysis of race*. Routledge.

Shapiro, L. (Ed.). (2007). *The correspondence between princess Elisabeth of Bohemia and René Descartes*. University of Chicago Press.

Sharp, G. (2005). *Waging nonviolent struggle: 20th century practice and 21st century potential*. Extending Horizons Books.

Sheehi, L. (2026). *From the clinic to the streets: Psychoanalysis for revolutionary futures*. Pluto Press.

Sheehi, S. (2018). The transnational Palestinian self: Toward decolonizing psychoanalytic thought. *Psychoanalytic Perspectives*, 15(3), 307–322.

Sheehi, L., & Sheehi, S. (2022). *Psychoanalysis under occupation: Practicing resistance in Palestine*. Routledge.

Sheehi, S., & Sheehi, L. (2024). The colonial republic of psychoanalysis: How psychoanalysis polices the psychic sovereignty of "Others". *Psychoanalysis, Culture & Society*, 1–20.

Sidanius, J., & Pratto, F. (1999). *Social dominance: An intergroup theory of social hierarchy and oppression*. Cambridge University Press.

Slife, B. D., Smith, A. F., & Burchfield, C. M. (2003). Psychotherapists as crypto-missionaries: An exemplar on the crossroads of history, theory, and philosophy. In D. B. Hill & M. J. Kral (Eds.), *About psychology: Essays at the crossroads of history, theory, and philosophy* (pp. 55–69). State University of New York Press.

Sloan, T. (1996). *Damaged life: The crisis of the modern Psyche*. Routledge.

Smith, B. (2020, February 10). I helped coin the term 'identity politics'. I'm endorsing Bernie Sanders. *The Guardian*. https://www.theguardian.com/commentisfree/2020/feb/10/identity-politics-bernie-sanders-endorsement

Smith, J. R., & Haslam, S. A. (Eds.). (2017). *Social psychology: Revisiting the classic studies* (2nd ed.). SAGE.

Smith, L. T. (2012). *Decolonizing methodologies: Research and Indigenous peoples* (2nd ed.). Zed Books.

Soler, C. (2015). *Lacanian affects: The function of affect in Lacan's Work*. Routledge.

Solomon, R. C. (2002). *Spirituality for the skeptic: The thoughtful love of life*. Oxford University Press.

Sontag, S. (2003). Regarding the pain of others. *Diogène*, 201(1), 127–139.

Sparks, G. (2018, May 11). We asked about Kanye in our poll and the results are not positive. *CNN*. https://www.cnn.com/2018/05/11/politics/kanye-west-favorability/index.html

Spivak, G. C. (1999). *A critique of postcolonial reason: Toward a history of the vanishing present*. Harvard University Press.

Stauffer, E.R. (1987). *Unconditional love and forgiveness*. Triangle.

Stavrakakis, Y. (2002). *Lacan and the Political*. Routledge.

Stavrakakis, Y. (2007). *The Lacanian left: Psychoanalysis, theory, and politics*. Edinburgh University Press.
Stevens, G. (2018). Raced repetition: perpetual paralysis or paradoxical promise?. *International Journal of Critical Diversity Studies*, 1(2), 42–57.
Stewart, J. (2007). "Breaking the power of the past over the present": psychology, utopianism, and the Frankfurt School. *Utopian Studies*, 18(1), 21–42.
Stoute, B. J., & Slevin, M. (Eds.) (2022). *The trauma of racism: Lessons from the therapeutic encounter*. Routledge.
Strauss, L. (1988). *Persecution and the art of writing*. University of Chicago Press.
Subzwari, V. (2024, June 6). One image, seen by millions: A social media effort to draw attention to Rafah surges. *AP News*. https://apnews.com/article/eyes-on-rafa-gaza-israel-hamas-fae6f49887637aaf4cbf548ce236dcb9
Swartz, S. (2018). *Ruthless Winnicott: The role of ruthlessness in psychoanalysis and political protest*. Routledge.
Swartz, S. (2023). *Psychoanalysis and colonialism: A contemporary introduction*. Routledge.
Szasz, T. S. (1960). The myth of mental illness. *American psychologist*, 15(2), 113–118.
Táíwò, O. (2022a). *Against decolonisation: Taking African agency seriously*. Hurst Publishers.
Táíwò, O.O. (2022b). *Elite capture: How the powerful took over identity politics (And everything else)*. Haymarket Books.
Tallis, R. (2018). *Logos: The mystery of how we make sense of the world*. Agenda.
Thiong'o, N.W. (1986). *Decolonising the mind: The politics of language in African literature*. Boydell & Brewer.
Tibi, B. (2013). European identity contested? In M. Tamcke, J. De Jong, L. Klein, & M. van der Waal (Eds.), *Europe – space for transcultural existence?* (pp. 47–56). Universitätsverlag Göttingen.
Togashi, K. (2020). *The psychoanalytic zero: A decolonizing study of therapeutic dialogues*. Routledge.
Tomšič, S. (2015). *The capitalist unconscious: Marx and Lacan*. Verso.
Toscano, A. (2009). Fanaticism as fantasy: Notes on Islam, psychoanalysis, & political philosophy. In J. Copjec (Ed.), *Umbr(a): Islam*. Umbr(a) Journal.
Tosquelles, F. (2024). Psychopathology and dialectical materialism. In M. Miguel & E. Vogman (Eds.), *Psychotherapy and materialism: Essays by Francois Tosquelles and Jean Oury* (pp. 47–88). ICI Berlin Press.
Tresilian, D. (2020, November 24). The Egyptian Oedipus: Remembering psychoanalyst Moustapha Safouan. *Ahram Online*. https://english.ahram.org.eg/NewsContentPrint/50/0/395496/AlAhram-Weekly/0/The-Egyptian-Oedipus-Remembering-psychoanalyst-Mou.aspx
Trotsky, L. (1939, December). *The ABC of materialist dialectics*. Marxists Internet Archive. https://www.marxists.org/archive/trotsky/1939/12/abc.htm
Trouillot, M. (1995). *Silencing the past: Power and the production of history*. Beacon Press.
Tuck, E., & Yang, K. W. (2012). Decolonization is not a metaphor. *Decolonization: Indigeneity, education & society*, 1(1), 1–40.
Tummala-Narra, P. (2022). Can we decolonize psychoanalytic theory and practice? *Psychoanalytic Dialogues*, 32(3), 217–234.
Ture, K., & Hamilton, C. V. (1967). *Black power: The politics of liberation in America*. Vintage.
Turner, L., & Neville, H. (Eds.). (2020). *Frantz Fanon's psychotherapeutic approaches to clinical work: Practicing internationally with marginalized communities*. Routledge.
Tutt, D. (2022). *Psychoanalysis and the politics of the family: The crisis of initiation*. Springer Nature.

UN Independent International Commission of Inquiry on the Occupied Palestinian Territory, including East Jerusalem, and Israel. (2025). *Legal analysis of the conduct of Israel in Gaza pursuant to the Convention on the Prevention and Punishment of the Crime of Genocide*. United Nations Human Rights Council. https://www.ohchr.org/sites/default/files/documents/hrbodies/hrcouncil/sessions-regular/session60/advance-version/a-hrc-60-crp-3.pdf

Uždavinys, A. (2008). *Philosophy as a rite of rebirth: From ancient Egypt to Neoplatonism*. The Matheson Trust.

Wahba, M. (1980). The paradox of Averroes. *ARSP: Archiv für Rechts-und Sozialphilosophie/Archives for Philosophy of Law and Social Philosophy*, 66(2), 257–260.

Wahba, M. (2004). مفارقة ابن رشد (R. K. Beshara, Trans.). الهيئة المصرية العامة للكتاب.

Wahba, M. (2006). Averroes as a bridge. *Think*, 4(12), 13–16.

Wahba, M. (2022). *Fundamentalism and secularization* (R. K. Beshara, Trans.). Bloomsbury.

Wai, F. (2013). Critical psychology is not psychology: An essay from the perspective of an ancient Chinese philosopher Gongsun Longzi written by a so-called Hong Kong psychologist. *Annual Review of Critical Psychology*, 10, 277–292.

Wai, F. (2021). Critical Deconstruction of "East meets West": The Lesson from Hong Kong. In R. K. Beshara (Ed.), *Critical psychology praxis: Psychosocial non-alignment to modernity/Coloniality*. Routledge.

Wallace, B. A. (2007). *Contemplative science: Where Buddhism and neuroscience converge*. Columbia University Press.

Wallerstein, I. M. (2004). *World-systems analysis: An introduction*. Duke University Press.

Walsh, R. T., Teo, T., & Baydala, A. (2014). *A critical history and philosophy of psychology: Diversity of context, thought, and practice*. Cambridge University Press.

Wapeemukwa, W. (2022). Oedipal empire: Psychoanalysis, indigenous peoples, and the Oedipus complex in colonial context. In S. George and D. Hook (Eds.), *Lacan and Race: Racism, Identity, and Psychoanalytic Theory*. Routledge.

Watkins, M., & Shulman, H. (2008). *Toward psychologies of liberation* (pp. 53–63). Palgrave Macmillan.

Ward, C. (1966). Anarchism as a Theory of Organization. *The Anarchist Library*.

Webster, J. (2018). *Conversion disorder: Listening to the body in psychoanalysis*. Columbia University Press.

Weiss, B. (2020). Resignation letter. https://www.bariweiss.com/resignation-letter

Wells, B. (2018). Nightmarish romanticism: The Third Reich and the appropriation of Romanticism. *Constellations*, 9(1), 1–10.

Wertz, F. J., Charmaz, K., McMullen, L. M., Josselson, R., Anderson, R., & McSpadden, E. (2011). *Five ways of doing qualitative analysis: Phenomenological psychology, grounded theory, discourse analysis, narrative research, and intuitive inquiry*. Guilford Press.

West-Eastern Divan Orchestra. (2009). *Statement of the West-Eastern Divan Orchestra musicians*. Fundación Barenboim-Said. https://barenboim-said.org/en/west-eastern-divan-orchestra/

Wetherell, M. (2012). The prejudice problematic. In J. Dixon & M. Levine (Eds.), *Beyond prejudice: Extending the social psychology of conflict, inequality and social change*. Cambridge University Press.

Wilderson III, F. B. (2020). *Afropessimism*. Liveright Publishing.

Wilson, A. N. (1993). *The falsification of Afrikan consciousness: Eurocentric history, psychiatry, and the politics of white supremacy*. Afrikan World Infosystems.

Wittig, M. (1992). *The straight mind: And other essays*. Beacon Press.

Wolfe, P. (2001). Land, labor, and difference: Elementary structures of race. *The American Historical Review*, 106(3), 866–905.

Wolfreys, J. (2018). *Republic of Islamophobia: The rise of respectable racism in France*. Oxford University Press.

Wolin, R. (2004). *The seduction of unreason: The intellectual romance with fascism from Nietzsche to Postmodernism*. Princeton University Press.
Workers Solidarity Movement (2009, Spring). Complex systems & anarchism. *Red & Black Revolution*, (15).
Wu, G. (2014). *The great dragon fantasy: A Lacanian analysis of contemporary Chinese thought*. World Scientific.
Wynter, S. (2003). Unsettling the coloniality of being/Power/Truth/Freedom: Towards the human, after man, its overrepresentation–an argument. *CR: The New Centennial Review*, 3(3), 257–337. https://doi.org/10.1353/ncr.2004.0015
Valentini, P., & Tourage, M. (Eds.). (2019). *Esoteric Lacan*. Rowman & Littlefield.
Viego, A. (2007). *Dead subjects: Toward a politics of loss in Latino studies*. Duke University Press.
Vinthagen, S. (2015). *A theory of nonviolent action: How civil resistance works*. Bloomsbury.
Virilio, P. (1983/2008). *Pure war: Twenty-five years later* (M. Polizzotti, Trans.). S. Lotringer (Ed.). Los Angeles, CA: Semiotext.
Virilio, P. (2006). *Speed and politics*. Semiotext(e).
Voloshinov, V. (1976/2014). *Freudianism: A Marxist critique*. Verso.
Von Kügelgen, A. (1996). A Call for Rationalism: "Arab Averroists" in the Twentieth Century/دعوة للعقلانية: الرشديون العرب في القرن العشرين. *Alif: Journal of Comparative Poetics* (16), 97–132.
Young, I. M. (1990). *Justice and the politics of difference*. Princeton University Press.
Zalloua, Z. (2024). Against exceptionalism. *Humanities*, 13(2), 50.
Zaretsky, E. (2004). *Secrets of the soul: A social and cultural history of psychoanalysis*. Vintage.
Žižek, S. (1989). *The sublime object of ideology*. Verso.
Žižek, S. (1997). *The plague of fantasies*. Verso.
Zizek, S. (Ed.). (1998a). *Cogito and the Unconscious*. Duke University Press.
Žižek, S. (1998b). A leftist plea for "Eurocentrism". *Critical Inquiry*, 24(4), 988–1009.
Žižek, S. (1999). *The ticklish subject: The absent centre of political ontology*. Verso.
Žižek, S. (2002). *For they know not what they do: Enjoyment as a political factor*. Verso.
Žižek, S., & Milbank, J. (2009). *The monstrosity of Christ: Paradox or dialectic?* MIT Press.
Zupančič, A. (2017). *What IS sex?* MIT Press.

Index